This collection of essays addresses, in a comprehensive and critical fashion, fundamental issues in the history of medicine in modern Germany. The essays also investigate important continuities and discontinuities in German history, and between Germany and the West. The central focus of the collection is on the professionalization of modern medicine and the medicalization of modern society. The problem of Nazi Germany is a common and prominent theme of many of the essays, partially because of its influence upon the debate over the nature of modern German government and society in relation to Western social, political, and economic development. Other topics include: the social place of hospitals in the early nineteenth century, the various forms of social Darwinism, the politics of state-run health insurance, the influence of eugenics on medicine and psychiatry, social control and "shell shock" in World War I, the history of sterilization and euthanasia, Nazi experimentation on humans, the abortion debate, and the role of former Nazis in the West German medical leadership.

PUBLICATIONS OF THE GERMAN HISTORICAL INSTITUTE
WASHINGTON, D.C.

Edited by Detlef Junker
with the assistance of Daniel S. Mattern

Medicine and Modernity

THE GERMAN HISTORICAL INSTITUTE, WASHINGTON, D.C.

The German Historical Institute is a center for advanced study and research whose purpose is to provide a permanent basis for scholarly cooperation between historians from the Federal Republic of Germany and the United States. The Institute conducts, promotes, and supports research into both American and German political, social, economic, and cultural history, into transatlantic migration, especially in the nineteenth and twentieth centuries, and into the history of international relations, with special emphasis on the roles played by the United States and Germany.

Other books in the series

Hartmut Lehmann and James J. Sheehan, editors, *An Interrupted Past: German-Speaking Refugee Historians in the United States after 1933*

Corol Fink, Axel Frohn, and Jürgen Heideking, editors, *Genoa, Rapallo, and European Reconstruction in 1922*

David Clay Large, editor, *Contending with Hitler: Varieties of German Resistance in the Third Reich*

Larry Eugene Jones and James Retallack, editors, *Elections, Mass Politics, and Social Change in Modern Germany*

Hartmut Lehmann and Guenther Roth, editors, *Weber's Protestant Ethic: Origins, Evidence, Contexts*

Catherine Epstein, *A Past Renewed: A Catalog of German-Speaking Refugee Historians in the United States after 1933*

Hartmut Lehmann and James Van Horn Melton, editors, *Paths of Continuity: Central European Historiography from the 1903s to the 1950s*

Jeffry M. Diefendorf, Axel Frohn, and Hermann-Josef Rupieper, editors, *American Policy and the Reconstruction of West Germany, 1945–1955*

Henry Geitz, Jürgen Heideking, and Jurgen Herbst, editors, *German Influences on Education in the United States to 1917*

Peter Graf Kielmansegg, Horst Mewes, and Elisabeth Glaser-Schmidt, editors, *Hannah Arendt and Leo Strauss: German Emigrés and American Political Thought after World War II*

Dirk Hoerder and Jörg Nagler, editors, *People in Transit: German Migrations in Comparative Perspective, 1820–1930*

R. Po-chia Hsia and Hartmut Lehmann, editors, *In and Out of the Ghetto: Jewish–Gentile Relations in Late Medieval and Early Modern Germany*

Sibylle Quack, editor, *Between Sorrow and Strength: Women Refugees of the Nazi Period*

Mitchell G. Ash and Alfons Söllner, editors, *Forced Migration and Scientific Change: Emigré German-Speaking Scientists and Scholars after 1933*

Medicine and Modernity

PUBLIC HEALTH AND MEDICAL CARE
IN NINETEENTH- AND TWENTIETH-CENTURY GERMANY

Edited by

MANFRED BERG AND GEOFFREY COCKS

GERMAN HISTORICAL INSTITUTE
Washington, D.C.
and

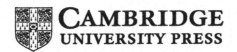

CAMBRIDGE
UNIVERSITY PRESS

PUBLISHED BY THE PRESS SYNDICATE OF THE UNIVERSITY OF CAMBRIDGE
The Pitt Building, Trumpington Street, Cambridge, United Kingdom

CAMBRIDGE UNIVERSITY PRESS
The Edinburgh Building, Cambridge CB2 2RU, UK
40 West 20th Street, New York NY 10011–4211, USA
477 Williamstown Road, Port Melbourne, VIC 3207, Australia
Ruiz de Alarcón 13, 28014 Madrid, Spain
Dock House, The Waterfront, Cape Town 8001, South Africa

http://www.cambridge.org

© German Historical Institute, Washington, D.C., 1997

First published 1997
First paperback edition 2002

A catalogue record for this book is available from the British Library

Library of Congress Cataloguing in Publication data
Medicine and modernity: public health and medical care in nineteenth- and
twentieth-century Germany / edited by Manfred Berg. Geoffrey Cocks.
p.   cm.
Includes index.
ISBN 0 521 56411 5 (hc)
1. Social medicine – Germany – History – 19th century.   2. Social
medicine – Germany – History – 20th century.   3. Medical policy –
Germany – History – 19th century.   4. Medical policy – Germany –
History – 20th century.   5. Medicine, State – Germany – History – 19th
century.   6. Medicine, State – Germany – History – 20th century.
I. Berg, Manfred, 1959– .   II. Cocks, Geoffrey, 1948– .
RA418.3.G3M43   1997
362.1′0943–dc20   96-15487   CIP

ISBN 0 521 56411 5 hardback
ISBN 0 521 52456 3 paperback

Contents

Contributors

Manfred Berg, research fellow, German Historical Institute, Washington, D.C.

Johanna Bleker, professor of the history of medicine, Free University of Berlin

Gisela Bock, professor of history, University of Bielefeld

Geoffrey Cocks, professor of history, Albion College, Albion, Michigan

Richard J. Evans, professor of history, Birkbeck College, University of London

Atina Grossmann, professor of history, Columbia University, New York City

Michael H. Kater, professor of history, Atkinson College, York University, Toronto

Alfons Labisch, professor of the history of medicine, Heinrich Heine University, Düsseldorf

Paul Lerner, member of the history department, Columbia University, New York City

Charles E. McClelland, professor of history, University of New Mexico, Albuquerque

Heinz-Peter Schmiedebach, professor of the history of medicine, Ernst-Moritz-Arndt University, Greifswald

Introduction

GEOFFREY COCKS

The Third Reich is a black hole in German history. Like hypothetical black holes in space, it draws everything toward itself. At the edges of black holes, massive gravitational forces slow time to a stop. Anything falling toward a black hole, therefore, would appear to an observer to fall forever. Similarly, since 1945 historians of Germany have found themselves gripped by the gravity of teleology. The pull exerted by the Third Reich has often led, in the words of Richard Evans, to a view of modern German history "from Hitler to Bismarck."[1] Although it was not the aim of the German Historical Institute conference on "Medicine in Nineteenth- and Twentieth-Century Germany: Ethics, Politics, and Law," from which the chapters in this book stem, to detail the already well-documented medical crimes of the Nazis,[2] it was the central purpose of the conference to place the medical crimes and collaborations of the National Socialist era into their larger German and Western contexts. In so doing, the papers, comments, and discussions attempted to pull the history of the Third Reich back into the history of Germany, Europe, and the West, rendering it less of a black entity unto itself than a part of other, broader constellations characterized as much by differentiation as by the historiographical problem of teleology.

This very task and result, of course, only underscores the reach and press on German history of the dark gravity of the Third Reich. But the heavy presence of Hitler's Germany also constitutes a vital opportunity for historians – and humanity – to confront the lessons of the German past for

1 Richard J. Evans, "From Hitler to Bismarck: 'Third Reich' and Kaiserreich in Recent Historiography," *Historical Journal* 26 (1983): 485–97, 999–1020.
2 See, among others, Alexander Mitscherlich and Fred Mielke, *Wissenschaft ohne Menschlichkeit: Medizinische und Eugenische Irrwege unter Diktatur, Bürokratie und Krieg* (Heidelberg, 1949); Alice Platen-Hallermund, *Die Tötung Geisteskranker in Deutschland* (Frankfurt/Main, 1948); Robert Jay Lifton, *The Nazi Doctors: Medicalized Killing and the Psychology of Genocide* (New York, 1986); Robert N. Proctor, *Racial Hygiene: Medicine under the Nazis* (Cambridge, Mass., 1988); and Henry Friedlander, *The Origins of Nazi Genocide: From Euthanasia to the Final Solution* (Chapel Hill, N.C., 1995).

1

the sake of the human present. The weight of moral gravity takes over from that of teleology. This is especially the case with the history of medicine. Questions of health and illness are universal. What is more, the modern history of medicine in the West reaches deeply and broadly into society and culture, as well as across national and temporal boundaries. The history of medicine – particularly in regard to the Third Reich – also raises monumental moral questions concerning modern human dispositions of the quality and quantity of life and death. Such lessons and questions have relatively rarely been confronted by physicians themselves. This reticence has been particularly marked at the highest – and oldest – levels of the German medical establishment with respect to the history of their profession between 1933 and 1945. That the German Historical Institute brought together physicians, as well as historians, from Germany, the United States, and Great Britain was especially salutary in helping to counter inertia of this kind. Again like a black hole, the Third Reich has often held light itself in its grip.

Parallel to the problem of teleology in German history lies the historical problem of continuity and discontinuity between the history of the Third Reich and the history of modern Germany as a whole. How does Nazi Germany fit into the history of the Germans and of the German nation? Before, during, and even after World War II, this question elicited some rather crude answers. Some charged that Nazism was the inevitable outcome of German society, culture, character, and history. Others contented themselves with the striking, though most often shallowly conceived, conundrum of the land of Goethe, Beethoven – and Hitler. Still others in the West, deeply influenced by the Cold War, equated German National Socialism with Soviet Marxism as manifestations of the uniquely modern form of rule of totalitarianism. Conservative and apologist Germans seized upon this interpretation, among others, to argue that Nazism was an accident in German history occasioned by modern secular revolutionary impulses in Europe. On the other hand, various Marxist models saw European fascism in general as symptomatic of the mortal crisis of late monopoly capitalism.

The predominant postwar paradigm among historians in the West, however, was the liberal idea of the German *Sonderweg* ("special path"). This was the thesis that, unlike France and Britain, Germany during the nineteenth century had not undergone a socially, politically, and economically modernizing bourgeois revolution; this failure allowed preindustrial feudal elites to lead the country down a uniquely German authoritarian path to Hitler.[3] The issue of the power of the Prussian-German state in

---

3 Ralf Dahrendorf, *Society and Democracy in Germany* (Garden City, N.Y., 1967); Jürgen Kocka, "Ursachen des Nationalsozialismus," *Aus Politik und Zeitgeschichte*, June 21, 1980, 9–13.

particular, therefore, has an important dual quality: not only the matter of government intervention unique in degree and kind to Germany but the *type* of government and the interests of its masters. Since the 1960s, however, historians have generated new varieties of sophisticated questions and answers about the nature of the Third Reich, its place in the history of Germany, and the course of modern German history as a whole. Many of these findings have come about as a result of work in other periods and aspects of the history of modern Germany. In particular, the study of the various stations and conditions of the modern industrial society Germany had become by the onset of the twentieth century has provided great insight into significant developments to and through the Third Reich. Arguments over the impact of modernization have therefore been especially important in evaluating the course and consequences of German history in the era of the two world wars. The "Bielefeld School" used social science methods to refine the *Sonderweg* model of the uniquely German authoritarian divergence from the evolution of modern democracy in the West.[4] Neo-Marxist approaches have been most persistent in posing the questions of the degree to which Germany had in fact undergone a transformation into a bourgeois state and society, the degree to which as a result "feudal" elites were in fact in control, and thus the extent to which it was in fact political and economic liberalism itself that was responsible for the conditions that led to the rise of the Nazis.[5]

Ongoing research into the social, economic, and political complexities of modern German history has significantly qualified both the *Sonderweg* approach and that of its critics. In the history of medicine, issues such as the professionalization of doctors, the "medicalization" of society, the role of the state in medical professionalization, health, and public hygiene, the political battles over health insurance, the relationships between medicine and Nazism before and after 1945, the rise of eugenic thinking, and the places of women and patients all engage the question of the respective roles of a unique German past and of a general Western pattern of development.[6] The various complex functions within the "polycracy" of a somewhat chaotic Nazi party and state, it has been argued,[7] created a continuity of such established systems.

4 Hans-Ulrich Wehler, *Das deutsche Kaiserreich 1871–1918* (Göttingen, 1973).
5 Geoff Eley, "What Produces Fascism: Pre-Industrial Traditions or a Crisis of the Capitalist State?" in Geoff Eley, *From Unification to Nazism: Reinterpreting the German Past* (Boston, 1986), 254–82; David Blackbourn and Geoff Eley, *The Peculiarities of German History: Bourgeois Society and Politics in Nineteenth-Century Germany* (New York, 1984).
6 On comparative policy implications, see Donald W. Light and Alexander Schuller, eds., *Political Values and Health Care: The German Experience*, MIT Press Series on the Humanistic and Social Dimensions of Medicine, vol. 4 (Cambridge, Mass., 1986).
7 Peter Hüttenberger, "Nationalsozialistische Polykratie," *Geschichte und Gesellschaft* 2 (1976): 417–42.

Moreover, distinctly modern technical capacities in medicine—as else-where—were required by Nazi policy, as well as preserved by Nazi political disorder. Medicine and public health in modern Germany in particular have been the subject of critical study for their role in furthering economic, polit-ical, and military demands for social productivity (*Leistung*) through the "practical utility" of various prophylactic policies and therapeutic methods.[8] Closer to the black core of Nazi ideology and policy—the singularity, to extend our astrophysical metaphor, of its biological racism and the resultant Holocaust—discontinuity takes on greater, though not exclusive, importance. In all of this, as in other specialized fields of German history, historians of medicine have had to consider the relative importance, particularly with regard to the rise of Nazism, of various traditional junctures: To what extent have long-standing German political, social, and cultural characteristics ante-dating the nineteenth century played a role? What is the relevance of the founding of a Germany dominated by Prussia in 1871? Was industrialization and its impact on the German economy, polity, and society most crucial? Or was it more the series of disastrous events after 1914 and 1918 that consti-tuted the more decisive elements?

The history of medicine in general has gone through distinct stages of evolution. In the nineteenth century, it displayed a Whiggish orientation that celebrated the advance of enlightened and progressive forces of science and humanitarianism against an ancien régime of obscurantism and persecution. Such histories were in line with the bourgeois ethos of the age, highlighting heroic men clearing away ignorance and helping impose the rational order of freedom upon a chaotic and superstitious society. In the course of the twentieth century, Marxist thought, similarly preoccupied with progress, gradually turned some historians to the history of the proletariat.[9] This tendency, ghettoized politically—and then also geographically during the Cold War—eventually contributed to a growing historical interest in social history in reaction to the traditional emphasis upon the ideas and activities of political leaders and cultural elites. Much of the initial interest of histori-ans of Europe centered on the working class, the most numerous class of

8 Michael Hubenstorf, "'Aber es kommt mir doch so vor, als ob Sie dabei nichts verloren hätten.' Zum Exodus von Wissenschaftlern aus den staatlichen Forschungsinstituten Berlins im Bereich des öffentlichen Gesundheitswesens," in Wolfram Fischer et al., eds., *Exodus von Wissenschaften aus Berlin: Fragestellungen – Ergebnisse – Desiderate: Entwicklungen vor und nach 1933*, Akademie der Wissenschaften-zu Berlin Forschungsbericht, no. 7 (Berlin, 1994), 368–9, 448; Alfons Labisch, *Homo Hygienicus: Gesundheit und Medizin in der Neuzeit* (Frankfurt/Main, 1992), 133.

9 Marxist historiography was no less a bourgeois heir of the Enlightenment in its preoccupation with progress. The only difference was that whereas liberals saw the bourgeoisie as a means to the future through its ongoing success, Marxists saw the bourgeoisie as a means to the future through its ulti-mate failure.

modern urban industrial society.[10] In the realm of health and illness, research demonstrated the close tie between disease and social class, living conditions, and occupational environment.[11] During the 1950s this historical school was dogmatized in East Germany and ignored in West Germany; it grew in the Federal Republic during the 1960s and was partially suppressed there in the 1970s; increasing academic exchange on the subject across the intra-German border characterized the 1980s; and unification brought even fuller collaboration but also some evaluation and weeding out of Marxist-Leninist historians in the former German Democratic Republic.

Increased interest in the history of the middle classes has spurred further work in the history of medicine.[12] Some of this recent research arose from structuralist critiques of the ethos of bourgeois "social control" seen to be manifested in nineteenth-century medicine and in Whiggish accounts of it. Much of the work has concerned itself with the medical profession and in particular the process of its professionalization during the late nineteenth and early twentieth centuries. The subject of professionalization was pioneered by sociologists in the 1930s and 1940s. This early work, however, merely validated "the normative claims of professionals and ... linked [them] to the advancement of modernization."[13] Beginning in the 1960s, more critical studies concentrated on the powerful organized self-interest manifested among the professions.[14] Historians of the German professions have highlighted the differences – in particular the greater role of the state in professionalization – as well as the similarities to the Anglo-American model.[15] Historians of Germany have also had to examine the whys and ways of the involvement of professionals with Nazism and the Third Reich, an issue particularly acute in the case of medicine.

Doctors in Germany and Europe during the nineteenth century moved from rather artless dependence upon rich clients toward autonomy based on some degree of specialized knowledge, standardized training, and the growing demand for medical services.[16] The medical profession was also

10 For an early classic example of the genre, see E. P. Thompson, *The Making of the English Working Class* (New York, 1964).

11 Dirk Blasius, "Geschichte und Krankheit: Sozialgeschichtliche Perspektiven der Medizingeschichte," *Geschichte und Gesellschaft* 2 (1976): 386–415.

12 See, e.g., Peter Gay, *The Bourgeois Experience: Victoria to Freud*, 4 vols. (New York, 1984–96).

13 Konrad H. Jarausch, "The German Professions in History and Theory," in Geoffrey Cocks and Konrad H. Jarausch, eds., *German Professions, 1800–1950* (New York, 1990), 9–10.

14 See, e.g., Margaret S. Larson, *The Rise of Professionalism* (Berkeley and Los Angeles, 1977); and Paul Starr, *The Social Transformation of American Medicine* (New York, 1982).

15 Claudia Huerkamp, "The Making of the Modern Medical Profession, 1800–1914: Prussian Doctors in the Nineteenth Century," in Cocks and Jarausch, eds., *German Professions*, 66–84.

16 Claudia Huerkamp, *Der Aufstieg der Ärzte im 19. Jahrhundert: Vom gelehrten Stand zum professionellen Experten: Das Beispiel Preussens* (Göttingen, 1985).

especially affected after 1871 by the social policy of Imperial Germany. Free trade sentiment, particularly among liberal Berlin physicians, had resulted in 1869 in medicine being legally designated by the North German Confederation as a trade rather than as a profession. This allowed doctors to practice almost without any restrictions, but also allowed unlicensed medical practitioners, or "quacks" (Kurpfuscher), the same freedom. Many doctors did not welcome this competition and objected as well on scientific grounds to the end of sanctions against quackery. In any case, Bismarck's policy of attempting to disarm Social Democracy through the introduction of state health insurance in 1883 changed the ground upon which doctors in Germany operated. The growth in the number of medical practitioners and "the constant expansion of the medical insurance system had the effect of... making competition keener."[17] An open conflict, unique in kind and degree to Germany, erupted between ever more professionally organized physicians – using union tactics such as boycotts, lockouts, and strikes – and the insurance companies. This, coupled with most doctors' political aversion to increasing socialist control over the Krankenkassen (sickness funds) system, laid the basis for further rightward radicalization among physicians after 1918.

The growth of the medical profession and of the state health bureaucracy grew into, as well as over, more general social dynamics involving health and illness. The "modernization" of Germany, whatever – like "tradition" – its roughness as a measure, brought with it a "medicalization" of society, that is, "the extension of rational, scientific values in medicine to a wide range of social activities."[18] The growing power and prestige of doctors, and of science in general, tended dangerously to convince many of them – and much of the public – of their expertise in a wide range of social, political, and philosophical matters.[19] But this process was not uniform, unidirectional, or unproblematic, confined to the professional aims of doctors, the ideals of social reformers, or the political and economic aims of elites. Doctors themselves were divided along political and intradisciplinary lines. And the health-care system in Germany as a whole, whatever its ultimate or inherent

17 Charles E. McClelland, The German Experience of Professionalization: Modern Learned Professions and Their Organizations from the Early Nineteenth Century to the Hitler Era (Cambridge, 1991), 86.
18 Paul Weindling, "Medicine and Modernization: The Social History of German Health and Medicine," History of Science 24 (1986): 277.
19 See, e.g., Eric J. Engstrom, "Emil Kraepelin and Public Affairs in Wilhelmine Germany," History of Psychiatry 2 (1991): 111–32; cf. Robert M. Veatch, "Scientific Expertise and Value Judgments: The Generalization of Expertise," Hastings Center Studies 1, no. 2 (1973): 20–40; and Max Weber, "Wissenschaft als Beruf" (1918), in Max Weber, Gesammelte Aufsätze zur Wissenschaftslehre (Tübingen, 1922), 524–55.

failings, was also possessed of features with contemporary comparative policy implications.[20]

But health and illness in general are matters of complex social influences. The most obvious trend of the nineteenth century was the increase in morbidity – the suffering and dying from chronic illnesses spawned by living and working conditions – over the earlier predominant mortality crises of plagues and epidemics. In Imperial Germany morbidity figures reflected significant short-term social inequality but were revealing not only of the effects of maldistribution of wealth but also of values and attitudes.[21] Although people from all social classes and regions sought medical care, there was also resistance and recourse to alternative therapies. In the nineteenth century, this stemmed not only from the persistence of traditions and mentalities but also from the fact of medicine's inability to treat and cure most illnesses. In the twentieth century, even though medical therapy eventually made great strides and patient reliance on doctors (and drugs) grew, individuals and groups found reasons to remain skeptical or opposed to modern scientific medicine and the burgeoning state medical bureaucracy.[22] Many, if not most, German doctors subscribed to the notion that "Der Patient bleibt stumm." But the words of George Bernard Shaw in the preface to his play *The Doctor's Dilemma* (1906) applied to Germany as well as to Britain and the West in general: "The doctor may lay down the law despotically enough to the patient at points where the patient's mind is simply blank; but when the patient has a prejudice the doctor must either keep it in countenance or lose his patient." There was some basis, for example, for one of the justifications offered by German industry for its preference for their own factory doctors over the free choice of doctors under the state health insurance scheme. Industrialists argued, among other things, that "inexperienced doctors could be fooled by patients and would indulge them because they feared losing them to competition."[23]

Some historians have argued that hygienic values were imposed by ruling elites for purposes of social control. Others maintain that such values more often simply percolate downward[24] – or even upward or at least

20 See, e.g., Jane Caplan, *Government without Administration: State and Civil Service in Weimar and Nazi and Nazi Germany* (New York, 1988).

21 Reinhard Spree, *Health and Social Class in Imperial Germany: A Social History of Mortality, Morbidity and Inequality*, trans. Stuart McKinnon and John Halliday (Oxford, 1988).

22 Edward Shorter, *Bedside Manners: The Troubled History of Doctors and Patients* (New York, 1985); for the effects among former soldiers, e.g., see Robert Weldon Whalen, *Bitter Wounds: German Victims of the Great War, 1914–1939* (Ithaca, N.Y., 1984); and James M. Diehl, *The Thanks of the Fatherland: German Veterans after the Second World War* (Ithaca, N.Y., 1993).

23 Martin H. Geyer, *Die Reichsknappschaft: Versicherungsreform und Sozialpolitik im Bergbau 1900–1945* (Munich, 1987), 239.

24 Norbert Elias, *The Civilizing Process*, trans. Edmund Jephcott (New York, 1978).

around – randomly. It is certainly the case, as Richard Evans has shown in his study of cholera in nineteenth-century Hamburg, that powerful economic, social, and political interests could influence or even determine medical policies, as well as privilege scientific theories compatible with these interests.[25] And institutions, such as hospitals and movements such as that for social hygiene, can be locations for the slippery slopes leading from progressive treatment to repressive mistreatment. This perspective has been particularly useful in the subfield of the history of psychiatry because mental illness was regarded as a direct threat to the moral and behavioral order prescribed for modern society.[26] In Germany at the end of the nineteenth century, what at the time was labeled "Imperial German psychiatry" displayed an authoritarianism that – somewhat ironically – admitted the ability only to classify rather than treat or cure mental illness.[27] In both medicine and psychiatry in Germany, these ambiguities culminated in the outright evil of exterminatory Nazi eugenics. But even with the atrocious instance of National Socialism, the history of medical treatment as a whole in the Third Reich cannot be reduced to the victimization of patients. Many dominant values and attitudes were internalized by the general population. Even (or especially) under the oppression and exhortation howled out by the Third Reich there were also widespread instances of what sociologist Michel de Certeau has labeled "antidiscipline" created by the "polytheism of scattered practices."[28] Nazi biopolitics made such responses particularly common in matters of health and illness because even in the best of times medical personnel regularly intrude more deeply into people's lives than other official and professional entities.[29]

The history of medicine in Germany has also had to address the sad and ultimately tragic phenomenon of anti-Semitism, specifically the fate of

25 Richard J. Evans, *Death in Hamburg: Society and Politics in the Cholera Years, 1830-1910* (Oxford, 1987).

26 Klaus Doerner, *Madmen and the Bourgeoisie: A Social History of Insanity and Psychiatry*, trans. Joachim Neugroschel and Jean Steinberg (Oxford, 1981); Michel Foucault, *Madness and Civilization: A History of Insanity in the Age of Reason*, trans. Richard Howard (New York, 1965); Roy Porter and Mark Micale, "Reflections on Psychiatry and Its Histories," in Roy Porter and Mark Micale, eds., *Discovering the History of Psychiatry* (New York, 1994), 3–36.

27 Hannah S. Decker, *Freud in Germany: Revolution and Reaction in Science, 1893-1907* (New York, 1977), 50–3.

28 Michel de Certeau, *The Practice of Everyday Life*, trans. Steven Rendall (Berkeley and Los Angeles, 1984), 47; see also Richard J. Evans, "In Pursuit of the Untertanengeist: Crime, Law and Social Order in German History," in Richard J. Evans, ed., *Rethinking German History* (London, 1987), 156–87. For a critique of the "historization" of the Third Reich, see Saul Friedländer, "Some Reflections on the Historization of National Socialism," *Tel Aviver Jahrbuch für deutsche Geschichte* 16 (1987): 310–24.

29 Geoffrey Cocks, "Partners and Pariahs: Jews and Medicine in Modern German Society," *Leo Baeck Institute Yearbook* 36 (1991): 191–206; see also Fridolf Kudlien, "Bilanz und Ausblick," in Johanna Bleker and Norbert Jachertz, eds., *Medizin im "Dritten Reich"*, 2d ed. (Cologne, 1993), 222–8; and Geoffrey Cocks, *Psychotherapy in the Third Reich: The Göring Institute* (New York, 1985).

Jewish physicians and patients in the Third Reich as well as the central role of doctors in implementing the "Final Solution."[30] Anti-Semitism among German physicians had been aggravated by a surplus of young doctors waiting to get into the national health insurance system during the Great Depression. The large numbers of Jewish doctors in metropolitan areas such as Berlin, Frankfurt, and Hamburg made them easy scapegoats. In the late nineteenth century, Jews had been shunted into less attractive medical specialties such as dermatology and internal medicine, which were now more highly developed and in greater demand. Moreover, Jews had long been widely caricatured as obsessed with money and sex, as well as being associated with mental and physical illness.[31] University medical faculties were closed to Jews unless they converted. And although Jewish physicians for the first time received field commissions during World War I, "[t]he prejudice that no Jew could fit the Prussian ideal of martial masculinity was difficult to dispel."[32] This observation reminds one, among other things, of Fritz Stern's judgment distinguishing Germany in this regard, as in others, from the rest of Europe: "In Germany there was no Dreyfus Affair because there was no Dreyfus."[33]

The study of prejudice and racism in the history of medicine in Germany also provides a link to recent methodological discussions concerning the relative value of linguistic and social science modes of explanation in history. Postmodernism, poststructuralism, and deconstruction have all challenged "the core premises of the Enlightenment project of emancipation – that is, abstract universalism, the unitary subject, and the (intelligible) social totality."[34] These movements – sometimes known collectively as "the linguistic turn" – argue that "knowledge" is an imposition of the powerful in the absence of any stable meaning "beyond the text." But postmodernist, poststructuralist, and deconstructionist thought all privilege the critical investigator at the expense of theory and subject matter: In this paradigm, it seems, everything but the work of the investigator is subject to the distorting volatility and fullness of language. Although the historian must not be naive about knowledge as a function of power, he or she also must not cynically abandon the search for what knowledge can be gained through painstaking thought and research. At the same time, however, the historian must be aware

30 Michael H. Kater, "Unresolved Questions of German Medicine and Medical History in the Past and Present," *Central European History* 25 (1992): 407–23.
31 Sander L. Gilman, "Jews and Mental Illness: Medical Metaphors, Anti-Semitism, and the Jewish Response," *Journal of the History of the Behavioral Sciences* 20 (1984): 150.
32 Kater, "Unresolved Questions," 414.
33 Fritz Stern, "The Burden of Success: Reflections on German Jewry," in Fritz Stern, *Dreams and Delusions: The Drama of German History* (New York, 1987), 108.
34 Jane Caplan, "Postmodernism, Poststructuralism, and Deconstruction: Notes for Historians," *Central European History* 22 (1989): 201.

of both the inevitability and, within limits, the utility of retrodiction (the historian's subjective and objective experience) and likewise the uses and limits of theory. And when it comes to National Socialism, how can the historian not know – and not judge – the Nazis through their recorded words and deeds as anything but definitively and irredeemably evil?

But the questioning of the power behind received and created "knowledge" has bolstered an appreciation for different "voices" previously written out of history by the Western "authoritarianism of truth-seeking." Although none of the chapters in this book adopts a wholly postmodern approach to its material, much of the subject matter consists of the voices of the previously ignored, undervalued, and victimized: the sick, the mentally ill, the handicapped, women, and ethnic and religious minorities. More generally, the rich and varied subject matter of the history of health and medicine introduces new phenomena into – and new ways of seeing old phenomena in – German history. This increase in the variety of the subject matter is a modest but appropriate way of "deconstructing" received truths and categories in German history by way of testing, modifying, enriching, or even confirming them. And the universal human quality of most of the subject matter of the history of medicine easily carries the historian across the many regional boundaries of political, cultural, and (too often) Prussian "Germany." Finally, although recognizing specific German historical contexts, this material has also been consistently comparative, taking the historian across the borders of Germany and back again. This can contribute to what Michael Geyer has deconstructively argued should be on the agenda for historians of Germany: the recognition of the "fragility and permeability of all (and not just the German) national constructions."[35] Geyer maintains that the noisy quests for national unity in the nineteenth century, especially those in Central Europe, were in fact frantic attempts to flee from the "internal heterogeneity of nations" in search of "fictions of... autonomy for the nation and hegemony for Europe."[36]

The ten chapters in this book discuss vital major aspects of the history of medicine in Germany during the nineteenth and twentieth centuries. The chapters are arranged in a generally chronological order and more or less grouped around shared subject matter: Johanna Bleker and Alfons Labisch both deal with the effects on patient groups of the institutional policy of hospitals and the government, respectively; Richard Evans analyzes the varieties of social Darwinist thought in Germany before 1930; Charles

---

35 Michael Geyer, "Historical Fictions of Autonomy and the Europeanization of National History,"
    Central European History 22 (1989): 341.
36 Ibid., 316, 317, 341.

McClelland and Geoffrey Cocks treat different aspects of the professional-ization of medicine; Heinz-Peter Schmiedebach, Paul Lerner, and Gisela Bock all discuss problematic and fateful aspects of the history of psychiatry; and Atina Grossmann and Michael Kater deal in different ways with issues of continuity in the history of medicine in Germany before 1933 and after 1945.

Johanna Bleker's study of hospitals in various regions of Germany in the fifty years before the country's first unification under Prussia argues that hos-pitals had a number of reasons for being and were not simply a function of the advance of medicine. Hospitals were one means of dealing with the social and economic problems brought by the new migratory labor required by the growth of manufacturing. Hospitals brought advantages and disadvantages to doctors, who were divided over their desirability. The advantages included greater technical capacities and control of patients; among the disadvantages was low pay. The latter was a common phenomenon in Europe in the early nineteenth century, as expressed in the words of Tertius Lydgate, the idealis-tic young doctor in George Eliot's *Middlemarch* (1873), a novel of England in the 1830s:

The highest object to me is my profession, and I had identified the Hospital with the best use I can at present make of my profession. But the best use is not always the same with monetary success. Everything which has made the Hospital unpopular has helped with other causes – I think they are all connected with my professional zeal – to make me unpopular as a practitioner. I get chiefly patients who can't pay me. I should like them best, if I had nobody to pay on my own side.

Lydgate's ambivalent attitude toward the hospital in the fictional town of Middlemarch also suggests Bleker's challenge to the traditional view that hospitals in the nineteenth century were simply places of contagion and oppression that patients avoided. Bleker offers evidence that hospitals more often were sought-after oases from a dangerous life and not just loci for the victimization of helpless patients. Her study is therefore typical of a "third wave" of research in the history of medicine, which draws from the "social control" critique of the Whiggish first wave while qualifying or con-testing the second wave critique through extensive documentation.[37]

Like Bleker, Alfons Labisch emphasizes the importance of the bourgeoi-sie's desire to control the newly mobilized industrial and commercial labor force, but the chief concern of his chapter is the "political patriarchalism" em-bodied in Bismarck's health insurance legislation. And although Bleker con-centrates more on the dynamics of patients' responses to the policies imposed upon – and created around – them, Labisch focuses on the aims and methods

---

37   For another example of this type of research, see W. F. Bynum et al., eds., *The Anatomy of Madness: Essays in the History of Psychiatry*, 2 vols. (London, 1985).

of governmental policymakers. Labisch argues that Bismarck's policy was a peculiarly mercantilist one arising from his *Junker* loyalties and designed to tie the workers to the state instead of to the Social Democratic Party or their employers. This was an effort, Labisch says, of "forming society by politics." One discerns in this analysis an emphasis upon traditional Prussian forms and attitudes that would seem to argue for the uniqueness of the German experience under Bismarck. The question is how decisive a role the reactionary aims and institutions of Bismarckian political and social policy played in the evolution of an increasingly industrialized state and society before 1914. At the very least, one can draw instructive contrasts to the history of medicine in other countries. It is clear, for example, that doctors in Germany were in the position of having to face (and exploit) an established state policy in the realm of health care, whereas elsewhere in Europe and in the United States, the state had to confront independently mobilized physicians advancing and securing their interests and control over the medicalization of society.

Richard Evans's chapter on the historiography of social Darwinism in Germany underlines the relatively recent mainstream consensus among historians that social Darwinism was, from its origins in the late nineteenth century, a politically and philosophically variegated phenomenon. According to this view, the radical and racist varieties of social Darwinism that presaged and animated the Nazis were in the minority and were only a part of a "transition from evolutionism to selectionism, from left to right, in the 1890s." Evans critiques various versions of, and challenges to, this consensus, arguing that the most important issue is why the authoritarian and racist variety won out; for Evans, this eventual, if temporary, ascendancy was due to more than just the consequences of Nazi political victory in 1933. Until 1914 varieties of social Darwinist thinking persisted among Social Democrats, Pan-Germans, and the emergent "racial hygienists." This last group had a major effect on what Evans calls "the welfarist discourse" before World War I. But, according to Evans, it took the slaughter of the war and the crises of the 1920s and 1930s to radicalize theory and practice along selectionist lines. More generally, Evans sees German history as much more than a *prologomena* to Hitler even in one of the realms of the history of ideas and of professional and public discourse often most closely identified with the roots of Nazi ideology.

Charles McClelland analyzes the professionalization of doctors in Germany during the first thirty years of the twentieth century. McClelland argues that there was no specifically German "fatal flaw" in this process. Rather, corporatist characteristics inherent in the structure of modern professions combined with a series of economic disruptions and political reverses after World War I to make National Socialism an attractive political option for many doctors. McClelland labels this process "interrupted professionalization" and does not consider it evidence for the inevitable evils of professionalization per se nor peculiar to the German experience of it. This interpretation differs from that of Konrad H. Jarausch, who sees a problematic "neocorporatist" strain of professionalization across all the professions in Germany. This arose, according to Jarausch, out of a more general tradition of illiberalism and a bourgeois shift from liberalism to nationalism during the German Empire.[38] Michael Kater, on the other hand, has emphasized discrete qualities of the culture and history of modern Germany by concentrating on certain characteristics, such as political conservatism, anti-Semitism, militarism, and male chauvinism, which he argues were common among German doctors. When combined with the military disaster that befell the German Empire in World War I and the economic and political crises that bedeviled the Weimar Republic after the war, these attitudes made many doctors receptive to the prejudices of the Nazis as well as to their promises.[39]

Heinz-Peter Schmiedebach investigates the social place of the mental patient as determined by the interests both of the state and of psychiatrists. Psychiatry was a creation of the nineteenth century: Johann Christian Reil of Halle coined the term "psychiatry" in 1808. Schmiedebach examines the social construction of mental illness through psychiatry and the asylum. The great theoretical and practical divide among German psychiatrists in the nineteenth century was between "mentalists," who argued for psychological causation and treatment, and "somaticists," who believed that mental illness was physical in origin. Schmiedebach shows, however, that both sides shared a conservative moral view of their patients. The mentalists wished to create "self-discipline" in their charges, whereas the somaticists imposed a "patriarchal philanthropism." In addition, Schmiedebach maintains, psychiatrists became ever more tractable when it came to government priorities, chiefly because of concern for their professional fortunes. The "therapeutic activism" of midcentury was gradually replaced by official insistence upon social order in the face of the growing urban masses and as a result of "therapeutic nihilism" among psychiatrists.[40] By the turn of the century, according to Schmiedebach, psychiatry was being significantly influenced by eugenic thought and the dual concern of the state over the cost of housing the mentally ill and cultivating the maximum number of men for labor and war.

---

38 Konrad H. Jarausch, *The Unfree Professions: German Lawyers, Teachers, and Engineers, 1900-1950* (New York, 1990), 22–4, 220–1.
39 Michael H. Kater, *Doctors Under Hitler* (Chapel Hill, N.C., 1989).
40 Bernd Walter, "Fürsorgepflicht und Heilungsanspruch: Die Überforderung der Anstalt? (1870–1930)," in Franz-Werner Kersting et al., eds., *Nach Hadamar: Zum Verhältnis von Psychiatrie und Gesellschaft im 20. Jahrhundert* (Paderborn, 1993), 66–97.

These trends culminated in the mass starvation of mental patients in German asylums during World War I.[41] And although more beneficent policies made headway under the Weimar Republic, these measures were doomed by the Great Depression. There was also a tragically ironic effect of distinguishing the curable from the incurable: For the latter, sterilization was an increasingly attractive alternative to psychiatrists and bureaucrats even before 1933.[42]

Paul Lerner focuses on the treatment of war neuroses during World War I. Although army psychiatrists were initially overwhelmed by the number and nature of what was at first called "shell shock," a variety of relatively effective treatment modalities were quickly developed and deployed. The traditional somaticist point of view insisted that these disorders were organic. But the psychogenic school of thought, which had been gaining adherents since the turn of the century, predominated over the course of the war. This was due largely to the efficacy of its various methods in returning soldiers to battle and reducing the pension obligations of the government. Lerner documents a significant degree of differentiation among psychiatrists in the first two decades of the twentieth century. Although there were complaints about the brutality of some of the methods, in particular Kaufmann's electrotherapy, the "therapeutic turn" of the war years laid the basis for a psychiatric reform movement during the 1920s. These reforms were of course cut short by economic and political catastrophe at the end of the decade, but Lerner also documents the social ambiguities of psychiatric therapies in and of themselves as agents both of healing and of control.

Gisela Bock seeks to place Nazi forced sterilization and "euthanasia" policies in the overall context of German history. In so doing, she offers a nuanced examination of the important historiographical issues. Some scholars see Nazi race hygiene as part of a process of modernization and rationalization; others view it in terms not of the outgrowth of modernization but of a crisis within it. Bock also weighs the arguments for the importance of ideas ("intentionalist") versus structure ("functionalist") in the implementation of Nazi racial policy. Finally, she considers the question of the historical origins of this policy: early or late nineteenth century? World War I? or 1933? Bock argues that the crucial transitions occurred with World War I and the

41   Approximately 40,000 mental patients starved to death under the Vichy government in France during World War II; see Max Lafont, *L'Extermination douce* (Nantes, 1987). On the German case in World War I, see Hans-Ludwig Siemen, *Die Menschen blieben auf der Strecke ... Psychiatrie zwischen Reform und Nationalsozialismus* (Gütersloh, 1987), 29–30. More research needs to be done to determine the extent to which the starvation of German mental patients in World War I was motivated out of eugenic considerations or was the "logical" extension of general popular privation to the asylums.

42   Hans-Ludwig Siemen, "Die Reformpsychiatrie der Weimarer Republik: Subjektive Ansprüche und die Macht des Faktischen," in Franz-Werner Kersting et al., eds., *Nach Hadamar*, 98–108.

Nazi assumption of power in 1933. Although she notes the fact that most of the agents of "euthanasia" under National Socialism came from the ranks of "progressive" doctors, Bock argues that Nazi policies can be viewed more effectively in ethical terms than in the terms of modernization, a theme taken up in conference discussions about the lack of ethics instruction in German medical education past and present. According to Bock, there are distinct continuities in this history but also distinct discontinuities. The crucial issues for Bock are: (1) the Nazi introduction of compulsion into the realm of social engineering; and (2) individual decisions one way or the other when it came to crossing ethical boundaries in the treatment of other human beings as "valuable" or as "unworthy."

My own chapter attempts to place the actions of the doctors tried at Nuremberg for medical crimes into the larger contexts of German and Western history before and after 1945. I argue that much of what motivated the doctors who carried out experiments on concentration camp inmates during World War II arose from various conditions set by the social place of medicine in modern Germany and the West. The Nuremberg Doctors' Trial is significant not simply as a further revelation of Nazi atrocities, of the successes and failures of international justice, or of the moral choices made or not made by doctors in Germany and, subsequently, by doctors in service to other nations at other times. The trial tells us a great deal about the historical contexts and structures of the history of medicine in modern German society and the West. And it also offers us a chance to reevaluate the place of German history in the history of the West. I attempt to show that an evolving corporate ethic, peculiarly strong in Germany and especially evident among professionals, was aggravated by Nazi policies and the military exigencies of World War II. The medicalization of German society during the twentieth century advanced, but also complicated, the position of doctors, patients, and the public health system. These complications were worsened by a series of genuine and perceived health crises as a result of military, political, and economic crises after 1914. The Nazis in turn intensified official and popular concern with matters of actual and "racial" health, while their policies of mobilization and war further aggravated problems of health and illness among almost all segments of the population.

The final two chapters also extend their analysis into the years after 1945. Atina Grossmann discusses the history of abortion in Germany from the late Weimar period through the Third Reich and the immediate postwar years and into the era of the two German republics. She shows that there has been significant continuity in German public policy concerning abortion, in particular a tendency to see abortion not in terms of individual (women's) rights but rather in terms of social and economic conditions or of individual "fitness." Attempts by feminists and communists in the late Weimar period to change the law criminalizing most abortions were defeated, and the Nazi government toughened the law against abortions for "Aryans," while advocating and even compelling abortions for women of "inferior" quality. In 1945 both the government of the collapsing Third Reich and postwar Allied administrations suspended the law to allow abortions for women who had been raped by Red Army soldiers. In the Soviet zone, reform of the law was pursued, although the underlying rationale of collective welfare prepared the way for the recriminalization of abortion in 1950. In 1972 the Democratic Republic relegalized abortion while also increasing pro-natalist benefits. Abortion remained illegal in the Federal Republic and reunification has left the issue a source of both compromise and conflict, with doctors continuing to play a major role in an ambiguous legal environment.

Michael Kater closes the book with a detailed examination of the so-called Sewering scandal of 1993. Like many of the preceding studies, Kater's chapter documents a continuity of personnel across traditional divides, in this case the oft-presumed chasm of 1945. And although Nazi racial policies were abandoned, Kater also shows that the conservative political and social culture of the Federal Republic permitted and even encouraged the persistence of provincialism and old prejudices, as well as perpetrating a blindness to the moral lessons of the immediate past and a concomitant tolerance – and even indulgence – of former Nazis. Recent research in the history of medicine in Germany – such as that presented at the German Historical Institute conference – has documented the major role played by doctors in all realms of the Third Reich. This knowledge renders the long-standing unwillingness of the German medical profession in particular to examine critically its own past that much more regrettable and reprehensible.

At the end of this book, therefore, we return to its beginning. The reticence of the German medical profession to acknowledge deeply troubling dimensions to its past testifies to the morally and intellectually darkening gravity of the Third Reich in German history. Against such inertia, historians like those whose work is contained in this book must continue to bring to bear the countervailing gravity of concerned and effective scholarship.

1

To Benefit the Poor and Advance Medical Science

Hospitals and Hospital Care in Germany, 1820–1870

JOHANNA BLEKER

In recent years historians of nineteenth-century medicine have traced the development of physicians' professional interests, concentrating on the interplay of professional ambitions and reasons of state that have led to the medical profession's control over private life. In discussions of the complex triangle of the state, physicians, and patients, the concepts of professionalization, medicalization, and hygienization have become dominant. Undoubtedly, these concepts have yielded fruitful insights into the role of physicians and public institutions, but they have contributed very little to our understanding of the patients' role in these processes. The patient appears only as the victim, indeed, one who would have been much better off without the so-called progress that destroyed his or her traditional medical system, discredited lay medicine and family help, and ended with the expropriation of his or her body.

I would first like to make some critical observations on writing and researching the history of patients. Patients' history will always suffer from a lack of adequate and appropriate sources. The dearth of good historical material makes it easy to transfer our own sentiments toward medicine back onto history, largely because of our feelings of impotence in the face of modern medicine, our postmodern disbelief in progress, and our longing for an intact world, one unimpaired by the alienating forces of modern society. Moreover, viewing the patient as simply the victim of medicalization overlooks the fact that most of the people subjected to medicalization had already been uprooted from their traditional surroundings. As a result of the enormous social changes of the nineteenth century – particularly the great migration and urbanization processes – the traditional support of family, neighborhood, and village community gradually disappeared.

To substantiate the preceding argument, in this chapter I concentrate on the development of hospital care over the course of the nineteenth century. Hospitals can be seen as paradigmatic cases of medicalization. They clearly

17

served as instruments of the state for maintaining public order and dealing with, although not solving, social problems. In this process patients who had never before considered consulting an academic physician were forced into the hospital, where they were isolated from their normal social surroundings and where their physical and moral conduct was supervised by medical experts.[1] Viewed in terms of medical professionalization, hospitals were, already at the beginning of the century, the spaces where doctors were able to establish a dominant position within the doctor–patient relationship. As the sociologist Ivan Waddington noted in 1973, "Perhaps for the first time, doctors were in the position to ignore the wishes of their patients in situations where to grant those wishes would run counter to their professional judgment."[2] The emergence of modern scientific medicine is clearly based on hospital medicine, for it was in the hospital that observation and experimentation could be performed without resistance.[3]

Furthermore, most historians are convinced that the patients never went to the hospital out of free will, but rather "avoided hospitals like the plague."[4] Because of their unsanitary conditions, hospitals have been labeled "gateways to death."[5] Although most of the evidence for the patients' negative attitude is taken from late eighteenth-century medical critics, it is maintained that this attitude remained unchanged through the end of the nineteenth century.[6] Moreover, it can be stated that we are still without a thoroughgoing historical analysis of hospitals and hospital care in Germany between 1800 and 1870.

The essential role of hospitals in the development of modern medicine is undisputed. Yet, authors dealing with the history of the German health-care system in the nineteenth century have concentrated almost exclusively on outpatient care, only occasionally including a few remarks on hospital facilities. Hence, we are led to believe that before 1870 – or, at the latest, 1880 – hospitals were of only marginal importance. To counter this misconception,

1 Ute Frevert, *Krankheit als politisches Problem, 1770–1880: Soziale Unterschichten in Preussen zwischen medizinischer Polizei und staatlicher Versicherungsordnung*, Kritische Studien zur Geschichtswissenschaft, vol. 62 (Göttingen, 1984), 78–82, 108–12, 263–7.

2 Ivan Waddington, "The Role of the Hospital in the Development of Modern Medicine: A Sociological Analysis," *Sociology: Journal of the British Sociological Association* 7 (1973): 211–24, esp. 217; Claudia Huerkamp, *Der Aufstieg der Ärzte im 19. Jahrhundert: Vom gelehrten Stand zum professionellen Experten: Das Beispiel Preussens*, Kritische Studien zur Geschichtswissenschaft, vol. 68 (Göttingen, 1985), 140–1; Frevert, *Krankheit als politisches Problem*, 74.

3 Övind Larsen, "Case Histories in Nineteenth-Century Hospitals – What Do They Tell the Historian? Some Methodological Considerations: With Special Reference to McKeon's Criticism of Medicine," *Medizin, Gesellschaft und Geschichte* 10 (1991): 127–48.

4 Frevert, *Krankheit als politisches Problem*, 75.

5 This label was first used by K. F. Helleiner in 1965. See Guenter B. Risse, *Hospital Life in Enlightenment Scotland: Care and Teaching at the Royal Infirmary of Edinburgh* (Cambridge, 1986), 386.

6 For criticism of this argument, see ibid., 4, 287–90.

it is necessary to begin this analysis with several facts concerning the role of hospitals within the process of medicalization.

The work of historian Claudia Huerkamp has shown that between 1820 and 1870 academic physicians succeeded in supplanting nonacademic physicians and barber surgeons. But the total number of medical professionals did not rise. Although in 1828 in Prussia there was 1 medical professional for every 2,877 inhabitants, by 1876 the ratio had actually deteriorated to 1 doctor for every 3,388.[7] This indicates that over the course of the century the intensity of outpatient care did not increase. In the same period the number of public hospitals in Prussia rose from 155 in 1822 to 1,122 in 1876. Even more noteworthy is the increase in the number of hospital patients as a proportion of the total population. Using the official Prussian statistics, Salomon Neumann ascertained that in 1843 only 1 out of 1,841 inhabitants were treated in a hospital once a year. In 1852 it was 1 out of 121, and three years later, in 1855, 1 out of 86.[8]

Even though the figures for 1843 are based on rough estimates, the statistics show a surprising shift toward hospital treatment by the early 1850s. There is little to suggest that this development was the result of medical achievements, because the years before 1880 witnessed no relevant discoveries that changed hospital medicine.[9] Despite the fact that physicians were involved in the construction and improvement of local hospitals throughout the century, this development on the whole took place largely without comment from the medical profession. Thus, we have to look beyond medicine when investigating the history of hospitals and hospital care in the midnineteenth century.

Historian Alfons Labisch has proposed looking at hospital history within the framework of diverging systems that aim at different ends.[10] In fact, the multiplicity of purposes and functions of the modern hospital can be traced to the original establishment of such institutions. When Bamberg's new general hospital opened in 1787, Adalbert Friedrich Markus, a medical reformer, philosopher, and personal physician, gave a loyal speech to his prince-bishop and outlined the functions of this institution. It was intended to serve the state in a twofold manner: by benefitting the poor and by providing

7   Huerkamp, *Der Aufstieg der Ärzte*, 149.
8   Salomon Neumann, "Die Krankenanstalten im preussischen Staate," *Archiv für Landeskunde der preussischen Monarchie* 5 (1859): 349–88, esp. 350, 357, 370, 373.
9   See Alfons Labisch, "Das Krankenhaus in der kommunalen Sozial- und Gesundheitspolitik," paper presented at the "Tagung Sozialgeschichte des Allgemeinen Krankenhauses in Deutschland (19. und frühes 20. Jahrhundert)," Düsseldorf, April 1993.
10 Alfons Labisch, "Krankenhauspolitik in der Krankenhausgeschichte," *Historia Hospitalium* 13 (1979–80): 217–33.

hospital training for physicians.[11] Thus, from the very start the modern hospital in Germany had two distinct functions that involved two separate social and political spheres. The social function fell within the framework of the poor relief system, and the educational function within the medical realm. My research suggests that, throughout the nineteenth century, these two systems remained distinct aspects of the development of modern hospitals. Apart from a short period during the 1840s, when the "Social Question" (*soziale Frage*) was discussed both as a public and as a medical problem, there is no evidence that doctors concerned themselves with the social dimensions of stationary care. The role of the hospital in the promotion of medical science and professional skills, in contrast, was the subject of continuous discussion and debate.

In the first part of this chapter, I consider the social forces that influenced hospital development. In the second, I outline the professional and scientific interests of the doctors and deal with the "Hospital Question" (*Krankenhausfrage*) within the medical reform movement of the 1840s. In the conclusion, I draw attention to hospital patients and to some new findings that might help to redefine their role in the process.

In the nineteenth century, most of the so-called public hospitals were administered by cities or local communities.[12] Some had developed under the aegis of charitable foundations; some were founded by religious organizations or by miners', railroad, or other workers' societies. All of these hospitals had their own statutes, but because most of them had assumed public functions and, therefore, also received public financial support, they had to accept a certain degree of governmental control.[13] The general legal and administrative issues involving hospitals were governed by the poor law well into the twentieth century. Hence, it can be assumed that the development of stationary care was linked to changes within the poor relief system. Unfortunately, historians who have dealt with the history of pauperism in Germany have not yet extended their analyses to the question of hospitals before the introduction of the national insurance system.[14] Therefore, I am able to present only a few general observations here.

---

11 Adalbert Friedrich Markus, *Von den Vortheilen der Krankenhäuser für den Staat: Rede zum Einweihungstage des neuen Allgemeinen Krankenhauses zu Bamberg, nebst 13 Beylagen* (Bamberg, 1790), 6.

12 The term "public hospital" is used here as it was understood at the time. It includes not only hospitals run by cities and towns but also those institutions run by workers or religious societies, or other nonprofit organizations. See Neumann, "Die Krankenanstalten," and Labisch, "Das Krankenhaus in der kommunalen Sozial- und Gesundheitspolitik."

13 Lorenz Stein, *Verwaltungslehre*, pt. 3 (Stuttgart, 1867), 121–3.

14 Christoph Sachsse and Florian Tennstedt, *Geschichte der Armenfürsorge in Deutschland* (Stuttgart, 1980) vol. 1, Florian Tennstedt, "Die Frühgeschichte der deutschen Sozialversicherung und das

According to regulations that were issued in most German states in the first decades of the nineteenth century, poor relief was defined as the responsibility of cities, communities, or districts, which had to set up a poor relief fund to pay for the most urgent needs of the registered poor. Moreover, it was decreed that poor relief must also provide for medical care – the doctors' fees and the costs for remedies were to be paid out of public funds.[15] In larger cities poor relief physicians were appointed who, in addition to their private practices, had to treat the resident poor and were compensated with a moderate annual fee. Although the contemporary academic physician hoped for a yearly income of 1,000 taler, poor relief work paid between 100 and 200 taler annually.[16]

In areas where a hospital was located, poor relief could also pay for stationary treatment. Hospital care would be granted when it was thought that the patient's illness could be cured (or at least that his or her condition would improve) and when living conditions at home were judged ill suited for recuperation.[17] The question of whether hospital care was more or less economical than outpatient care was frequently discussed. In Berlin outpatient care was said to be cheaper than the fees charged by the Charité, the most important Berlin hospital.[18] But more often it was maintained that the costs for food, remedies, and numerous doctors' visits would exceed the allowance for a hospital stay.[19] A complaint often heard was that the bureaucratic procedure that a pauper had to endure before hospital admission lasted from between one and three weeks.[20]

In addition to the resident poor, there existed another group that relied on public funding when they fell ill. These people earned their living within the community but lacked the support of home or family. In preindustrial decades this group mainly consisted of servants and journeymen. In large

öffentliche Krankenhauswesen," paper presented at the "Tagung Sozialgeschichte des Allgemeinen Krankenhauses in Deutschland"; Labisch, "Das Krankenhaus in der kommunalen Sozial- und Gesundheitspolitik."

15 Stein, *Verwaltungslehre*; Labisch, "Das Krankenhaus in der kommunalen Sozial- und Gesundheitspolitk."
16 Salomon Neumann, *Die öffentliche Gesundheitspflege und das Eigenthum* (Berlin, 1847), 54; W. Fischer, J. Krengel, and J. Wietog, eds., *Sozialgeschichtliches Arbeitsbuch*, vol. 1: *Materialien zur Statistik des Deutschen Bundes, 1815–1870* (Munich, 1982), 122–6.
17 Eva Brinkschulte and Pascal Grosse, "Die Patienten des Juliusspitals: Aufnahmewege und Aufnahmebedingungen," in Johanna Bleker, Eva Brinkschulte, and Pascal Grosse, eds., *Kranke und Krankheiten im Juliusspital zu Würzburg, 1819–1829: Zur frühen Geschichte des Allgemeinen Krankenhauses in Deutschland*, Abhandlungen zur Geschichte der Medizin und der Naturwissenschaften, vol. 72 (Husam, 1995), 43–74; "Über die Armenpflege in Köln," *Allgemeines Volksblatt: Populärer Monatsbericht über die wichtigsten Zeitfragen* (1845): no. 3, 18–20; no. 5, 37–9; no. 8, 59–62.
18 Frevert, *Krankheit als politisches Problem*, 108–9.
19 Joseph Hermann Schmidt, *Die Reform der Medicinal-Verfassung Preussens* (Berlin, 1846), 193.
20 Brinkschulte and Grosse, "Die Patienten des Juliusspitals"; "Über die Armenpflege in Köln."

cities students also had to be given medical care and nursing. In the second half óf the century, more and more factory workers flooded into large cities and industrial areas. By law these people, when they became ill or destitute, were forced to rely on the resources of their place of origin. But often it would be impossible or utterly inhumane to send them home. In such cases they were cared for by the community where they resided, which in turn tried to recoup the costs from the sick person's place of birth.[21] By the beginning of the century, moreover, the traditional order, according to which patrons had to care for their sick workers, was already crumbling.[22]

At the end of the eighteenth century, special funds for sick journeymen and servants had been established that were connected to local hospitals and provided stationary care in case of illness.[23] Initially, servants, masters, and guilds could join voluntarily, but membership soon became compulsory in most places. By the midnineteenth century, insurance funds for servants and journeymen could be found wherever there was a general hospital. When a community decided to build a new hospital, insurance funds were established at the same time.[24] It is evident that these institutions had many advantages. The community was spared the trouble of retrieving the costs, and patrons no longer felt obliged to care for their workers. Servants and journeymen, who often had no bed of their own, had a place to rest when they were sick. Additionally, these funds helped cover the operating costs for the hospital. In many hospitals nonresident workers formed the largest group of patients, and insurance funds covered most of the annual expenditures.[25]

The Prussian poor laws were reformed in 1842. The principle that a person's place of birth was responsible for poor relief was discarded. Now, the communities where a person found himself or herself were obligated to care for newcomers. This was a response to the growing mobility of the working population, but it created enormous problems for the rapidly growing

21 Eva Brinkschulte, "Historische Vorläufer der Krankenversicherung und das Krankenhaus – am Beispiel des Würzburger Juliusspitals, 1776–1830," paper presented at the "Tagung zur Sozialgeschichte des Allgemeinen Krankenhauses in Deutschland."

22 Ibid.; Schmidt, *Die Reform der Medizinalverfassung,* 177–8; Christian Pfeufer, *Geschichte des Allgemeinen Krankenhauses zu Bamberg* (Bamberg, 1825), 77–8.

23 Brinkschulte, "Historische Vorläufer"; Frevert, *Krankheit als politisches Problem,* 263.

24 Eberhard Wormer, "Das Leben der Oberpfälzer in Gesundheit und Krankheit an der Schwelle zum Industriezeitalter: Nach den Physikatsberichten der Bezirksärzte, 1858–1861," Med. diss., University of Munich, 1986, 91–3, 154; Eva Berger, *Wer bürgt für die Kosten? Zur Sozialgeschichte des Krankenhauses: 125 Jahre Stadt-Krankenhaus Osnabrück, 180 Jahre Städtische Gesundheitspolitik,* Beiträge zur Kunst- und Kulturgeschichte der Stadt Osnabrück, vol. 4 (Bramsche, 1990), 17–21; Philipp Franz von Walther, *Über klinische Lehranstalten in Krankenhäusern: Eine Prinzipienfrage* (Freiburg, 1846), 32–3; Reinhard Spree, "Quantitative Aspekte der Entwicklung des Krankenhauswesens im 19. und 20. Jahrhundert," paper presented at the "Tagung Sozialgeschichte des Allgemeinen Krankenhauses in Deutschland"; Frevert, *Krankheit als politisches Problem,* 265.

25 Walther, *Über klinische Lehranstalten,* 32–44; Spree, "Quantitative Aspekte."

industrial areas and cities.[26] The construction of hospitals was perhaps one response to this situation. According to Neumann's statistics, in 1855, when on average 1 out of 86 inhabitants were treated at a hospital, within cities 1 out of 27 received stationary care. The most favorable ratio appeared in large cities and in those areas that industrialized early, such as Upper Silesia and Cologne.[27] Along with this development went the increase of insurance funds whose chief purpose was to provide hospital care for servants and workers.[28] In short, the rise of the public hospital system in Germany during the nineteenth century was linked to the growing presence of working migrants who, having lost their traditional support system, were in need of new sources of social assistance and local medical care.

At the beginning of the nineteenth century, the idea that hospital training would make better physicians was by no means widely shared. It is true that in the first decades of the century state regulations came into effect requiring all medical students to take clinical courses.[29] But authorities within the profession, such as Christoph Wilhelm Hufeland, disputed the usefulness of hospitals for clinical education.[30] Their objection can be explained in terms of the professional status of the academic physicians. The physicians' source of income came from the small group of upper-middle-class citizens who could afford to pay a family doctor. A family doctor had to know the individual dispositions of his patients, their ways of life, and their joys and sorrows. He had to act in accordance with their social expectations and conform to their tastes. Whereas diagnosis and treatment of particular diseases were still uncertain, the doctor based his medical advice on the individual characteristics of the patient. This approach was called "individualizing," and this type of medical practice was generally called "private practice." Hufeland argued that the best

26 Sachsse and Tennstedt, *Geschichte der Armenfürsorge*, 195–203, 277–80; see also Otto Mugdan, "Spezielle Krankenversorgung: Für Arbeiter: Im Krankheitsfall," *Handbuch der Krankenversorgung und Krankenpflege*, vol. 2, pt. 2 (Berlin, 1902), 1–17; Labisch, "Das Krankenhaus in der kommunalen Sozial- und Gesundheitspolitik."

27 E.g., the ratio in Breslau was 1:12, in Oppeln, 1:13, and in Cologne, 1:16; Neumann, "Die Krankenanstalten," 370.

28 Frevert, *Krankheit als politisches Problem*, 263–66.

29 Johanna Bleker, "Medical Students to the Bed-side or to the Laboratory? The Emergence of Laboratory Training in German Medical Education, 1870–1900," *Clio Medica* 21 (1987–88): 35–46; Johanna Bleker, "'Der einzig wahre Weg, brauchbare Männer zu bilden': Der medizinisch-klinische Unterricht an der Berliner Universität und an der Charité, 1810–1850," in P. Schneck and H. U. Lammel, eds., *Die Medizin an der Berliner Universität und an der Charité zwischen 1810 und 1850*, Abhandlungen zur Geschichte der Medizin und der Naturwissenschaften, vol. 67 (Husum, 1994), 90–100.

30 Christoph Wilhelm Hufeland, "Nachrichten von der Medicinisch-Chirurgischen Krankenanstalt zu Jena nebst einer Vergleichung der klinischen und Hospitalanstalten überhaupt," *Journal der practischen Arzneykunde* 3 (1797): 528–66.

school for private practice was the polyclinic, where students visited poor patients in their homes.[31]

In many ways hospital practice was the complete antithesis of private practice. Hospital patients could be controlled and ordered about. Hospital medicine could not, however, ameliorate the unsanitary circumstances that produced disease among the poor. Instead, it concentrated on diagnosing and treating special types of diseases, with little interest in the patient's individual disposition. Although it was agreed that hospital medicine would contribute to the advancement of science, it was – as most German doctors decided – completely worthless for treating the private patients who comprised the clientele.[32] Moreover, there was no financial gain in treating hospital patients. Medical visits to the hospital, which were often requested only once or twice a week, were usually an uncompensated duty for the municipal doctor or, at university hospitals, the clinical professor.[33]

University medicine did not overcome its reservations about training students in hospitals until the 1830s. The change is associated with the name of Johann Lukas Schönlein, who, between 1819 and 1832, had been a professor of clinical medicine in Würzburg, where he made use of the medical ward of a large general hospital, the renowned Juliusspital. His new "natural history" approach linked systematic bedside observation to pathological anatomy, which became basic to medical research and teaching.[34]

Because most university hospitals were too small to allow for systematic observation, academics sought access to the general hospitals. In Berlin there was a long-lasting fight over the right of the university to use Charité patients for medical instruction.[35] In Saxony doctors claimed that Dresden's new city hospital should be opened to students from Leipzig.[36] In Munich the famous surgeon Franz Philipp von Walther stressed in 1846 that the establishment of clinical schools within general hospitals was a natural process that could be observed everywhere.[37]

Not surprisingly, the rush of university medical students into general hospitals resulted in conflicts with hospital administrators. In Munich critics

31 Ibid.; See also Johanna Bleker, "Biedermeiermedizin – Medizin der Biedermeier? Tendenzen, Probleme, Widersprüche 1830–1850," *Medizinhistorisches Journal* 23 (1988): 5–22, esp. 9. Bleker, "Der einzig wahre Weg."
32 See also Ursula Geigenmueller, "Aussagen über die französische Medizin der Jahre 1820–1847 in Reiseberichten deutscher Ärzte," Dent. Med. diss., Free University Berlin, 1985, 139–46.
33 Walther, *Über klinische Lehranstalten*, 44.
34 Bleker, "Biedermeiermedizin," 11–16.
35 Bleker, "Der einzig wahre Weg."
36 Hermann Eberhard Richter, "Über die Benutzung des neuen Stadtkrankenhauses zu Dresden für den klinischen ärztlichen Unterricht (1846)," in Hermann Eberhard Richter, *Schriften zur Medicinalreform* (Dresden, 1865), 41–56.
37 Walther, *Über klinische Lehranstalten*, 9.

argued that the doctors "considered the hospital as their property" and "behaved as absolute rulers."[38] The prescriptions written by these academic intruders were too expensive. And professors tried to admit or retain "interesting" patients, who, according to the poor law, had no right to hospital care. In short, clinical activities were said to ruin hospital finances, which in the 1840s had become precarious. One pamphlet actually labeled the clinical school "the cankerous evil of the hospital."[39]

Von Walther did not dispute the fact that the interests of hospitals differed from those of the medical profession. But he claimed that all improvements in hospitals had been achieved by physicians and that without the scientific energy of doctors hospitals would be ruled by dirt, indifference, and lazy routine. Nevertheless, von Walther did not approve of having full-time doctors in hospitals. They would become either depressed or callous by the unchangeable human misery surrounding them. And, he continued, of course no physician of skill and ability could be persuaded to work for the miserable fees paid by hospitals.[40]

According to von Walther the best way to handle hospital medicine was to achieve a balance of interests. As was the case with free "international trade," each party involved should benefit when it allowed the other side to prosper.[41] But, in the 1840s, many doctors thought that the balance had been upset. Moreover, liberal economic ideas no longer seemed appropriate for solving political and social problems. In turning toward the "Social Question," physicians and hospitals trod common ground, although not for very long.

At midcentury Germany stood on the threshold of its industrial age. Thousands were leaving rural districts and settling in cities and towns. They migrated from the eastern provinces to the west, and soon the poverty rates on the Rhine were twice as high as in eastern Prussia.[42] In 1830 five *Armenärzte* (doctors for the poor) were working within Cologne's system of poor relief to care for the 6,584 registered poor; by 1846 that number had climbed to more than 21,000.[43] Whereas the poor law reform of 1842 had burdened this city with new financial liabilities, its system of medical care within the poor relief system altogether collapsed.

In 1842 the medical society of Cologne published the following complaint:

38   Ibid., 3.
39   Ibid.
40   Ibid., 44–6.
41   Ibid., 25.
42   Johann Schwarz, *Das Armenwesen der Stadt Köln vom Ende des 18. Jahrhunderts bis 1918* (Cologne, n.d.), 197.
43   Ibid., 207.

Among the 75,000 inhabitants of Cologne 21,000 are so poor that medical advice and remedies have to be paid out of public funds. Another part of the population is able to pay for the remedies or obtains them with the help of a benefactor, but cannot afford to pay the doctor. Among these are craftsmen, lower government officials, and commercial clerks, and their total amounts to at least another 10,000 souls.[44]

In 1845 the city of Cologne had about sixty medical doctors and twenty surgeons.[45] But only 4,000 families had an annual income of more than 400 taler and were thus able to pay the doctor what he was actually due for his services.[46]

In this situation the so-called *Kurierzwang* (compulsory provision of medical services) added to doctors' financial problems. In Prussia, and in other German lands as well, every doctor was obliged to give medical aid to a poor person if the situation was urgent. Afterward he could apply to the public relief funds to reimburse his costs, but most often the doctor's claims were rejected. This was because only a small portion of destitute individuals was legally registered as paupers. In the course of the 1840s, the public relief funds proved insufficient to cope with the growing number of unemployed, hungry, and homeless.[47] For the doctors this meant that their sources of income became smaller, while their uncompensated workload increased.

In this context the question of public health assistance became a major concern of the medical reform movement of the 1840s. The main goal of the professional discourse was to improve the social conditions of physicians; but apart from mere professional concerns, quite a number of physicians realized the broader context of the problem. Some even went so far as to argue that the question of medical help could only be solved through the "abolition of pauperism."[48]

Within the medical reform movement, hospitals were not seen as playing a major role. Radical reformers considered them stopgap measures within the larger poor relief system. According to Rudolf Virchow, it was the moral duty of the state to guarantee the "equal right of all to a healthful existence."[49] He

44 *Die Reform der Medizinal–Verfassung Preussens: Bericht eines Ausschusses des Ärztlichen Vereins zu Köln* (1842), quoted in Rüdiger Müller, "Die Medizinalreformbewegung in Rheinpreussen, 1840–1849," Med. diss., Universität Münster, 1979, 257.

45 Carl Moritz Sponholz, *Allgemeine und specielle Statistik der Medicinalpersonen der Preussischen Monarchie* (Stralsund, 1845), 309–10.

46 Karl Obermann, "Karl d'Ester, Arzt und Revolutionär, seine Tätigkeit in den Jahren, 1842–1845," in Deutsche Akademie der Wissenschaften Berlin, ed., *Aus der Frühgeschichte der deutschen Arbeiterbewegung*, Schriften des Instituts für Geschichte, sec. 1, vol. 1 (Berlin, 1965), 102–200, esp. 127.

47 Schwarz, *Das Armenwesen der Stadt Köln*, 72–4; "Über die Armenpflege in Köln," 39.

48 Bleker, "Biedermeiermedizin," 18.

49 Rudolf Virchow, "Die öffentliche Gesundheitspflege" (1848), in *Gesammelte Abhandlungen zur öffentlichen Medicin und der Seuchenlehre* (Berlin, 1879), 1:14–30, esp. 17: "Die gleichmässige Berechtigung aller auf gesundheitsgemässe Existenz."

also claimed that, for the time being, "admission to a hospital must be possible for anybody who stands in need of it, no matter if he has money or not, if he is Jewish or a heathen."[50] But with the abolition of pauperism, every patient would have access to the doctor of his or her choice, and there would be no need for hospitals. (This idea was favored by Virchow until the 1860s.[51])

Thus, it is not surprising that the most comprehensive text on hospitals was written by a conservative, Joseph Hermann Schmidt. The author was commissioned by the Prussian government to present plans for medical reform. He later worked for the Ministry of Education and Cultural Affairs.

Schmidt was a strong supporter of the monarchy and believed that patriotism grew out of subordination and charity. In order to solve the "Social Question," he advocated the "principle of charity" and not the "unnatural principle of democracy."[52]

He argued that it was in the interests of both the state and the wealthy that poor workers and their families should not fall into complete misery on account of illness. But the indigent infirm not only needed medicines, they also needed good food, clean dwellings, a healthy environment, and proper medical care. Accordingly, insurance funds and good hospitals should be provided. To achieve this goal, the state's function should be to issue the necessary regulations, the local administration's role should be to implement them, and it should be the task of private charity to supply hospitals with the proper equipment. Schmidt depicted his vision of the project as follows:

Only in recent times have all sides begun to realize that a hospital is the best and the cheapest tool to help the sick poor. But when this fact has been realized, all will compete to support the work of charity. Masters will insure their servants, guilds their journeymen and apprentices, children will scrape lint, scholars will write books and art societies will give concerts, all to the best of the new hospital – *Singula collecta iuvant* (for small gifts help).[53]

As Erwin H. Ackerknecht has pointed out, many physicians approved of Schmidt's ideas.[54] But there was also a lot of criticism from those who claimed that poor relief should no longer be based on the principle of charity but on the principle of equal rights.

A third group of reformers hoped to reconcile the principle of equal rights with the new scientific interest in hospital medicine. They argued that

50 Ibid., 27.
51 Rudolf Virchow, "Über den Fortschritt in der Entwicklung der Humanitätsanstalten" (1860), in *Gesammelte Abhandlungen aus dem Gebiet der öffentlichen Medicin und der Seuchenlehre* (Berlin, 1879), 2:3–6, esp. 3.
52 Schmidt, *Die Reform der Medicinalverfassung*, 188.
53 Ibid., 199–200.
54 Erwin H. Ackerknecht, "Beiträge zur Geschichte der Medizinalreform von 1848," *Sudhoffs Archiv für Geschichte der Medizin* 25 (1932): 61–109, 113–83, esp. 146.

heretofore a physician had to base his advice on the individual needs of his patient. As long as this subjective approach prevailed, private practice had been superior to hospital practice. But with the introduction of objective scientific medicine, the art of "individualizing" had become obsolete. Hospital medicine could now be as good as private medicine. In 1848 Carl Reclam, a young doctor from Leipzig, wrote: "There are certain achievements in the sciences that are no less precious than those of political life. The principle 'All Germans are equal before the law' is tantamount to another achieved by a tremendous effort: 'Natural laws are equally valid under all conditions.'"[55]

Therefore, as another author put it, medicine would "no longer be rooted in the subjective interests of private medicine but in objective facts, based on natural history and statistics."[56] In a hospital that was to be managed according to the new physiological medicine, the hitherto existing discrimination of hospital patients would be abolished.[57]

The concept of scientific objectivity, one that would know no difference between rich and poor, private and hospital patients, naturally resulted in the complete neglect of social problems. When doctors in the 1860s and 1870s busied themselves with the task of improving hospitals, it was hospital architecture and sanitary conditions, such as air circulation and plumbing, that occupied their minds. The period in which reflection on medicine, social politics, and hospitals found a common aim came to a close in the early 1850s.[58] But, from the professional point of view, the concept proved successful. The characteristics of hospital medicine that had been the source of general disapproval among doctors at the beginning of the century were now considered advantageous. In 1880 a professor of surgery, König, pronounced that hospital medicine was superior to all other forms of medical practice because it granted the unchallenged authority of the physician and the complete isolation of the patients from their social background.[59]

But, in the 1840s, the state and its medical advisors were not the only ones to show an interest in the "Hospital Question." Hospitals were also discussed in left-leaning circles, as reflected by the coverage in their newspapers. In a text that deals ironically with physicians as servants of the rich, the

55 Carl Reclam, "Zweiter Bericht Über die Medicinische Reformbewegung in Leipzig," *Allgemeine Medicinische Central-Zeitung* 17 (1848): 601.
56 Hermann Eberhard Richter, "Über Medicinalreform und ihr Verhältnis zum Staat" (1844), in Hermann Eberhard Richter, *Schriften zur Medicinalreform* (Dresden, 1865), 1–17, esp. 8.
57 Richter, "Über die Benutzung des neuen Stadtkrankenhauses," 45.
58 See also Norbert Klinkenberg, "Die sozialpolitische Isolierung des Krankenhauses im 19. Jahrhundert auf dem Hintergrund der katholisch–bürgerlichen Sozialbestrebungen," *Historia Hospitalium* 15 (1983-84), 213–25.
59 König, "Der Arzt und der Kranke: Mit besonderer Berücksichtigung des Krankenhausarztes," *Zeitschrift für sociale Medicin* 1 (1895): 1–11.

anonymous author demands among other changes "the improvement, the embellishment, and the expansion of hospitals in every respect."[60] Another author meditates on a thorough reform:

Social conditions as a whole are unfavorable to a normalization of hospital practice. They depend on family life and the life of the individual. So, as a matter of fact hospitals are only needed when family assistance and domestic happiness are destroyed. Poverty breaks up these domestic conditions by force and fills the hospitals. ... In our present social order the hospitals are nothing but institutions of charity. They are not an asylum for all who are ill and suffering, but exclusively for the destitute who are ill and suffering. If these preconditions were changed, a comparison between hospital practice and private practice would show that the first had great advantages over the latter.[61]

For only when the hospital would serve rich and poor alike would the patient be sheltered from the noxious influences of his daily reality. He would get the nourishment and nursing his illness required and the constant presence of a doctor. To achieve this the author proposed to end private practice entirely and to transfer all medical care and physicians to the hospital.

Along with this optimistic picture of stationary care came harsh criticism of its reality. Through the end of the nineteenth century, whenever hospital conditions were subjected to political critique from the working-class point of view, the same objections were raised. Hospitals were too small or overcrowded, they were too dirty, the food was bad, admission procedures were too bureaucratic, the staff was rude, the administration or the religious nurses tried to interfere in the patient's personal belief system or moral standards. The medical care was insufficient because doctors lacked sympathy, and methods of treatment ignored the social causes of illness.[62] But such authors accepted at the same time the principle that hospitals were useful, as did the craftsmen's and workers' societies when they offered stationary care to their individual members.[63]

Yet, the fact that inpatient treatment met the needs of patients who had no other alternatives does not imply that they were happy with that care. However, there is in fact some evidence of positive reactions. Barbara Elkeles, who has recently analyzed autobiographies of working-class people who

60   XYZ, "Arzt und Nichtarzt," *Deutsch-Brüsseler-Zeitung*, no. 70 (Sept. 2, 1847), 1–3, esp. 3.
61   "Über die Armenpflege in Köln," 59–60.
62   Ibid.; Barbara Elkeles, "Das Krankenhaus um die Wende vom 19. zum 20. Jahrhundert aus der Sicht seiner Patienten," *Historia Hospitalium* 17 (1986–88): 89–105, and Arbeiterautobiographien als Quelle der Krankenhausgeschichte," *Medizinhistorisches Journal* 23 (1988): 342–58; Alfons Labisch, "Das Krankenhaus in der Gesundheitspolitik der deutschen Sozialdemokratie vor dem Ersten Weltkrieg," *Medizinsoziologisches Jahrbuch* 1 (1981): 126–51; Berger, *Wer bürgt für die Kosten?* 66–82.
63   Frevert's deduction, that married workers who preferred receiving money to getting hospital care did so because they hated the hospital, is not convincing. Most likely they wanted the money for their families. Frevert, *Krankheit als politisches Problem*, 263, 292.

experienced hospital treatment in the second half of the nineteenth century, found that most of the authors remembered the rest, food, and care as benefits that they did not experience in normal life. They often departed the shelter of the hospital with resentment because the doctor declared them recovered or because the insurance funds refused to pay any longer.[64] Sometimes workers' societies complained because their members stayed longer than was necessary.[65]

The strongest argument for the general aversion of patients to hospital care is based on the high death rates that are said to be typical for German public hospitals, at least before the era of antiseptics. As evidence for this thesis, scholars usually cite the case of the Charité in Berlin,[66] where indeed one-third of the patients died in the eighteenth century and where the mortality rate was still at 17 percent in the 1830s.[67] But the Charité was notorious for its overcrowding and bad sanitary conditions and must be considered an exception. In most of the German hospitals, death rates were much lower. Robert Lee has pointed out that, of all the patients treated in the available hospitals in Bavaria in 1851–52, less than 5 percent died.[68] In 1841 the Katharinen Hospital in Stuttgart reported a death rate of 3.2 percent.[69] In the Juliusspital in Würzburg, less than 6 percent of the patients admitted between 1819 and 1829 died while at the hospital.[70]

These figures do not support the thesis that patients saw hospitals as death traps; however, the reliability of these percentages must be examined. Hospital administrators and doctors might have been eager to publish positive results. But at least the death rate of the Juliusspital has been calculated on the basis of unpublished records, compiled by the leading physician, Schönlein. They did not serve any official purpose but were kept solely for scientific reasons; there would have been no point in falsifying these numbers to achieve happier

64 Elkeles, "Arbeiterautobiographien."
65 Berger, Wer bürgt für die Kosten? 20.
66 Frevert, Krankheit als politisches Problem, 75–7, 266.
67 Arthur E. Imhof, "Die Funktion des Krankenhauses in der Stadt des 18. Jahrhunderts," Zeitschrift für Stadtgeschichte, Stadtsoziologie und Denkmalpflege 4 (1977): 215–42, esp. 237; Conrad Heinrich Fuchs, "Über die Sterblichkeit der Stadt Würzburg vom 1. Juli 1819 bis zum 30. Juli 1829," Zeitschrift für die Staatsarzneikunde 25 1833): 369–403, esp. 391.
68 Robert S. Lee, "The Mechanism of Mortality Change in Germany, 1750-1850," Medizinhistorisches Journal 15 (1980): 244–68, esp. 253.
69 Georg Cless, "Fünfzehnter Jahresbericht über die innerliche Abteilung des Katharinenhospitales in Stuttgart vom 1. Juni 1841 bis 30. Juni 1842," Medicinisches Correspondenz-Blatt des Württembergischen ärztlichen Vereins 2 (1842): 281–301, esp. 282.
70 This and what follows are based on an analysis of the hospital records of the Juliusspital, 1819–29, covering more than 10,000 patients who were admitted to the medical ward. Additional information could be drawn from thirty-seven case histories that were published in dissertations between 1820 and 1835. The complete analysis is published in Bleker, Brinkschulte, and Grosse, eds., Kranke und Krankheiten. The final report of the project was sponsored by the Deutsche Forschungsgemeinschaft (DFG).

results. The fact that the calculated mortality rate corresponds with figures in contemporary publications shows that there is no reason to doubt the favorable figures published by other contemporary hospitals.[71]

Another possible explanation for these favorable results could be that general hospitals might have excluded incurable cases. But, at least for Würzburg, research indicates that this was not the case. Quite a number of patients were accepted with clearly fatal diseases, such as cancer or pneumophthisis, and were cared for until death. Moreover, the diagnoses show that the patients who died in the Juliusspital died not because of adverse hospital conditions, but rather of fatal diseases.[72]

On the contrary it can be demonstrated that the high percentage of patients who left the hospital in relatively good health was due to the fact that most of them were young journeymen and female servants. Because of the existence of insurance funds, these people had quick and uncomplicated access to stationary care. Acute diseases and minor health problems, such as indigestion, common cold, headaches, lumbago, and skin diseases, were the most frequent complaints. The Juliusspital, moreover, was on a sound financial footing. It supplied good food and clean beds, and the treatment was moderate.[73] In view of the working and living conditions of the hospital-bound classes, hospital care may well have contributed to their recovery.[74]

A comparison of different groups of patients with respect to their differing rights of access shows that the servants, who were accepted nearly without formalities, more frequently suffered from less serious ailments than the journeymen, whose admissions procedure was slightly more complicated. Compared to both groups, the registered poor, who were accepted only after a thorough consideration of their bodily and social situation, were generally in a bad state of health.

The spectrum of diagnoses suggests that the class of people who had both the right to enter hospitals and relatively easy access to them did so frequently – even when they suffered from disorders that might have been easily cured without medical attention. There were also a number of cases of psychosomatic disease. The most intriguing phenomenon involves the several hundred patients admitted to hospitals between 1819 and 1929 suffering from "hysteria." Schönlein used the term "hysteria" for disorders whereby patients'

---

71 See, e.g., Fuchs, "Über die Sterblichkeit der Stadt Würzburg."

72 The main causes of death among the young were acute pneumonia, tuberculosis, typhus, and typhoid fever. Old people died most often of dropsy, heart disease, apoplexia, and cachexia. Bleker, Brinkschulte, and Grosse, eds., *Kranke und Krankheiten*. See also Lee, "Mechanism of Mortality Change."

73 Schönlein, the leading physician of the medical ward, obviously thought that in most cases improving diet worked better than purging and bloodletting.

74 Pfeufer, *Geschichte des Allgemeinen Krankenhauses*, 77–9.

complaints did not correspond to the objective signs of disease. Most of these patients recovered within one or two weeks – all of them were female servants. A possible explanation lies in the circumstance that these working-class women had learned to express bodily exhaustion and social stress in terms of illness.[75] If this was the case, then the process of medicalization brought about by the rise of hospital care was not a one-way street; it was met by a response from the patients' side, which until now has been largely over-looked in historical studies.

Of course, we must be careful because the patients' attitude must have depended on the condition of the nearest hospital.[76] Moreover, different attitudes arose based on the hopes that patients set on the treatment. In Würzburg, for example, evidence exists that moribund patients pleaded to be sent home. Thus, on the one hand, people may well have approved of stationary care when they needed rest and cure for everyday illnesses. On the other hand, they were frightened of the prospect of dying in the hospital, without friends or family, and by the distressing image of anatomical dissection after death.

In summarizing the arguments I have articulated in this chapter, I would like to submit three theses:

1. Between 1820 and 1870 hospital care became an important compo-nent of the health care system for a discrete class of patients. The majority of the patients were not the registered poor but rather working migrants such as journeymen, servants, miners, and factory workers. To cover their basic needs while sick, insurance funds were created, which provided for station-ary care and also contributed to the operating costs of public hospitals. The increase in stationary facilities in the late 1840s was closely tied to changes in the poor law concerning the working migrants and met the urgent needs of the early industrializing period.

2. Meanwhile, the main interest of the medical profession lay in the educational and scientific possibilities of hospital medicine. Only after the concept of scientific medicine had been generally adopted (in the 1850s and 1860s), did physicians decide that hospital treatment could be as successful as private practice. There is no doubt that on the local level physicians con-tributed a great deal to the establishment and improvement of hospitals. Little evidence exists, however, that the medical profession exerted a substantial influence on the shaping of the hospital as a social institution.

---

75 Johanna Bleker, "Hysterie – Dysmenorrhoe – Chlorose: Diagnosen bei Frauen der Unterschicht im frühen 19. Jahrhundert," *Medizinhistorisches Journal* 29 (1993): 345–74.

76 See also Dietrich, "Die Bedeutung der Krankenhäuser im Gesundheitswesen," *Gesundheit: Zeitschrift für öffentliche und private Hygiene* 13, no. 1 (1888): 3.

3. Concerning the history of hospital patients, a number of currently held opinions need to be revised. The belief that patients hated hospitals "like the plague" or feared them as "gateways to death" can no longer be maintained. With the exception of Berlin's Charité hospital, the average death rate in hospitals was far lower than has been generally claimed. We also find evidence that patients agreed to hospital care, at least when hospitals were administrated properly. Newer research even suggests that patients may have responded to inpatient facilities by medicalizing their bodily and social problems.

2

From Traditional Individualism to Collective Professionalism

State, Patient, Compulsory Health Insurance, and the Panel Doctor Question in Germany, 1883–1931

ALFONS LABISCH

In all industrialized societies, doctors have become exemplary professionals. In different industrial countries, however, the relationship between patients and doctors is arranged differently. In Germany it was Bismarck's social policy and, especially, the advent of health insurance for workers that created the special historical conditions shaping this relationship. As a consequence, in the center of my inquiry lies the rise of compulsory health insurance, as it developed in Germany in the dynamic triangle of the (publicly insured) patient, the panel doctor, and the state between 1871 and 1931. In this chapter I shed light on how doctors first opposed the "collective patient," as the laborers' *Krankenkassen* organization was called, and then eventually came to accept this new health care system.

DOCTORS AND THE STATE BEFORE BISMARCKIAN SOCIAL POLICY

The history of academically trained doctors from the beginning of the nineteenth century to the founding of the German Reich in 1871 is characterized by two developments: the formation of a uniform professional group and their liberation from direct state control.[1] The state was largely responsible for the homogenization of doctors as a group: Training was standardized and controlled; so was the examination, registration, and the supervision of doctors. The role of the state can be seen as marking the historical difference between the professionalization of medicine in Germany and that process in the United Kingdom or the United States.

* Daniel Sanford, Düsseldorf, translated this chapter from German. I would also like to thank him for his further help and advice.

1 Claudia Huerkamp, *Der Aufstieg der Ärzte im 19. Jahrhundert: Vom gelehrten Stand zum professionellen Experten: Das Beispiel Preussens* (Göttingen, 1985); Annette Drees, *Die Ärzte auf dem Weg zu Prestige und Wohlstand: Sozialgeschichte der württembergischen Ärzte im 19. Jahrhundert* (Münster, 1988).

The state also enforced quality control over medical care, which subjected nonregistered healers, including the surgeons of those days, to doctors' control or even ousted them from their practice.[2] The cost of this intervention was that doctors were understood, and understood themselves, to be the auxiliary staff of the state. It was a doctor's duty, for example, to treat the sick, especially the poor (*Kurierzwang*, or compulsory caregiving). Thus, doctors were a fixed item in the late absolutist welfare state.

Regardless of the usefulness of the state's protection and promotion of the social rise of doctors, who were commissioned by the state in the senses of being both authorized and ordered to serve, for individual physicians it was a high price to pay. Even before the 1848 bourgeois revolution, the professional agenda of doctors was aimed at extracting themselves from state control. This goal was attained in the 1869 laws governing trade and industry (*Gewerbeordnung*) within the North German Confederation. Only the title "physician" (*Arzt*) remained regulated, effective for all of Germany after 1871.

The price paid for the status of free entrepreneurs, though, was high. Doctors had to compete with lay healers on an equal basis; they lacked institutionalized influence over state health policy; and they had no control over their own profession. Thus, just a few years after their liberation from state control, doctors' professional agenda took a new direction; namely, revision of the *Gewerbeordnung* (Trade and industry regulations) of 1869 – without, however, affecting their status as a "free profession." Owing to the dramatic increase in the number of academically trained doctors, this agenda soon gained considerable importance.

In 1871 the Reich became responsible for policy-making in the area of medicine. As a reaction, the Federation of German Medical Associations (*Deutscher Ärztevereinsbund*, or DÄVB) was founded at the first Congress of German Doctors (*erster Deutscher Ärztetag*), held in Wiesbaden on September 17, 1873. According to the statutes of the DÄVB, the organization's goal was "to unite the scattered medical associations in Germany for the purpose of mutual encouragement and concerted use of the scientific and practical, even social connections of the medical profession."[3] The DÄVB, therefore, was composed of associations; that is, it consisted of juridical and not natural persons. To the extent that scientific problems were delegated to the numerous specialist societies, the DÄVB concentrated "more or less on the representation of doctors' interests in the narrower sense, as its actually central function."[4]

---

2 Sabine Sander, *Handwerkschirurgen: Sozialgeschichte einer verdrängten Berufsgruppe* (Göttingen, 1989).
3 Huerkamp, *Aufstieg*, 249.
4 Ibid.

The exchange of *Kurierzwang* (compulsory caregiving) for *Kurierfreiheit* (freedom to chose patients) in the *Gewerbeordnung* of 1873 remained controversial. Gradually, those doctors who demanded official representation got the upper hand. In this diverse development, which differed from state to state, a new form of professional representation, recognized by the state yet self-organized, the *Ärztekammern* (doctors' chambers), emerged in Prussia and elsewhere. These chambers were part of a general attempt on the part of the states to organize trade, agriculture, business, and the free professions. The Royal Prescription of May 25, 1887, forced all doctors to enroll in doctors' chambers, the function of which was the "discussion of all questions and problems relating to the medical profession or to the interest of public health care, or which are directed toward the observation and representation of professional interests of doctors."[5]

Nevertheless, a doctors' chamber had very little power to impose discipline on its members. Only the active and passive voting rights in the organization could be suspended. Therefore, the advocates of a state-protected representative body judged the power of professional self-regulation to be weak. As a result a public discussion of health policy appeared necessary, one that emphasized the significance of doctors—as had happened in the mercantilist welfare policy and its "medical police." It was Bismarck's social policy that sparked the public's interest, the necessary counterpart of the well-directed and effective effort to further doctors' professional interests.

THE REICH BEFORE BISMARCK'S SOCIAL POLICY (1871–1881)

It is impossible to understand German social policy without understanding the contemporary political situation in the Reich. The German Reich had been established in 1871 in the course of Prussia's deliberate policy under Otto von Bismarck, the Prussian minister president, of seeking hegemony in Germany. Bismarck secured the newly gained unity of the various German states by means of a foreign policy that was based on a complex system of alliances. This "external founding of the Reich" was complemented by an "internal founding"—the standardization of the laws and economic structures (e.g., monetary and postal systems) across the traditionally independent German states.

One problem of domestic policy that remained unresolved was the political and social position of labor. The fate of workers was inextricably tied to both industrial development and economic policy. Economic policy had been generally liberal since the early nineteenth century. Driven by the fear

5 Ibid., 263.

of a "red revolution," however, a policy of restriction and exclusion was implemented against the constantly growing laboring classes. In towns and in the individual states, labor was excluded from political participation by means of weighted voting, a three-class electoral system, which was based on the amount of taxes paid. If laborers could not provide for their families – due to illness or accident, for example – and had to apply for public relief, they fell under the jurisdiction of the poverty laws and thus lost their few civil rights. What was the social position of the constantly growing "fourth estate," or industrial labor, to be in a society that grew to be the second most powerful industrial and trading power in the world, yet still saw itself as a society organized corporatively and according to authoritarian principles?

The relatively powerless Reichstag was, in contrast, elected by universal manhood suffrage. The percentage of votes received by the Social Democratic Party continued to increase from 3.2 percent in 1871 to 9.1 percent in 1877. On October 18, 1878, the parliament passed the anti-Socialist laws, which banned the party press and party organizations. Social Democrats were, however, still permitted to be elected to the Reichstag. Despite the attempt to subdue the political labor movement by police force, which was ardently pursued from 1878 until 1881, its representation in the Reichstag kept growing. By 1887 the Social Democrats had 10.1 percent of all votes. Only in this historical context – "external founding of the Reich," "internal founding of the Reich," authoritarian-corporative notions of the society in the minds of the leading bourgeois and Junker classes, and legal and police exclusion of the labor movement – can the development of Germany's social policy be understood.

An offspring of old conservative Brandenburg nobility, Bismarck revived the patronizing poverty policy of the preindustrial mercantilistic welfare state. The goal of Bismarck's integrationist labor policy was to bind to the nation those needy subjects who had been expelled by the liberal economic policy. They were, however, to remain second-class citizens. On the one hand, this policy was directed against economic liberalism and its, as it were, "natural" exclusion of labor and the poor. On the other hand, it was clearly also directed against the socialist labor movement, which, as a "party of rebellion," was engaged in turning labor against society and the state.

As a consequence of this philosophy, the sociopolitical reasons for Bismarck's labor policy and his aims can be summarized as follows: (1) The liberal notion of private subsistence of the propertyless by work-for-pay alone is neither "natural" nor is it sufficient in the case of sickness, accident, or old age; (2) Subsidization of the poor according to liberal concepts promotes alienation from the public institutions of the ruling system; (3) The private subsistence of labor has to be augmented by a public and legally and politically nondiscriminatory social policy, which should create new social attachments to the state; and (4) The Reich's social policy should affect workers directly, not indirectly, and thus be conspicuous to them.[6] In the famous imperial decree of November 17, 1881, this program was presented to the Reichstag.

With this policy, which was based on a conservative, patriarchal view of the state, Bismarck simultaneously took on industrialists, Junkers, and the socialist labor movement alike. In practice, he had to make substantial concessions. Nevertheless, this constellation of opposing interests is necessary in order to understand the construction of the German social security system. This applies especially to the health insurance system, which was to become the key to the social integration of labor, although in a totally different way than anyone could have expected.

FROM THE HEALTH INSURANCE LAW (1883) TO ITS AMENDMENT (1892)

The Law Concerning Health Insurance of Laborers (*Gesetz betr. die Krankenversicherung der Arbeiter*, hereafter referred to as the Health Insurance Law) passed the Reichstag on June 15, 1883, as the first of the proposed social welfare laws. The Health Insurance Law fell into an area that traditionally had been the site of political strife.[7] Some of the existing health insurance institutions could be traced to the mutual insurance of medieval guilds, some to the health insurance of miners' guilds, some to the company health insurance created by industrialists, some to the voluntary, self-organized workers' insurance, and some to the local community insurance for the poor. Since 1854 employers had been required to pay part of the premiums of (industrial) auxiliary insurance.

As a result of this history, three elements of health insurance institutions developed: compulsory health insurance or compulsory membership in local or in trade health insurance organizations; financial participation of employers in their employees' insurance payments; and the extraordinary

---

6   Florian Tennstedt, "Vorgeschichte und Entstehung der Kaiserlichen Botschaft vom 17. November 1881," *Zeitschrift für Sozialreform* 27 (1981): 663–710.

7   Florian Tennstedt, "Sozialgeschichte der Sozialversicherung," in Maria Blohmke et al., eds., *Handbuch der Sozialmedizin* (Stuttgart, 1976), 3:385–492; Florian Tennstedt, *Geschichte der Selbstverwaltung in der Krankenversicherung von der Mitte des 19. Jahrhunderts bis zur Gründung der Bundesrepublik Deutschland* (Bonn, 1977); Florian Tennstedt, "Die Errichtung von Krankenkassen in deutschen Städten nach dem Gesetz betr. die Krankenversicherung der Arbeiter vom 15. Juni 1883: Ein Beitrag zur Frühgeschichte der gesetzlichen Krankenversicherung in Deutschland," *Zeitschrift für Sozialreform* 29 (1983): 297–338; Ute Frevert, *Krankheit als politisches Problem, 1770–1880: Soziale Unterschichten in Preussen zwischen medizinischer Polizei und staatlicher Sozialversicherung* (Göttingen, 1984).

political significance for labor of the independent management of their health insurance funds.

On April 7, 1876, the "independent health insurance organizations" (*freie Hilfskassen*), organized by trade unions, became regulated by law. They began to form in the 1860s and freed workers from compulsory membership in the aforementioned local or trade health insurance organizations. Health insurance was still compulsory, but as opposed to the locally or administratively prescribed insurance organizations, the *Hilfskassen* were self-managed by labor.

In this sociopolitically highly sensitive area of public policy, the Health Insurance Law felt like an imposition. Nevertheless, the law contained the structural principles – still inherent in the present-day health insurance system in Germany – that insurance is compulsory, and premiums are paid as advance concessions; that members have a legal claim to services without a preliminary check of neediness; that rates are not dependent on risk factors (such as age, sex, or preexisting conditions), but on gross income (social leveling among different earnings); that a health certificate is not required when joining the insurance; that services rendered need not be paid back; and that employers partially pay premiums.[8]

Accordingly, health insurance organizations became juridical persons under public law and were called "compulsory insurance funds" (*gesetzliche Krankenkassen*).The services of these funds consisted mostly of cash payments: money in cases of sickness (paid after a three-day waiting period and making up 50 percent to a maximum of 75 percent of lost income), money in cases of death, and maternity support (only for female members, and not for uninsured wives of members). Material support consisted of free medical treatment, medication, glasses, trusses, and other remedies. Fees were compulsorily paid as a percentage of income (beginning with slightly less than 2 percent). One third was aid by the employer, two thirds by the employee. Self-management by labor was intended to help integrate this group socially. The seats in the self-management organs of the health insurance organizations were distributed according to the portion paid. Thus, labor always took two thirds of the seats.

The main goal of the Health Insurance Law was to prevent economic disadvantages on account of illness, and thus to prevent laborers and their families from falling under the jurisdiction of the poverty laws. The economic situation of labor families in cases of illness was to be improved, and the burden of public support for the poor was to be alleviated. Here we clearly

8 Tennstedt, "Sozialversicherung," 386; Florian Tennstedt, *Sozialgeschichte der Sozialpolitik vom 18. Jahrhundert bis zum 1. Weltkrieg* (Göttingen, 1981), 169–70.

see the connection between labor policy and poverty policy. The Health Insurance Law was not a part of health policy as such, but of labor and poverty policies. At the center of health insurance services was not medical aid, but securing income, that is, sick money. Thus, the relationship between funds for doctors and sickness played a subordinate role for the legislature, and was not regulated by the Health Insurance Law. However, health insurance organizations were required to guarantee medical services according to the principle of material support. In addition, doctors had to attest to an illness by their professional report, for instance, in the form of a certificate of illness (*Krankenschein*). Thus, insurance organizations were dependent on the cooperation of the doctors. Health insurance organizations – and, through their self-management, labor as well – and doctors were forced to cooperate in a field where all sorts of sociopolitical and professional aims and goals interacted.

Thus, in health insurance, social compensation of poor living conditions, and not the individual health risk, was dominant. Moreover, membership in compulsory *Krankenkassen* had to meet labor law and social policy criteria, not medical or health policy criteria. The labor movement especially criticized the political intentions of the law. Political labor thus immediately started agitation against the Health Insurance Law and its newly created *Krankenkassen*. The labor movement's goals were then concentrated in independent health insurance organizations.

In light of the battles to come, doctors paid little attention to the Health Insurance Law. In the last years of the nineteenth century, the role of insurance-affiliated doctors was restricted to attesting to illness and thus providing access to sick money and other monetary services. Medical treatment was not the rule. In 1899 a committee of the Prussian chamber of doctors stated, "[B]y far the greater part of members of health and accident insurance organizations now in medical treatment never used to make use of doctors' services without suffering any lasting harm from it."[9]

Cooperation of doctors and health insurance organizations was, therefore, burdened by quite ordinary financial and organizational difficulties. This relationship toppled mainly because of two developments.[10] The number of licensed doctors grew rapidly during this time, leading to dramatic competition. At the same time, the compulsory health insurance led to a significant rise in the number of insured patients. The various laws and ordinances brought about an increase in the percentage of the state-insured population from 9.2 percent in 1885 to 23 percent in 1914, excluding family members.

9 Tennstedt, "Sozialversicherung," 388.
10 Huerkamp, *Aufstieg*, 151, 198.

If one includes family members and people insured in nonstate organizations, one third of the German population was compulsorily insured before World War I. A clientele hitherto unknown to doctors and, as far as poor-house doctors go, rather disliked, grew considerably, whereas the middle-class clientele diminished.

Caught between competition and the compulsorily insured, it became clear that the treatment of the latter type of patient would become increasingly important for the medical profession. Perhaps the classical ideal of the independent physician would have to be dropped in favor of the more or less dependent panel doctor. The boards of the various *Krankenkassen* approached doctors as monopolistic suppliers, whereas doctors competed individually for positions as panel doctors. Thus, the boards could determine the fundamental conditions of the contracts. These developments alone would have provided enough cause for future dispute.

On June 15, 1892, the Prussian parliament passed a Law Concerning Amendment of the Law on Health Insurance of Laborers (hereafter referred to as the Health Insurance Amendment Law). This law was an attack on the independent aid health insurance organizations (*freie Hilfskassen*), which were run by labor. It generalized the principle of material services for all compulsory insurance organizations. It also gave preference to the hitherto universal (not trade-restricted) local insurance organizations, which in some cities were developing into larger general insurance funds (*Allgemeine Ortskrankenkassen*).

Only now, because escape into independent insurance organizations was precluded, the organized labor movement started to "turn away from founding and managing independent health insurance organizations (*Hilfskassen*) in favor of membership and self-management in the local health insurance organizations. Thus begins the 'rule of Social Democracy in Health Insurance,' which was strongly opposed to by all supporting powers in the kaiser's Reich."[11] Here, too, we must bear in mind the general sociopolitical situation. Under the auspices of Kaiser Wilhelm II's "new course," the anti-Socialist laws were not renewed in 1890. The labor movement was now able to expand their political and social organizations without impediment, and no longer needed the *Hilfskassen*.

THE "RULE OF SOCIAL DEMOCRACY" IN THE KRANKENKASSEN

The distribution of free medical services based on the Health Insurance Law (§ 6) created difficult contractual conditions between doctors and

11   Tennstedt, "Sozialversicherung," 390.

compulsory health insurance organizations.[12] The contracts usually had one of the following forms: Mainly small *Krankenkassen* had only one contracted doctor (so-called fixed panel doctors, or *fixierte Kassenärzte*); larger *Krankenkassen* had several doctors spread out over the organization's area of operation (so-called district physician system).

Ideal contractual conditions were to be found in the "free choice of/by doctors" (*freie Arztwahl*), although interpretations of what this meant varied widely. From the beginning of health insurance in the 1840s, the term *freie Arztwahl* had meant that workers were not forced to visit any specific doctor. For doctors, it meant that any doctor could work on behalf of the health insurance organizations if he wished to do so. Thus, the idea of a doctor's free choice was truly realized only with the passage of the Health Insurance Law. In the broadest sense, it was supposed to secure a collective contract between *Krankenkassen* and doctors so that all doctors could participate in treatment of the compulsory insured patients.

In any case, a new triangular relationship resulted in the compulsory health insurance system. Into the traditionally "classical" mutual relationship between doctors and patients,

the health insurance organization inserted itself as a third player. It had to influence the extent and type of medical treatment, if it wanted to remain efficient. The heretofore existing "liberal and individual" profession of doctors, who liked to view themselves as the "epitome of the liberal bourgeoisie" and pioneers of the "educated classes," was confronted with a new situation. Doctors, insofar as they worked for insurance organizations, felt cast into the role of employees, an idea unbearable to doctors who insisted on their academic education.[13]

A difficult situation arose. Members of *Krankenkassen* had an interest in extending the number and type of insurance services. Doctors in turn profited from this development. The potentially solvent clientele was constantly growing by means of compulsory insurance membership. However, the ideal of medical action was seen in the supposedly classical relationship between family doctor and private patient. It mattered little that this glorified view had nothing to do with historical fact.[14]

After 1895 the influential role that Social Democracy played in the *Krankenkassen*, which was fiercely discussed in the press, added to the problems.[15] Essentially, it meant that the elite of Social Democratic labor and

12 Huerkamp, *Aufstieg*, 194–240.
13 Hans-Werner Niemann, "Der Kampf der deutschen Ärzte gegen die gesetzlichen Krankenkassen (1883–1914)," *Niedersächsisches Jahrbuch für Landesgeschichte* 52 (1980): 267–8.
14 Huerkamp, *Aufstieg*, 22–24.
15 Florian Tennstedt, *Vom Proleten zum Industriearbeiter: Arbeiterbewegung und Sozialpolitik in Deutschland, 1800–1914* (Cologne, 1983), 432–70.

trade unions constituted the boards and the membership of the local insurance organizations in industrial regions. Accordingly, the ubiquitous hassle
between insurance boards and their contracted doctors was sociopolitically
heated.

This conflict between doctors and labor's *Krankenkassen* contributed
substantially to the unification of the medical profession. To the extent that
competition among doctors increased during the 1880s and 1890s, the
established doctors' chambers proved to be inadequate in enforcing unified
representation of doctors' interests. Young doctors, in particular, would not
easily be disciplined by collective professional representation.

Thus, conservative policymakers within the profession demanded – in
addition to the doctors' chambers, which were recognized by public law – an
independent professional tribunal.[16] It was much harder, however, to win
approval for this demand from the doctors' professional organization and from
the state. For the first time, proponents of this professional agenda utilized
the argument that even doctors had to become active against the "poison of
Social Democracy." The noble appeal to "public health care" was exchanged
for something more substantial: The panel doctors took the bourgeois/avant-
garde position in the central sociopolitical conflict of their time. In Prussia
medical professional tribunal legislation became law on April 1, 1900. These
medical tribunals proved to be effective instruments with which to discipline
nonconformist doctors.[17] Doctors practicing alternative medicine or those
who held politically incorrect views were brought up on charges, typically
because of supposed "unfriendly collegiality." At the beginning of the twentieth century almost every fifth doctor in Prussia faced such a suit.

Around 1900 doctors were obligated to join the doctors' chambers,
although differences existed among the various states, and they were subject
to disciplinary action by professional tribunals. Thus, the regulations on trade
and industry (*Gewerbeordnung*) of 1869–73 had been revised in certain
respects – but not by the state, whose intrusive power was resented, but by
newly won influence of the medical profession.

16 Please note that the professional agenda of German doctors united numerous traditions, which have
    hitherto not been properly investigated. Toward the end of the nineteenth century, and especially
    during the Weimar era, they were slowly absorbed by more conservative traditions. See Michael
    Hubenstorf, "Von der 'freien Arztwahl' zur Reichsärzteordnung: Ärztliche Standespolitik zwischen
    Liberalismus und Nationalsozialismus," in Johanna Bleker and Norbert Jachertz, eds., *Medizin im
    Dritten Reich* (Cologne, 1989), 112–22; Michael Hubenstorf, "Deutsche Landärzte an die Front!"
    Ärztliche Standespolitik zwischen Liberalismus und Nationalsozialismus," in Christian Pross and
    Götz Aly, eds., *Der Wert des Menschen: Medizin in Deutschland, 1918–1945* (Berlin, 1989), 200–23.
17 Ernst Luther, "Die Herausbildung und gesellschaftliche Sanktionierung der ärztlichen
    Standesauffassung in der zweiten Hälfte des 19. Jahrhunderts," *Wissenschaftliche Zeitschrift der Martin-
    Luther-Universität Halle-Wittenberg, Mathematisch-Naturwissenschaftliche Abteilung*, ser. 24, no. 2
    (1975): 23–4; Huerkamp, *Aufstieg*, 270–2.

FROM THE "LEIPZIGER VERBAND" (1900) TO THE BERLIN AGREEMENT (1913)

Beginning in 1894 health insurance organizations had started to organize on the provincial, then on the national level.[18] The panel doctor question was one of the main subjects at the organizations' meetings. In general, the drafting of contracts was left to the individual *Krankenkasse*. Thus, individual contracts with doctors were the rule. Structurally, the doctors were at a disadvantage compared to insurance organizations. Especially loathsome was the position of fixed panel doctors, who were bound to the insurance organization by contract and—in the words of doctors—degraded to the position of subordinate officials subject to the former's directives. This "proletarianization" to a status even below that of the laboring classes was, of course, the exact opposite of the independent family doctor.

In 1900 some doctors in Leipzig, Freiburg, and Ludwigshafen started to organize behind the economic interests of panel doctors collectively in imitation of the tactics used by trade unions.[19] The rather reserved policy ("befitting to the social standing of medicine") of the DÄVB, which called for legislation regarding resolutions and petitions, was evaded—despite the doubts, and even in the face of the loud protest, of many doctors. And yet, how else should the necessary collective action of doctors working in their individual offices be organized? The tactics borrowed from the labor movement had to be utilized here, too, against two sides: and against the insurance organizations as the actual opponents; and against the colleagues, who had to be welded together out of amorphous and anarchic individuality into an organization united for battle.

On September 13, 1900, the panel doctor Hermann Hartmann, of Leipzig, founded the Association of German Doctors for the Defense of Their Economic Interests, commonly referred to as the Leipziger Verband.[20] According to the statutes of this organization, the society aimed "to improve the economic situation of doctors in the whole Reich and to provide the same with effective protection from inconsiderate exploitation on the part of the *Krankenkassen* and from the infringements of the funds' boards."[21] The

---

18 Tennstedt, *Selbstverwaltung*, 83–104.
19 A number of alternative solutions regarding professional policy and the panel doctors' question were either in public discussion or had already been implemented on the local level. With few exceptions, these alternatives in theory and practice have heretofore escaped the attention of historians of medicine. See Hubenstorf, "Deutsche Landärzte"; and Daniel S. Nadav, *Julius Moses und die Politik der Sozialhygiene in Deutschland* (Gerlingen, 1985).
20 Huerkamp, *Aufstieg*, 279–302; Rolf Neuhaus, *Arbeitskämpfe, Ärztestreiks, Sozialreformer: Sozialpolitische Konfliktregelung 1900 bis 1914* (Berlin, 1986).
21 Tennstedt, *Selbstverwaltung*, 77.

association's immediate goal was the organized free choice by doctors – of course in the doctors' version, with general, unlimited access to panel doctors' positions. The long-term goal was to retain the individual position of the (family) doctor even within the framework of collective compulsory health insurance.

In spite of the mistrust and even disapproval of the DÄVB, the Leipzig association pursued a clever course against the health insurance organizations. Single boycotts and strikes now were uniformly organized and were carried out with extreme severity. The association succeeded in organizing strikes by collective canceling of contracts, in which gradually all doctors participated. This even worked against large *Krankenkassen*, such as in Cologne in 1904 and in Leipzig in 1905. The successes of 1904–5 gained the Leipzig association the respect of many doctors, which it had previously lacked. In September 1903 the association was incorporated into the DÄVB as its economics division. In 1905 almost 60 percent of all doctors were organized in the Leipzig association; in 1911, more than 75 percent – and as opposed to the Federation of German Medical Associations these were all individual memberships.[22] Even trade unions never reached this degree of organization. The united front of doctors affected the action of funds' boards. According to Florian Tennstedt, the Leipzig association participated in a total of 1,700 disputes and conflicts between September 13, 1900, and September 23, 1913, "of which only eighteen had no satisfactory conclusion for its members."[23]

Thus, the constellation of power between doctors and insurance organizations had been turned around in just a few years. The reason was mainly the predicament into which the Health Insurance Law placed the *Krankenkassen*. The *Krankenkassen* had the legal obligation to provide their members with medical care. Doctors, however, were by no means obliged to provide their services to *Krankenkassen*. The policy of the Leipzig association was criticized not only by health insurance organizations and the societies supporting them; there was also a great deal of criticism from doctors themselves. In addition, the Supreme Court of the Reich accused the association of "immoral action."[24] Nevertheless, the association gained increasing influence upon the collective action and the professional orientation of doctors. For instance, the system of organized free choice of doctors became standard – against the protest of some doctors. The self-regulation of panel doctors by medical controllers also was established, a necessary system

22 Huerkamp, *Aufstieg*, 283.
23 Tennstedt, *Selbstverwaltung*, 81.
24 Tennstedt, "Sozialversicherung," 394. Criticism from inside the medical profession and from beyond its boundaries is discussed in Huerkamp, *Aufstieg*, 301; and Neuhaus, *Arbeitskämpfe*.

developed by the Leipzig association to check the efficiency of numbers and dues of panel doctors.

The discourse on the panel doctor question contributed decisively to the formation of a uniform medical profession, regarding the right of self-determination, and to the creation of the predominant view of the doctor as a free and independent (although collectively organized) panel doctor. The position of panel doctors – disagreeable, unavoidable, and certainly profitable – was integrated into the classical medical career of a private doctor in a bearable fashion. Social security altogether, and especially health insurance, thus became the decisive counterpart, against which doctors were able to achieve their professional independence within a mass society, that is, as a guild (*Stand*) or professional group. Ideologically, the representatives profited from acting like a bourgeois spearhead against social democracy, while using social democratic and trade unionist tactics for doing political battle. Moreover, the Leipzig association succeeded in "projecting the total social problem of doctors onto health insurance organizations as scapegoats."[25]

The unity of doctors was demonstrated in the discourse on the Reich insurance laws (*Reichsversicherungsordnung*, or RVO) from 1909 to 1911. Although the clientele of panel doctors was extended considerably by this law, it passed without taking into account the demands of the doctors, which had been vehemently expressed. The panel doctor question was not dealt with by the RVO. An extraordinary doctors' congress decided on October 26, 1913, "with thunderous applause" and near unanimity "to go on general strike with the coming into effect of the RVO on January 1, 1914."[26] The existing contracts with insurance organizations were canceled as of December 31, 1913. A nationwide general strike of panel doctors seemed unavoidable.

Faced with this threat, involved ministries, insurance organizations, and doctors' associations reached a compromise on the basis of a draft by Otto Heinemann, the secretary of the association of company *Krankenkassen*.[27] In this so-called Berlin Agreement, numerous arrangements were agreed upon: The employment autonomy of *Krankenkassen* was eliminated; in a regulated procedure, representatives of all panel doctors shared responsibility with the *Krankenkassen*; contracts between *Krankenkassen* and their doctors were individually based yet collectively drawn up.[28] The contract committee (*Vertragsausschuss*), the elected representative body of doctors facing the

25 Tennstedt, "Sozialversicherung," 394.
26 Huerkamp, *Aufstieg*, 302.
27 Tennstedt, *Selbstverwaltung*, 81–2; Neuhaus, *Arbeitskämpfe*, 351–6.
28 Tennstedt, *Selbstverwaltung*, 82.

Krankenkassen, was in effect an acknowledgment of collective contracts. The elimination of employment autonomy indirectly promoted the free choice of doctors, at least the way doctors understood the term. For every 1,350 individuals with compulsory insurance, one panel doctor was to be contractually employed.

In the Berlin Agreement, the doctors had achieved the position of equal partners in negotiations between ministries and *Krankenkassen* associations and of equals in contracts with *Krankenkassen*. This was due only to the high degree of organization and the aggressive policy of the Association for the Representation of Economic Interests of German Doctors. This association, in turn, had benefitted from having taken a front-line position against social democracy. In addition, and prompted mainly by the labor problem, doctors had finally established themselves as a professional group with a united appearance, in fact if not yet in law.

MEDICAL PROFESSIONAL INTERESTS, THE DEMOCRATIC WELFARE STATE, AND THE EMERGENCY DECREES OF 1924 AND 1931

The nationalist and conservative Reich collapsed in November 1918. In the aftermath, the Social Democrats, these "fatherlandless fellows" (*vaterlandslose Gesellen*), had shown themselves to be guarantors of law and the state. Their aim was no longer social revolution but a social welfare state. The first results of successful cooperation between insurance organizations and doctors were, however, destroyed by the inflation of 1922–3. The Berlin Agreement, which had fulfilled the function of providing a contractual framework for insurance organizations, was set to expire on December 31, 1923. Negotiations on the renewal of the agreement failed, mainly because representatives of health insurance organizations wanted to legislate the relationship between doctors and insurance organizations, which the representatives of doctors rejected.[29]

In this hopeless situation, the Reich Labor Ministry (*Reichsarbeitsministerium*, or RAM) employed a coercive legal instrument. On October 30, 1923, emergency decrees concerning doctors and insurance organizations and aiding the sick were enacted. The first decree gave the formerly voluntary mutual (Berlin) agreement the force of law. The formerly rather loosely organized Central Committee of Doctors and Insurance Organizations was converted into a mandatory cooperative. The main objective of this Reich committee was to work out guidelines for uniform and appropriate arrangements between doctors and health insurance organizations. The formerly private contract relationship between doctors and health insurance organiza-

29 Ibid., 133–49.

tions was slowly infiltrated by public law; the personal and local leeway was narrowed for doctors and health insurance organizations as well; and the power and influence of representative bodies were broadened.

In the decree on aiding the sick, doctors were made responsible for the economic risks of their prescriptions. Thus, panel doctors were compelled to consider the economic situation and capability of individual health insurance organizations. In the case of continued "breach of trust," panel doctors could be suspended and barred from treating compulsorily insured clientele for two years. These measures enraged the Leipzig association, and they organized a general strike. As of December 1, 1923, all doctors were called on to abrogate their existing contracts.[30]

This dispute was resolved on January 24, 1924, when the government, representatives of health insurance organizations, and the Leipzig association reached an agreement. All laws concerning doctors were to be discussed with the Leipzig association; the decree on aiding the sick was voided; and the legal situation ante was reestablished. On May 12, 1924, guidelines for the general content of contracts were enacted; they had not been drawn up by the government but by the Reich committee of doctors and health insurance organizations. On the whole, the procedures in the Berlin agreement were confirmed. This regulation increased the power of the regional and central organizations. The autonomy of the individual health insurance organization, as well as the autonomy of the individual panel doctor, had once and for all passed to its collective representatives.

Under the influence of the world economic crisis, several attempts were proposed to reduce costs. A bill on modification of the health insurance system was promoted, which included a rigid control of panel doctors by independent examining doctors (*Vertrauensarzt*), the possibility of malpractice suits against panel doctors, and flat-rate payment for services provided by panel doctors. The discourse about this law in the heated political situation toward the end of the Weimar Republic, however, became a stumbling block for the whole development of relations between doctors and health insurance organizations.

On July 26, 1930, an emergency decree was proclaimed that confirmed the aforementioned bill on modification of the health insurance system. This emergency decree mainly limited services rendered to holders of insurance and also limited payment and working conditions of panel doctors. The postliminary examination by "independent doctors" became compulsory, and medical examination offices were opened. It became apparent that under

30 Eckhard Hansen et al., eds., *Seit über einem Jahrhundert: Verschüttete Alternativen in der Sozialpolitik* (Cologne, 1981), 154.

the influence of health insurance organizations these "independent doctors" would attain some sort of power over panel doctors. The income and the rights of panel doctors would have been drastically cut by this emergency decree. Still, for the first time, doctors' representatives seemed to have realized how much their status and their income depended on the despised compulsory health insurance system. Membership in compulsory health insurance had jumped from 16 million in 1919 to 20 million by 1929. Including family members, who were also covered by insurance, two thirds of Germany's population was compulsorily insured before the onset of the world economic crisis. Social court verdicts had introduced family insurance as a common service. It could be seen that compulsory health insurance was developing from a health insurance system for the laboring classes to one for the whole population. If the system was endangered, then not only the panel doctors but all doctors were endangered. For in 1929, 37,246 of 49,974 doctors, or 75 percent, worked in independent – that is, private – practice.

Negotiations in the following months between doctors' representatives and health insurance representatives produced an agreement between the Main Association and the General Association of German Health Insurance Organizations and the two doctors' associations on October 17, 1931. When the other insurance representatives rejected the agreement, Reich President Paul von Hindenburg enforced it legally through the emergency decree of December 8, 1931. According to Otto Heinemann, the government changed course "because the Reich government had to count on doctors' votes in the Reichstag."[31]

The emergency decree of December 8, 1931, replaced that of July 26, 1930. In exchange for a lump sum (always a certain percentage of the insurance organizations' revenues), the panel doctors agreed to secure the medical treatment of insurance members. The responsibility was assumed by the regional representatives, the unions of panel doctors (*Kassenärztliche Vereinigungen*, or KV), which had been created by an emergency decree of November 8, 1931. The commission for securing treatment (*Sicherstellungsauftrag*) transferred the responsibility to provide medical treatment from insurance organizations to panel doctors.

As a reward for this financial and organizational risk, panel doctors were able to organize and supervise their work themselves, including their economic efficiency, through the KV. As representatives of the panel doctors, the KV became institutions of public law and membership became mandatory. In addition, the regionally organized unions, or KV, were mostly identical

31 Tennstedt, *Selbstverwaltung*, 132n. 64.

with the Leipzig association. The self-management of local health insurance organizations was mostly abolished. The individual contract between doctors and health insurance organizations was superseded by collective contracts and agreements on lump payments on the level of their representations. The ratio of doctors to insurance members was raised to 1:600.

Nonetheless, the individual panel doctor no longer had to hassle with insurance organizations. Instead, he was subject to strict control and sometimes examination by the panel doctor union. That was noticed in the struggle for positions as panel doctors; the positions were distributed by a licensing committee established by the KV. It was also noticed in the payment of fees to the individual panel doctor. They could be cut, depending on the money that had to be distributed and the services rendered by all panel doctors. A medical functionary commented that "a doctor who has been able to observe the situation from close up has established that doctors rid themselves of the rule of insurance organizations in 1931, but traded it in for the tyranny of an oligarchy of their own profession."[32] The classic relationship of conflict between doctors and health insurance organizations had toppled over in favor of the panel doctors. The three-way relationship of insured patient, insurance organization, and panel doctor, which had been typical for the system of compulsory health insurance since 1883, was broadened in 1931 to a four-way relationship both typical of, and unique to, Germany. It consisted – and still consists – of panel doctor, insured patient, insurance organization, and panel doctor unions. The health insurance organizations had found a counterpart in the KV, which was responsible for the provision of medical treatment, its organization and its efficiency, and for representation of panel doctors vis-à-vis insurance organizations.

Thus, doctors had managed to counter the "collective patient" of the labor health insurance organizations with an appropriate collective representation in the form of the panel doctor union. In the legal and economic realms, insured patients and panel doctors met, so to speak, as juridical persons in the form of insurance organizations and KV. The doctors' side was structurally superior: The KV were organized in public law and within the borders of the German states, or *Länder*, and were opposed by a number of separate health insurance organizations in private law, assembled in provincial and *Länder* associations, but lacking political consensus.

32 Julius Hadrich, *Die Arztfrage in der deutschen Sozialversicherung: Ihre soziologischen und wirtschaftlichen Probleme* (Berlin, 1955), 121.

THE STATE, THE PATIENT, THE PHYSICIAN: SOCIAL POLICY, LABOR, PANEL DOCTORS

Already conflict laden, the relationship between doctors and compulsory health insurance organizations had become one of the principal sociopolitical issues of the time. Moreover, beyond the mere socially disciplining aspect that was intended politically, the problem of compulsory health insurance became part of the secular civilizing process in industrial society.

Bismarck's social policy was a means of shaping society through politics. The first goal was to keep the laboring classes, which had evolved from the earlier crafts, above the poverty line. At the same time, labor was to be molded into an industrial population that was predictable with regard to productivity and behavior. All this was to be achieved with methods conforming to society and the market; methods and conditions of production were not to be fundamentally altered. Rather, assistance was offered, for which employers could plan and which made the reproduction of labor stable in method and price. In addition, this aid was, at least, to compensate for existential threats to labor by sickness, accident, old age, and death. Regarding conformity to the market, these compensatory services were organized as either cash payments or as actual services. This required the laborers to come to terms with the prevailing conditions of production and to balance their effects privately and in conformity with social norms, that is, through individual reproduction and market-oriented consumption.

Within this strategy, called "social security as social discipline," other mechanisms were effective that were neither planned nor predicted.[33] The socially disciplining effect of wants and needs, which had only been created by social security, was apparent. As a result of health insurance, a demand for medication and other aids, as well as medical consultation, had been generated. The satisfaction of basic needs such as food, clothing, housing, and education was to contribute to Social Democracy's development of pragmatic policies that conformed to societal norms under the cover of their revolutionary objectives.[34]

Here, a general civilizing development took place.[35] In the universal rationalization of all spheres of thinking and action during the period of industri-

---

33 Christoph Sachsse and Florian Tennstedt, eds., *Soziale Sicherheit und soziale Disziplinierung: Beiträge zu einer historischen Theorie der Sozialpolitik* (Frankfurt/Main, 1986).

34 Alfons Labisch, "Die Entwicklung der gesundheitspolitischen Vorstellungen der deutschen Sozialdemokratie von ihrer Gründung bis zur Parteispaltung, 1863–1917," *Archiv für Sozialgeschichte* 16 (1976): 325–70; Tennstedt, *Vom Proleten*; Alfons Labisch, "The Role of the Hospital in the Health Policy of the German Social Democratic Movement before World War I," *International Journal of Health Services* 17 (1987): 279–94.

35 Alfons Labisch, *Homo Hygienicus: Gesundheit und Medizin in der Neuzeit* (Frankfurt/Main, 1992).

alization, the concept of health was defined in medical scientific terms, and thus neutrally. Labor understood the scientific and technological definition of health: In everyday life, they were confronted on the job with the same type of thought and action they were accustomed to in the scientific-technological world. A scientific concept of health seemed ideologically neutral. This was obvious when compared to the religiously or morally oriented attempts at disciplining labor. They changed course "from Christian morals to secularized health."[36] The Social Democratic self-management of health insurance organizations became an independent movement, a socially and culturally based Social Democratic "health insurance movement" (*Kassenbewegung*).[37]

To the extent that manpower became scarce after the turn of the century, health became a value accepted by all social groups – by the high officials, politicians, industrialists, military officers, and finally by the individuals themselves. This development led to the general acceptance of the good "health" of society as a goal of political, social, and individual action. Only the means to this end were open to debate. At the same time, action and conduct conveyed by medical science conformed to the rules of society. Thus, health as a social good guaranteed the achievement of conformist behavior by way of scientifically defined behavioral codes; the "refinement of labor" was pursued actively and passively in terms of promoting "healthful behavior."[38]

This secular development affected labor as well as doctors and, accordingly, the health insurance problem discussed previously. With the self-management of social security institutions, an intended and purposeful element of labor participation had been created: Participation, however, was on the social margin and apart from the classical careers in secondary schools, universities, administration, or the military. And participation with double-edged effects. On the one hand, the elite of labor was tied into social security and integrated. The leading Social Democratic politicians of the Weimar Republic came from the trade union offices or from the self-management of insurance organizations. On the other hand, the social control of labor was effected by the self-management of insurance organizations, and thus by labor itself. That was how the class of labor elite, integrated into the (authoritarian class) society, was created.

Bismarck's immediate goal – to subdue the oppositional political labor movement by repressing social democracy, on the one hand, and by his integrative social policy, on the other – had failed. A disagreement over future

36 Tennstedt, *Sozialpolitik*, 147–51.
37 Tennstedt, *Vom Proleten*, 448–70.
38 Tennstedt, *Sozialpolitik*; Tennstedt, *Vom Proleten*; Alfons Labisch, "Doctors, Workers and the Scientific Cosmology of the Industrial World: The Social Construction of 'Health' and the 'Homo Hygienicus,'" *Journal of Contemporary History* 20 (1985): 599–615.

labor policy caused Bismarck's dismissal in 1890. That same year the newly reconstituted Social Democratic Party (*Sozialdemokratische Partei Deutschlands*, or SPD) received 19.7 percent of the votes in national elections, which was the highest percentage of all parties. Bismarck's fall over the question of labor policy (of all things) should not, however, mislead us. In the long run, Bismarck's social security laws, and especially his health insurance laws, contributed to the socialization of the labor movement into industrial society. His policies also changed social democracy from a revolutionary movement into one that only uttered revolutionary rhetoric.

Social security, and especially health insurance, had a similar secular significance for doctors. The rise of health to a social value created a space in society that they could fill with meaning and that they could claim as their domain. This civilizing process was common to all industrial societies. In Germany the Health Insurance Law made the cooperation of doctors in health insurance indispensable. After the amendment of 1892 and its effects on labor, doctors were drawn into the sociopolitical calculation of German social policy. But they quickly became caught between the millstones of a revolutionary labor movement and conservative social policy. Nevertheless, they achieved a social position where they had to be taken into account in the field of social policy. From this position they were able to assert their own interests, which were superficially of a financial or organizational nature, but upon closer inspection rather represented the interests of their professional status. This is the point where the position of doctors in Germany diverges from that of doctors in other industrial nations. Since 1913 doctors were collectively accepted as an equal bargaining partner. Since 1931 the numerous and divergently oriented health insurance organizations have been faced with the union of panel doctors as a monopolistic representation of all panel doctors. The ideal view of doctors in this struggle was, and has remained, that of the "doctor as a free professional," even though the panel doctor's medical practice was dependent on compulsory health insurance.

3

In Search of German Social Darwinism

The History and Historiography of a Concept

RICHARD J. EVANS

I

At a lunchtime meeting held on August 20, 1942, to mark the occasion of the appointment of Otto-Georg Thierack as Reich justice minister and Roland Freisler as president of the "People's Court," Hitler launched into one of his characteristic monologues. The judicial system, he said, was soft. Criminals were being allowed to get away with far too much on the home front. Looting and petty crime were being punished with mere prison sentences instead of death. The results of this in the longer term would be disastrous:

> Every war leads to a negative selection. The positive elements die in masses. The choice of the most dangerous military service is already a selection: the really brave ones become airmen, or join the U-boats. And even in these services there is always the call: who wants to volunteer? And it's always the best men who then get killed. All this time, the absolute ne'er-do-well is cared for lovingly in body and spirit. Anyone who ever enters a prison knows with absolute certainty that nothing more is going to happen to him. If you can imagine this going on for another three or four years, then you can see a gradual shift in the balance of the nation taking place: an over-exploitation on the one side; absolute conservation on the other.[1]

In order to reestablish the balance, Hitler declared, the "negative" elements in the German population had to be killed in much larger numbers. In the following months, Thierack and his officials redefined the role of penal policy to achieve this end. Punishment, the new Reich minister of justice told German judges on June 1, 1943, "in our time has to carry out the popular-hygienic task of continually cleansing the body of the race by the ruthless elimination of criminals unworthy of life."[2] The judges did not

---

1 Bundesarchiv Koblenz R22/4720: Abschrift, Aug. 20, 1942; Werner Jochmann, ed., *Adolf Hitler: Monologe im Führer-Hauptquartier, 1941–1944: Die Aufzeichnungen Heinrich Heims* (Hamburg, 1980), 347–54; Lothar Gruchmann, ed., "Hitler über die Justiz: Das Tischgespräch von 20. August 1942," *Vierteljahreshefte für Zeitgeschichte* 12 (1964): 86–101.

2 Heinz Boberach, ed., *Richterbriefe: Dokumente zur Beeinflussung der deutschen Rechtsprechung, 1942–1944* (Boppard/Rhein, 1975), 132.

demur. By the end of the war, thousands of offenders, many of them guilty of extremely trivial misdemeanors, had been sentenced to death by Hitler's courts, making a total of over 16,000 from the beginning of the Third Reich to the end; untold thousands more had been handed over to the Gestapo for "elimination," or transferred from Germany's prisons to the concentration camps of the SS for "extermination through labour."[3] By 1944, such a fate was reserved for all "community aliens" who showed themselves unworthy of belonging to the German race by their immorality, laziness, or even "frivolity,""disorderliness while drunk," or even their "irritability."[4] After all, as Hitler had remarked on another occasion,"apes trample outsiders to death as community aliens. And what holds good for apes, must hold good for humans to an even greater extent."[5]

Hitler's espousal of a ruthless policy of negative eugenic selection – even more, perhaps, the analogy he drew between the natural world and human society, between apes and people – reflected deeply held views. It found expression in other areas besides the judicial, most notoriously, perhaps, in the extermination of the mentally and physically handicapped and the chronically ill in Germany carried out from 1939 under the code name of "Action T4."[6] Hitler, as is well known, believed that world history consisted of a struggle for survival between races. The Jewish race was plotting to undermine the German; "inferior" groups such as the Slavs were also threatening the future of the Aryan "master-race"; and degenerative tendencies within the German race itself had to be countered if disaster was not to ensue. His views on these subjects have often been called social Darwinist. Yet historians have signally failed to agree on what social Darwinism was, or on how it developed from its scientific beginnings in the nineteenth century into a central component of an ideology of mass murder and racial warfare in the twentieth. The debate about social Darwinism and its relation to Nazism involves wider questions about the relationship of science and society, medicine and politics, about historical continuity, and about the

---

3 Richard J. Evans, *Rituals of Retribution: Capital Punishment in Germany, 1600–1987* (Oxford, 1996), chap. 16.

4 Detlev J. K. Peukert, "Arbeitslager und Jugend-KZ: die Behandlung 'Gemeinschaftsfremder' im Dritten Reich," in Detlev J. K. Peukert and Jürgen Reulecke, eds., *Die Reihen fast geschlossen: Beiträge zur Geschichte des Alltags unterm Nationalsozialismus* (Wuppertal, 1981), 416; see also Norbert Frei, *Der Führerstaat: Nationalsozialistische Herrschaft 1933 bis 1945* (Munich, 1987), 202–8; and P. Wagner, "Das Gesetz über die Behandlung Gemeinschaftsfremder: die Kriminalpolizei und die 'Vernichtung des Verbrechertums,'" in Wolfgang Ayass et al., eds., *Feinderklärung und Prävention: Kriminalbiologie, Zigeunerforschung und Asozialenpolitik* (Berlin, 1988), 75–100.

5 Henry Pickler, ed., *Hitlers Tischgespräche im Führerhauptquartier* (Stuttgart, 1976), 302 (April 15, 1942).

6 Michael Burleigh, *Death and Deliverance: "Euthanasia" in Germany, c. 1900-1945* (Cambridge,1994), is now the best study of these events.

problems and possibilities of tracing back Nazi ideology to its (real or imagined) nineteeth-century roots.

II

Ever since the early 1960s, social Darwinism has played a central role in arguments among historians about the ideological origins of Nazism. Hans-Günter Zmarzlik was the first serious German historian to tackle a subject that had hitherto been dominated by propagandists, polemicists, and philosophers.[7] Zmarzlik began his seminal article, published in 1963, by pointing out:

Darwinism has been claimed as an authority for very different interpretations of social processes. Proponents of altruistic ethics have rested their case on it, but so too have the spokesmen of a brutally elitist morality; liberal-progressive thought has called on it for legitimation, but so too has crass historical fatalism. Pioneers of the theory of socialist egalitarianism have employed it, but so too have the authors of manifestoes of racial inequality.[8]

Subsequent historians who have made Zmarzlik responsible for a teleological approach that reads back the whole of Nazi ideology into the configurations of social Darwinism before World War I are therefore wide of the mark.[9] From the very beginning, the modern historiography of social Darwinism made its links with nonracist and progressive ideologies absolutely clear. Of course, Zmarzlik did not stop at establishing social Darwinism's political diversity. He went on to argue that, subject to these reservations, the varieties of social Darwinism could be roughly subsumed under two headings. First, there was evolutionary social Darwinism, in which ideas of mutual aid were often as prominent as ideas of competition. Popular among liberals and on the left in the 1860s and 1870s, this variant began to be superseded in the 1890s by a second, stressing the struggle for the survival of the fittest. From

7 For the attempt of one of Germany's most senior philosophers of the immediate postwar years to come to terms with social Darwinism, see Hedwig Conrad-Martius, *Utopien der Menschenzüchtung: Der Sozialdarwinismus und seine Folgen* (Munich, 1955). This work stands apart from the more strictly historical literature on the subject. For a phenomenological approach to the subject, see Gunter Mann, "Biologie und der 'Neue Mensch': Denkstufen und Pläne zur Menschenzucht im Zweiten Kaiserreich," in Gunter Mann and Rolf Winau, eds., *Medizin, Naturwissenschaft, Technik und das Zweite Kaiserreich: Vorträge eines Kongresses vom 6. bis 11. September 1973 in Bad Nauheim* (Göttingen, 1977), 182–88.

8 Hans-Günter Zmarzlik, "Der Sozialdarwinismus in Deutschland als geschichtliches Problem," *Vierteljahreshefte für Zeitgeschichte* 11 (1963): 247. For an English version, see Hans-Günter Zmarzlik, "Social Darwinism in Germany: Seen as a Historical Problem," in Hajo Holborn, ed., *From Republic to Reich: The Making of the Nazi Revolution* (New York, 1972), 435–74. The translation above, however, is mine, as are all in the present essay. See also Hans-Günter Zmarzlik, "Social Darwinism in Germany: An Example of the Sociopolitical Abuse of Scientific Knowledge," in Günter Altner, ed., *The Human Creature* (Garden City, N.Y., 1974).

9 Dieter Groh, "Marx, Engels und Darwin: Naturgesetzliche Entwicklung oder Revolution," in Günter Altner, ed., *Der Darwinismus* (Darmstadt, 1981), 217–41. For Richard Weikart's criticisms of Zmarzlik, see subsequent discussion in this chapter.

about the turn of the century, racist and imperialist ideas entered the mixture
as well, and some social Darwinists began to think of racial and social engineering in the interests of the nation. This chronology, of course, was only
approximate, and Zmarzlik was careful to point out that older, evolutionary
forms of the ideology continued to be held – for example, among the social
Democrats – well after the turn of the century. He also differentiated carefully between the social Darwinism of racial anthropologists, racial hygienists,
and other scientific groups, many of whom, he said, made "valuable contributions" to social and scientific theory and practice, and the vulgarization,
popularization, and political exploitation of social Darwinism by imperialists
and Pan-Germans, who took up "more or less isolated slogans, without applying the Darwinist explanation of nature to the interpretation of political-
social processes in a consistent way."[10] Hitler and others like him, he argued,
only adopted vulgarized elements of "certain Darwinisms," not the whole
ideology, and the Nazis only purveyed a "primitive version" of social
Darwinism.[11] Zmarzlik warned against either making social Darwinism
responsible for the Nazi "descent into barbarism" or confusing the social
Darwinist slogans adopted by Hitler with the social and political programs of
more thoroughgoing social Darwinists, many of whom wanted their aims
to be realized humanely and without violence or coercion.[12]

Zmarzlik's central points – the existence of different varieties of social
Darwinism, the supersession of liberal-leftist, evolutionary variants by
rightist, selectionist variants from the 1890s, the vulgarized, sloganizing
oversimplifications of the Nazis, and the dangers of drawing a straight line
from social Darwinism per se to Nazism – have been echoed by many subsequent writers on the subject. In 1974, for instance, Hans-Ulrich Wehler
insisted in almost identical terms to those employed by Zmarzlik on "the
enormous, many-sided variety of social Darwinism as a kind of kaleidoscope,
which could be shaken into place according to purpose."[13] In the 1860s and
1870s, it helped form the ideology of the Social Democrats, and justified the
competitive capitalism of early German industrialization. Later on, a "vulgarized social Darwinism" brought the concept of the "struggle for existence" to the fore in political discourse, reducing it to warfare and violence
in the process.[14] Whereas Zmarzlik saw the shift in social Darwinist ideology

10 Ibid., 262.
11 Ibid., 246–7, 262.
12 Ibid., 266–9.
13 Hans-Ulrich Wehler, "Sozialdarwinismus im expandierenden Industriestaat," in Imanuel Geiss and
    Bernd-Jürgen Wendt, eds., *Deutschland in der Weltpolitik des 19. und 20. Jahrhunderts*, 2d ed.
    (Düsseldorf, 1974), 139.
14 Ibid., 138–9.

that occurred in the 1890s as a reflection of the wider political shift to the
era of Wilhelmine *Weltpolitik*, Wehler added his own inimitable twist to the
argument by suggesting that the adoption of a vulgarized, inegalitarian, and
selectionist version of the ideology reflected instead "the so-called feudaliza-
tion of the bourgeoisie, the influence of neo-aristocratic modes of behavior,
norms, values, and aims in life" that made the German middle classes more
receptive to such an interpretation than were their counterparts in the United
States.[15] The influence of selectionist social Darwinism in Germany could
thus be seen as an aspect of Germany's "special path" (*Sonderweg*) to modernity, reflecting the historic weakness of the German bourgeoisie. This was
not a particularly plausible argument; it lacked any credible evidence to
back it up and rested on a series of assumptions about the dominance of
aristocratic values and the "bourgeois" nature of egalitarianism in the late
nineteenth century that have not been confirmed by subsequent research.[16]
Nevertheless, Wehler was persuasive when, like Zmarzlik, he stressed the
many-faceted nature of social Darwinism and emphasized the shift in
the dominant Darwinian discourse from evolutionism to selectionism in
the 1890s. Another member of the "Bielefeld school," Hans-Walter Schmuhl,
has also followed Zmarzlik in pointing out that

Social Darwinism allowed its name to be lent to very diverse interpretations of
social processes, according to which aspect of the Darwinist theory of evolution and
selection was placed at the center of social Darwinist doctrine. Both Social
Democrats and "social aristocrats" claimed the authority of Darwinism, as did both
adherents of laissez-faire liberalism and champions of the modern interventionist
state, protagonists of altruistic ethics on the basis of "social instincts" and apologists
for a "morality of the master race" that emphasized the right of the stronger, as did
both militarists and pacifists.[17]

Schmuhl supported the consensus view and concurred with other historians
that social Darwinism had undergone a rightward shift in the 1890s.[18]
However, Schmuhl's view, typical for the Bielefeld school, that social

15 Ibid., 142. More recently, Wehler has described social Darwinism in the form it took in Wilhelmine
    Germany as a "Rechtfertigungsideologie der Oberklassen," in Hans-Ulrich Wehler, ed., *Deutsche
    Gesellschaftsgeschichte*, vol. 3: *Von der "Deutschen Doppelrevolution" bis zum Beginn des Ersten
    Weltkrieges, 1848–1914* (Munich, 1995), 1,081–5. But of course the idea of the "survival of the
    fittest" in no way committed its proponents to the view that the aristocracy were the fittest to sur-
    vive; on the contrary, social Darwinists of the radical right could just as easily claim that the aris-
    tocracy were by and large degenerate, effete, and lacking in eugenic vigor.
16 See esp. David Blackbourn, "The Discreet Charm of the Bourgeoisie: Reappraising German History
    in the Nineteenth Century," in David Blackbourn and Geoff Eley, eds., *The Peculiarities of German
    History: Bourgeois Society and Politics in Nineteenth-Century Germany* (Oxford, 1984), 159–292; and
    David Blackbourn and Richard J. Evans, eds., *The German Bourgeoisie: Essays on the Social History of
    the German Middle Classes from the Late Eighteenth to the Early Twentieth Century* (London, 1990).
17 Hans-Walter Schmuhl, *Rassenhygiene, Nationalsozialismus, Euthanasie* (Göttingen, 1987), 72.
18 Ibid., 53.

Darwinism on the whole served the interests of "system-stabilization" after the turn of the century, is not only unsupported by evidence, but demonstrably wrong.[19] Insofar as social Darwinist views were held by radical groups of the right and the left in Wilhelmine Germany, it seems clear enough that they operated against the stability of the political system rather than in its favor.[20]

Writing not about social Darwinism in general but rather about the ideological origins of Nazism, Michael Burleigh and Wolfgang Wippermann also insisted that "social Darwinism was not an exclusively right-wing concern. ... social Darwinians ... could be conservative, liberal, socialist, or fascist."[21] In their delineation of the prehistory of Nazi racism, they were careful to distinguish between the "collectivist and state interventionist variety" of social Darwinism that eventually triumphed in Germany, and other varieties, and to delimit all of the variants of social Darwinism from "racial anti-semitic theories."[22] Similarly, although the medical historian Gerhard Baader's rather simpleminded Marxism made him want to deny the label "social Darwinist" to what he admitted was the labor movement's espousal of a Darwinian "theory of descent," he too devoted some space to outlining the liberal, laissez-faire, and especially anticlerical affiliations of social Darwinism in the 1860s and also in the 1870s, the time of the *Kulturkampf.* He followed existing orthodoxy in pointing to a change of direction by social Darwinism in the 1890s, although the new, selectionist social Darwinists, he cautioned, were, initially at least, "nationalistic writers, who used Darwinist concepts like the struggle for existence, to embellish their arguments."[23] Baader's article, though rather brief and in some ways not very satisfactory, does not present a monolithic view of social Darwinism as leading to Nazism, but on the contrary, points out its varieties – laissez-faire and nationalist, moderate and extreme, scientific and vulgar – in what had, by the time he wrote it, become a thoroughly orthodox manner.

Not only did historians after Zmarzlik customarily emphasize the diversity of social Darwinism, they were also well aware of its role and the wider role of biological ideas, in informing movements of sexual liberation on the left. Writing about the feminist movement in Wilhelmine Germany in 1976, I

19 Ibid., 74–5.
20 For the general context, see Geoff Eley, *Reshaping the German Right: Radical Nationalism and Political Change after Bismarck* (New Haven, Conn., 1980).
21 Michael Burleigh and Wolfgang Wippermann, *The Racial State: Germany, 1933-1945* (Cambridge, 1991), 28.
22 Ibid., 132–3.
23 Gerhard Baader, "Zur Ideologie des Sozialdarwinismus," in Gerhard Baader and Ulrich Schultz, eds., *Medizin und Nationalsozialismus: Tabuisierte Vergangenheit – Ungebrochene Tradition?* Forum für Medizin und Gesundheitspolitik, Sonderband 15 (Berlin, 1980), 42, 50.

commented that Helene Stöcker's League for the Protection of Motherhood "attempted to ally liberalism, social Darwinism and Nietzscheanism into a new social ideology that would preserve the most libertarian and individualist elements in all three creeds and translate them into the practical demand that the individual woman should be allowed to dispose over her own body without interference from the state."[24] Correspondingly, the League rejected the more authoritarian variants of social Darwinism, despite their growing influence in public discourse, in the first years of its existence. Although "all the *Mutterschutz* enthusiasts believed to some extent in some form of racial hygiene,"[25] the pacifist views of the majority made them reject the argument that racial hygiene should be administered by the state using a form of legal compulsion. The feminist Maria Lischnewska, for example, "whose strong nationalism distinguished her from the bulk of the leading radical feminists and gave her social Darwinist views a strongly authoritarian tint,"[26] had little influence at this time. The League's failure to persuade the mainstream feminist movement to adopt its radical policies in 1908 led to a serious crisis in its affairs that resulted in the resignation of many of its leading members. This opened the way to the triumph in both the League and the feminist movement as a whole of a more right-wing variant of social Darwinism, in which racial hygiene was administered by the state against "degenerate" elements in the population in order to "improve" the German race in the struggle for survival against the Latins and the Slavs.[27] Such views were only one variant of social Darwinism among many. "Social Darwinism," I wrote, "had of course its progressive aspects. In the early years of the *Mutterschutz* movement, it clearly provided support for the movement's radical ideas about marriage, contraception and abortion." But "the variety of social Darwinism that took root in the German women's movement in the years 1908–1914 contained a strong element of authoritarianism."[28]

24   Richard J. Evans, *The Feminist Movement in Germany, 1894-1933* (London, 1976), 138.
25   Ibid.
26   Ibid., 160.
27   Ibid., 133–4, 136–7, 159.
28   Ibid., 158-69. Pointing out in the orthodox fashion that "speakers of all political persuasions drew on the stock vocabulary of social Darwinism," Ann Taylor Allen has argued, however, that Stöcker and her movement used eugenics only in a radical, progressive way. This constituted an attempt to argue for greater control by women over their own bodies. Unfortunately, she fails to distinguish between the rapidly changing phases of the movement's development, dismissing other historians' attempt to do so as mere "narrative history." She accuses my own writing on Stöcker of arguing that "the use of eugenic theory by the women's movement was in itself a symptom of a more general conservative revolution," and claims that this "fails to take into account the popularity of these social-radical theories among left-wing and progressive circles in Germany and elsewhere." Yet this accusation confuses the two periods in the movement's history, and ignores everything that I and others have written about the different varieties and shadings of social Darwinism and eugenics. The examples of progressive and emancipatory eugenic ideas that Allen presents from the feminist

The orthodox line was usefully summed up in 1982 by Ted Benton, who concluded: "Feminists and anti-feminists, revolutionaries and revisionists, socialists, liberals and conservatives, imperialists and internationalists: all, or almost all, seemed to find something in Darwinism and the idea of evolution which benefited their cases."[29] Rolf-Dieter Sieferle's emphasis on social Darwinism's complex and contradictory nature underscores this generally accepted point.[30] It has been repeated most recently by Paul Crook, who has emphasized the "cultural malleability" of German social Darwinism, which precludes any "correct" reading of the implications of Darwin's ideas, or those associated with him, for human society. Crook too concludes that in the early years German social Darwinism was "mainly influential on the left half of the political spectrum," but that "as liberalism weakened, there came to the fore an organicist and authoritarian" version of "social Darwinism marked by eugenic proposals to save the nation or race," fusing eventually with Gobineau's race theories to create a dangerous new mix.[31] This line of argument has also been followed by Paul Weindling, who, like Zmarzlik, has emphasized that "social Darwinism gave legitimacy to a variety of interests in an expanding industrial society, and cannot be identified as an exclusively right-wing racist ideology."[32] Like Zmarzlik, Weindling has posited a "transition in Darwinism from being a liberal and secular ideology of social reform during the 1860s" to meshing with "the social imperialism of the 1890s" so that "from the turn of the century, the doctrine of the survival of the fittest

movement's literature almost all date from the period before 1908, a period for which no historian has disputed their hegemony. But she altogether fails to demonstrate their continuity significantly beyond this point. Her confusion is underlined by her description of such ideas as "responses" to a series of authoritarian, male-dominated initiatives in reproductive policy that her footnotes indicate mostly dated from a later period! See Ann Taylor Allen, "Mothers of the New Generation: Adele Schreiber, Helene Stöcker, and the Evolution of a German Idea of Motherhood, 1900–1914," *Signs* 10 (1985): 435, 438. See also her articles, "German Radical Feminism and Eugenics, 1900–1908," *German Studies Review* 11 (1988): 31–56; and "Maternalism in German Feminist Movements," *Journal of Women's History* 5 (1993): 99–103; and her book, *Feminism and Motherhood in Germany, 1800–1914* (New Brunswick, N.J., 1991). For the location of the origins and early development of authoritarian discourses on sexuality and birth control in the direction taken by social Darwinism and eugenics before 1914, see Anna Bergmann, *Die verhütete Sexualität* (Hamburg, 1992). For further criticisms of Taylor's work, see Nancy M. Reagin, *A German Women's Movement: Class and Gender in Hanover, 1880–1933* (Chapel Hill, N.C., 1995).

29 Ted Benton, "Social Darwinism and Socialist Darwinism in Germany, 1860 to 1900," *Rivista di Filosofia* 23 (1982): 93–7.

30 Rolf-Dieter Sieferle, "Sozialdarwinismus," in Bodo-Michael Baumunk and Jürgen Riess, eds., *Darwin und Darwinismus* (Berlin, 1994), 134–42.

31 Paul Crook, *Darwinism, War and History: The Debate over the Biology of War from the "Origin of Species" to the First World War* (Cambridge, 1994), 31. The consensus is usefully summarized in the standard work by Peter Weingart, Jürgen Kroll, and Kurt Bayertz, *Rasse, Blut und Gene: Geschichte der Eugenik und Rassenhygiene in Deutschland* (Frankfurt/Main, 1992), 114–21.

32 Paul Weindling, *Health, Race and German Politics between National Unification and Nazism, 1870–1945* (Cambridge, 1989), 28.

became increasingly useful to doctrines of racial superiority."[33] Yet in his book on the cell biologist Oskar Hertwig, Weindling showed how Hertwig attacked militarists, such as Friedrich von Bernhardi, as being "social Darwinists" using Darwin's theories to justify war; accused social Darwinism of contributing to the overheated, militaristic political atmosphere before 1914; and criticized social Darwinists for advocating selective breeding. Hertwig's tract against social Darwinism, published in 1918,[34] "stands," in Weindling's view,

as an important commentary on the strength of social Darwinism and the racial hygiene movement. By 1918 it was possible to see these as fundamental threats to German liberal ideals and the international community....Hertwig's achievement was to demonstrate that there was already a concerted body of opinion which could be described as "social Darwinism."[35]

There is not much mention here of the varied and diverse nature of social Darwinism, nor of its differential political implications. Yet elsewhere Weindling claims that "the positive side to Darwinism" has been "overlooked by historians,"[36] who have tended to provide "schematic accounts of social Darwinism as a proto-fascist ideology."[37] Not only does he fail to provide convincing evidence that such accounts really have been widespread in the literature, but, as we have seen from his own account of Hertwig, the assumption that social Darwinism by World War I was a uniform doctrine that was mainly or even exclusively racist, nationalist, and militarist seems to be present not least in the work of Hertwig but indeed in the writings of Weindling himself.

In fact, as we have seen, the positive side to Darwinism has not been overlooked by historians. The only historian of whom this could plausibly be claimed is Daniel Gasman, who argued in 1971 that all forms of social Darwinism were part of the "scientific origins of National Socialism," to borrow the title of his book on Ernst Haeckel. Haeckel, a leading German popularizer of Darwin's views, had long been regarded as a liberal, but Gasman went to the other extreme and portrayed him instead as a fascist *avant la lettre*. Haeckel, for example, supported capital punishment because, as he said "it has a directly beneficial effect as a selection process" by "rendering incorrigible criminals harmless," and for good measure he added that

33 Ibid., 25; Paul Weindling, *Darwinism and Social Darwinism in Imperial Germany: The Contribution of the Cell Biologist Oscar Hertwig (1849–1922)*, Forschungen zur neueren Medizin- und Biologiegeschichte (Stuttgart, 1991), 3:302.
34 Oskar Hertwig, *Zur Abwehr des ethischen, des socialen, des politischen Darwinismus* (Jena, 1918).
35 Weindling, *Darwinism*, 270–87, 302, quotation on 287.
36 Ibid., 11.
37 Paul Weindling, "Theories of the Cell State in Imperial Germany," in Charles Webster, ed., *Biology, Medicine and Society, 1840–1940* (Cambridge, 1981), 101.

modern methods such as chemical injections and electrocution should be used and should also be applied to the mentally ill, because psychological disturbances were the expression of a physical degeneracy of the brain that could hold up human progress unless it was eliminated from the chain of heredity.[38] These views undoubtedly bore a close resemblance to those taken up later by the Nazis. Yet Haeckel also believed that war was wrong because it meant the slaughter of the best and bravest of the nation's youth, which would be a eugenic disaster. The "Monist League," which he founded, was therefore a pacifist organization, as far removed from Nazism in this respect as it was possible to be. Here is a classic example of how some aspects of an ideologue's thought can legitimately be regarded as precursors of aspects of Nazi thought, whereas others cannot. It was quite wrong of Gasman, therefore, to reduce Haeckel in toto to the originator of "the scientific origins of National Socialism."[39] This was recognized by other historians right away, however. In 1976 I reflected a widespread view when I wrote that "Gasman's account, though a valuable corrective to earlier works, is in general disappointingly one-sided."[40] Three years later, Robert Bannister added that "Gasman's definition of 'social Darwinism' compounds every confusion in the literature of the subject."[41] In 1981 Alfred Kelly added to the chorus of disapproval of Gasman's work. "If Haeckel and the Monist League can be forerunners of Nazism," he commented, "then so can most any other thinker or organization."[42] Further opprobrium came from Piet de Rooy in 1990, who pointed out that Haeckel's works were removed from German libraries by the Nazis in 1935.[43]

---

38 Alfred Fried, "Die Todesstrafe im Urteil der Zeitgenossen," *Der Zeitgeist: Beiheft zum Berliner Tageblatt*, Dec. 2, 1901, copy in Geheimes Staatsarchiv Preussischer Kulturbesitz, Berlin-Dahlem, Rep. 84a/7784, Bl. 203–5; and the *Deutsche Juristen-Zeitung* 16, no. 1 (Nov. 1, 1911), copy in Bundesarchiv, Abteilung Potsdam, Auswärtiges Amt IIIa Nr. 51, vol. 10, 135–6.

39 Daniel Gasman, *The Scientific Origins of Nazism: Social Darwinism in Ernst Haeckel and the Monist League* (New York, 1971). Moreover, Gasman went on to identify even the mutualist and evolutionist forms of social Darwinism espoused by Engels and the ideologues of the German Social Democratic Party as part of the intellectual heritage of Nazism as well! All this was achieved only by suppressing many aspects of social Darwinism, misrepresenting Haeckel's thought, and distorting the historical record. Haeckel was portrayed in positive terms by officially sponsored historians in the former German Democratic Republic. See Erika Krause, *Ernst Haeckel* (Leipzig, 1983); and Georg Uschmann, *Ernst Haeckel: Eine Biographie in Briefen* (Leipzig, 1983). For a recent, more negative assessment, see Jürgen Sandmann, *Der Bruch mit der humanitären Tradition: Die Biologisierung der Ethik bei Ernst Haeckel und anderen Darwinisten seiner Zeit* (Stuttgart, 1990).

40 Evans, *Feminist Movement*, 173n. 47.

41 Robert C. Bannister, *Social Darwinism: Science and Myth in Anglo-American Social Thought* (Philadalphia, 1979), 133.

42 Alfred Kelly, *The Descent of Darwin: The Popularization of Darwinism in Germany, 1860–1914* (Chapel Hill, N.C., 1981), 114.

43 Piet de Rooy, "Of Monkeys, Blacks and Proles: Ernst Haeckel's Theory of Recapitulation," in Jan Breman, ed., *Imperial Monkey Business: Racial Supremacy in Social Darwinist Theory and Colonial Practice* (Amsterdam, 1990), 7–34.

Gasman's interpretation in fact ultimately derives from Allied wartime propaganda, which cannot really be considered serious in scholarly terms. Books such as William McGovern's *From Luther to Hitler*, published in 1941 and containing a chapter on "Social Darwinists and their Allies," or Rohan Butler's *The Roots of National Socialism*, published the previous year, trawled German writings in the past, from Novalis to Nietzsche, not only in the search for antecedents of Nazism, but also in the attempt to prove that all German "ideology" had always been Nazi in one way or another, and that Nazism, in essence, was not new. Such arguments were related to the anti-German racism that was prominent in Allied propaganda during World War II and that early postwar German historians such as Gerhard Ritter attempted to counter by arguing that the Nazis got most of their ideas from other countries – racism from France (through Gobineau), anti-Semitism from Austria, and so on. Ritter in particular saw the origins of National Socialism not in a long-term continuity of German values, but in their collapse after World War I. He did not have anything to say in detail about social Darwinism and made no specific reference at all to any putative links with Nazi exterminism. Where he did draw a link, rather oddly, was between Hitler's geopolitical doctrine of *Lebensraum* – the claim for more territorial "living space" for the Germans – and "Darwinian theories which had been influencing the political literature of Europe for many years, and which caused disturbing symptoms in the writings of other countries too." Here Ritter was trying both to attribute the idea of *Lebensraum* to a non-German source, detaching it from the specificities of Germany's historical development in the process, and to suggest that other countries were as prone to territorial aggrandizement (above all, in World War I) as Germany was.[44] The Christian-conservative Ritter went on to argue that social Darwinism was an aspect of the materialist worldview of the Weimar Republic, which encompassed Marxism and atheism as well and displaced the religious values that he thought had dominated in the imperial period and that alone could guarantee political stability in the age of the masses. Historians on both sides of this dispute thus paid scant attention to the nuances of ideology or the historical context of

44 See Gerhard Ritter, "The Historical Foundations of the Rise of National Socialism," in *The Third Reich*, International Council for Philosophy and Humanistic Studies (London, 1955), 392–3, 415–6. The writings of Hansjoachim W. Koch on social Darwinism, published in the course of the "Fischer Controversy" over the origins of World War I, fall into the same context; their main argument is that social Darwinism was a general European ideology, rather than a specifically German mode of thought. See Hansjoachim W. Koch, "Social Darwinism as a Factor in the New Imperialism," in Hansjoachim W. Koch, ed., *The Origins of the First World War: Great Power Rivalry and German War Aims* (London, 1972), 329–54, paradoxically manages to deal with the subject without mentioning a single German social Darwinist. See also Hansjoachim W. Koch, *Der Sozialdarwinismus: Seine Genese und sein Einfluss auf das imperialistische Denken* (Munich, 1973).

ideas in their desire to heap collective historical blame upon the Germans for Nazism or to absolve them from responsibility for it. It was precisely this kind of unhistorical approach from which the more differentiated search for the origins of Nazi ideology undertaken from the 1960s onward was trying to escape.[45] In this respect Gasman's work represented a throwback to an earlier style of writing about ideas in German history, not the historiographical orthodoxy of the last thirty years. It is not surprising that it has had little or no influence among historians.

III

Nevertheless, the prevailing orthodoxy on the history of social Darwinist ideology in Germany has not gone unchallenged. A number of historians have been dissatisfied with it for a variety of reasons. The feminist historian Gisela Bock, for example, rejected the term "social Darwinism" in the context of her work on compulsory sterilization in the Third Reich, as "partly unjustified, partly unsatisfactory, partly unnecessary."[46] This was because, according to Bock, social Darwinism was essentially a liberal ideology. "If liberalism and the competitiveness of modern industrial society were the godparents of Darwin's interpretation of 'nature,'" she claimed, "this certainly did not hold good for the racial hygiene movement."[47] Racial hygiene and biology, Bock pointed out, were unknown to Darwin. The idea that natural selection had to be replaced by deliberate policy was alien to Darwin's thought. Racial hygiene, in fact, according to Bock, was

> less a movement in the history of ideas, than above all a sociopolitical movement with practical aims. Its theories did not address themselves, as Darwin's does, to the past, but to the present. Its interest was directed not toward the socioeconomic "struggle for existence," but to the socio-sexual "struggle" for reproduction. In this sphere it demanded not the "right of the stronger" in free competition, but its regulation by the state; practical racial hygiene. ... For these reasons it seemed advisable not to define racial hygiene or eugenics as social Darwinism, as thought and action that could be more or less reduced to Darwin, but instead to treat them as independent innovations.[48]

Feminist historians in general seem rather uncomfortable with the concept of social Darwinism, perhaps because it does not of itself imply sufficient

---

45   See the critique in Richard J. Evans, *Rethinking German History* (London, 1987), chaps. 1–2; also John C. G. Röhl, ed., *From Bismarck to Hitler: The Problem of Continuity in German History* (London, 1970).
46   Gisela Bock, *Zwangssterilisation im Nationalsozialismus: Studien zur Rassenpolitik und Frauenpolitik* (Opladen, 1986), 28.
47   Ibid., 29.
48   Ibid., 35–6.

sharpness of focus on the issues that concern them, above all, the "politics of the body" and women's reproductive role. Cornelie Usborne made no use of the term in her book on reproductive politics in the Weimar Republic, mentioning it only once, in passing, at the very beginning. Nor did Ann Taylor Allen use the concept in her work in this area, except in a purely marginal way.[49] But this austere disdain for the concept of social Darwinism, its restriction to what Darwin himself thought, does not convince. Darwin himself, as has long been recognized, took common social ideas of his time – above all, the competitiveness of early industrial capitalism – and applied them to nature.[50] Other ideas described as Darwinian even in his own day, including the "survival of the fittest," may have derived originally not from Darwin himself, but from others (in this case, Herbert Spencer).[51] After his death, different people interpreted Darwin, as historians have noted, in their own way and in the process, produced combinations of ideas that Darwin himself might not have recognized. But none of this made these ideas any less "Darwinian." Karl Marx, after all, is said to have complained, on reading the work of some of his disciples: "All I know is, I am not a Marxist"; and it is well known that Lenin, Kautsky, Plekhanov, and even Engels introduced new ideas or variant readings that radically changed the nature of Marx's original thought.[52] Nevertheless, it would be foolish and pedantic to deny them the label "Marxist" because of this. In a similar way, if social Darwinism means the application to human society, however crudely or loosely, of concepts ultimately derived from Darwin, or approved by him as conforming to his theories, or appealing to his authority – principally evolution, the struggle for existence, and the survival of the fittest – then the policy of the compulsory sterilization of the "unfit," the subject of Bock's work, was certainly social Darwinist.

More recently, Richard Weikart has also criticized Zmarzlik's two-stage model of the transition of social Darwinism from liberal competitiveness to radical-reactionary selectionism because, he says:

From the earliest expressions of social Darwinism in the 1860s until the turn of the century, numerous German scholars used the Darwinian theory to defend individualist economic competition and laissez faire, others emphasized a collectivist struggle for existence between societies, while *most upheld both simultaneously.* A synthesis of individualism and collectivism had great appeal to German liberals in the 1860s

---

49 Cornelie Usborne, *The Politics of the Body in Weimar Germany: Women's Reproductive Rights and Duties* (London, 1992), 4.

50 Wehler, "Sozialdarwinismus," citing observations by Engels.

51 Adrian Desmond and James Moore, *Darwin* (London, 1991), is the latest and fullest general account of Darwin's life and ideas.

52 David McLelland, *Marxism after Marx*, 2d ed. (London, 1979).

and 1870s, since the long-standing twin ideals of German liberalism were individual liberty and German national unity. While the idea of individualist struggle may have faded after 1890 as classical liberalism declined in Germany, it would be incorrect to speak of a shift from stress on individualist to collectivist struggle, since collective competition received emphasis from the start.[53]

In practice, therefore, on a close reading of this passage ("may have faded after 1890"), it *does* appear that Weikart conceded there was a shift in emphasis. Moreover, an inspection of his footnotes reveals that most of his references to "collectivist" social Darwinism, insofar as it applied to German society, date from 1890 onward, further undermining his basic point. He also shows that many early social Darwinists were National Liberals. They applied their advocacy of a society based on free competition between individuals to Germany, while transposing it onto the global scale by making analogies with the competition between races. In an age of imperialism, a cause to which National Liberals became strongly attached, this was not surprising. It has long been recognized that the emergence of Wilhelmine *Weltpolitik* provided the context for such views to be turned back on German society itself; and if we accept the connections between National Liberalism and social Darwinism, then the context also included the precipitate decline of the National Liberals from the mid-1880s and their turn toward more aggressive forms of nationalism and a more authoritarian view of society.[54] Weikart points out that even if laissez-faire social Darwinism was not important in the United States before the last years of the nineteenth century,[55] the same cannot be said of Germany, for "Darwinism had its greatest impact in Germany."[56] Although he pays insufficient attention to the Social Democratic version of social Darwinism, on the whole, Weikart confirms rather than overthrows the existing orthodoxy on the subject, despite his rhetorical sallies against it.[57]

Perhaps the most radical attempt to restrict the concept of social Darwinism was undertaken some years ago by Alfred Kelly. According to Kelly, "the common historical treatment of German social Darwinism as a theoretical rehearsal for Nazism is a mistake. ... Cast in the role of

---

53   Richard Weikart, "The Origins of Social Darwinism in Germany, 1859-1895," *Journal of the History of Ideas* 54 (1993), 471 [italics in original].

54   For a summary, see Larry Eugene Jones and Konrad H. Jarausch, *In Search of a Liberal Germany* (Oxford, 1992); Dan H. White, *The Splintered Party: National Liberalism in Hessen and the Reich, 1867–1918* (Cambridge, Mass., 1976) is an important regional study.

55   David Bellomy, "Social Darwinism Revisited," *Perspectives in American History*, n.s., 1 (1984): 1, 100.

56   Weikart, "Origins," 471.

57   It is a different matter when Weikart argues that nineteenth-century German liberals in general had an "organic conception of society" (ibid., 472). Weikart provides no evidence in support of this view, however, and in fact, virtually all varieties of German liberals in the midcentury decades (roughly from the 1840s to the 1870s) were more inclined to favor a contractual than an organic view of society.

proto-Nazism, social Darwinism almost inevitably takes on not only a malevolence, but also a prominence, coherence, and direction that it lacked in reality." Kelly argued that the "rhetoric of struggle," which (in his view) was usually equated with social Darwinism, antedated Darwin. Militarists did not need Darwinian language to tell themselves and the world that war was a good thing. The occasional appropriation of "a Darwinian phrase or two" did not make someone a social Darwinist. The real social Darwinists, according to Kelly—that is, "those who undertook a sustained and detailed application of Darwin to human society"—were few in number and relatively without influence. Historians in his view had failed to distinguish between the earlier, moderate phase of social Darwinism and the later, radical phase from the 1890s when "ominous changes" in the ideology took place, mainly because "many Darwinists had come under the influence of August Weismann's germ plasm theory," which implied a need to preserve the "best" germ plasm in the race and ensure it was passed on to the next generation.

Social Darwinism thus became mixed up with racism and eugenics in the writings of people such as Schallmayer, Ploetz, and Ammon. "The full dehumanizing brutality of radical social Darwinism," Kelly noted, "becomes evident in the work of Alexander Tille," who advocated the killing of the mentally and physically disabled. But these radical social Darwinists were few in number. They were "largely unread figures." Many racists and anti-Semites were not social Darwinists, and many eugenicists, such as Fritz Lenz, rejected anti-Semitism. Of the alleged ideological precursors of Nazism, Houston Stewart Chamberlain only "flirted with Darwinism," whereas the leader of the Pan-German League, Heinrich Class, did not use Darwinian language at all. Social Darwinism was not popular among the German middle classes, and social Darwinism in no sense "caused" Nazism.[58] In a similar vein, Britta Rupp-Eisenreich has recently attacked Zmarzlik, Wehler, and other historians for allegedly reading Nazism back into social Darwinism by expanding the concept and making it so imprecise that it has become a kind of "negative myth." She too has argued that the term can only legitimately be applied to a small group of individual scientists such as Ploetz, Schallmeyer, and Gumplowicz.[59]

But there are a number of problems with these arguments. In the first place, although Kelly conceded at the beginning of his treatment of the subject that Darwinism was applied to human society in terms of evolution as well as selection, he ignored this "progressive" aspect in the rest of his

58 Kelly, *Descent of Darwin*, 101–22.
59 Britta Rupp-Eisenreich, "Le Darwinisme social en Allemagne," in Patrick Tort, ed., *Darwinisme et société* (Paris, 1992), 169–236.

analysis.[60] Second, Kelly confused the search for the ideological origins of Nazism with the equation of earlier thinkers with Hitler. The point is simple but fundamental. Zmarzlik argued over a third of a century ago that the Nazis only took certain ideas from social Darwinists, vulgarizing them and combining them with other crude political doctrines in the process. No sensible historian has argued that the total package of Nazism was present in earlier social or political movements or ideologies. What historians have tried to do is to find out where the different parts of Nazi ideology came from. Crucial distinctions are being blurred here, not only between the part and the whole, but also between the embryonic and the fully grown. Similarly, nobody is really claiming that social Darwinism "caused" Nazism. Kelly presented no evidence in support of this odd assertion, nor could he; virtually everyone who has written on Nazism knows that its causes did not lie exclusively in the realm of ideas, let alone medical or biological ideas. Finally, Kelly's criterion for the popularity of social Darwinism, Darwinism, and indeed by extension any idea in history was extremely simplistic: He measured popularity exclusively in terms of book sales. A writer such as Haeckel, whose books sold widely, Kelly described as popular; a writer such as Ploetz, whose books did not, he described as unpopular. Then, crucially, Kelly transferred these assessments to the ideas the books purveyed. But all this is deeply implausible. Ideas, rhetoric, concepts were and are spread by many means other than books. Magazines, newspapers, speeches, parliamentary debates, court cases, conversations, political manifestoes, voluntary associations, pressure groups – all these were means of forming "public opinion" in Imperial Germany and the Weimar Republic, and all of them were ignored in Kelly's account. One can see why Kelly did not investigate these mechanisms of popularization, which would have involved a substantial amount of additional research. But the result is that the question of popularization is left largely unanswered by his book, despite the promise contained in its subtitle.

The major point at issue here is whether or not the kind of social Darwinist ideas that were developed by the theorists Kelly mentioned were taken up in wider public debate. Zmarzlik and the orthodox view that he did so much to shape argued that they were, even if in a crude, vulgarized, and unsystematic manner. Kelly said that they were not. But no one should suppose that elaborate scientific or even pseudoscientific theories were or are ever adopted wholesale in public debate. Kelly's criteria for popularization were thus too strict. When scientific ideas enter the realm of public political discourse, they inevitably do so in an imprecise, crude, and highly selective manner.

60 Kelly, *Descent of Darwin*, 100–1.

This is then the form in which they equally inevitably get discussed by general historians seeking to explain the broad contours of Germany's social and political development. This may be annoying to the specialist historian of science or the author of a detailed study in intellectual history, but it is nonetheless a reasonable enough procedure. In the political world, concepts of race and ethnicity were – still are, indeed – defined not by anthropological societies, university professors, or research scientists, but by politicians, demagogues, and the average citizen. This, therefore, is where most historians have located them.

The late Tim Mason, for example, advocated a materialist account of social Darwinism in a broad historical context, as part of his long and ultimately unsuccessful search for a Marxist reading of the Third Reich that overcame the greatest weakness of Marxism in this area – its inability to incorporate racism and exterminism into an integrated historical explanation of National Socialism.[61] Mason called for a study of Nazism and capitalism linked through the concept of social Darwinism as the ideology of struggle. In summing up the debates of the 1970s between "intentionalists" and "functionalists" – not his terms, but epithets already bandied about by participants – Mason's intention was to transcend them and move research onto "a Marxist approach, which attaches pre-eminent weight to the processes of capital accumulation and class conflict."[62] It was not his fault that this plea went largely unheeded. Intellectual and political developments since Mason wrote have placed racism increasingly at the core of historians' appreciation of the Nazi phenomenon, pushing the idea of class struggle increasingly onto the periphery. Marxist approaches have become less rather than more influential. In the 1980s and 1990s, with the coming of postmodernism and the growing influence of thinkers such as Foucault, intellectual history has enjoyed something of a renaissance, forcing "materialist history" into the background. Moreover, in making his plea for a materialist history of social Darwinism, Mason narrowed the concept down to the idea of struggle, which, following Engels' original critique of Darwinism, he saw as an expression of the competitive ethos of capitalist society. Yet few historians have accepted this extremely narrow definition. As we have seen, the application of Darwin's ideas, or what were taken to be his ideas, to human society could equally involve a stress on evolution and mutuality, ideas that exercised a strong fascination over the

61 Tim Mason, *Social Policy in the Third Reich: The Working Class and the "National Community"* (Providence, R.I., and Oxford, 1993). See esp. the "General Introduction" by Ursula Vogel, vii-xv, and Mason's own "Introduction" and "Epilogue," 1–18, 275–369.
62 Tim Mason, "Intention and Explanation: A Current Controversy about the Interpretation of National Socialism," in Gerhard Hirschfeld and Lothar Kettenacker, eds., *The "Führer State": Myth and Reality: Studies on the Structure and Politics of the Third Reich* (Stuttgart, 1981), 37, 39.

German Social Democrats at the turn of the century. Social Darwinism cannot simply be equated with the principle and practice of struggle in capitalist society, as Mason tried to do. Nor, for that matter, can racism. Historians nowadays would be far more prepared than Mason ever was to recognize that ideas have a force of their own. Yet in one respect at least, Mason's comments are worth heeding. Social Darwinism, he thought, was involved in competition between states, national and ethnic conflict, and many other areas of society. It was a protean and many-sided phenomenon. It was not simply part of medical and scientific discourses, but reached far beyond them into the worlds of domestic and international politics. This, indeed, is where much of the historical discussion on social Darwinism has been located, rather than in the more specialized areas of the history of medicine and science; and with good reason, as we shall now see.

IV

In Germany before 1914, social Darwinist concepts can be found in three major areas of public debate.[63] First, there was the Social Democratic labor movement, where evolutionary concepts were being applied to historical change in a manner that strengthened the movement's already existing tendency to political immobilism. Darwinism had an appeal not only as a means of allegedly refuting the ideological premises of Christianity, but also as a way of bolstering the Social Democrats' conviction that the future was theirs. In substituting an evolutionary for a dialectical view of human history, the majority of Social Democrats convinced themselves that there was a scientifically proven "law of evolution" of society toward socialism, so that the end of capitalism would come, as it were, of its own accord, without the party having to do very much about it. Industrialization would simply continue until the working class formed the majority of the population, and the Social Democrats would then win a majority of seats in the Reichstag and come to power. By giving the labor movement the assurance that revolution would come peacefully, the Darwinian, evolutionary element in German Marxism played an integrating role in the Social Democratic Party and helped bind it together as the world's largest and most cohesive socialist organization before 1914. Beyond this, too, it also informed the party's views on class struggle and welfare. It is possible to argue that faith in social Darwinism and the habit of using Darwinian language laid some Social Democrats at least open to the

---

63 This seems an appropriate point to note that the attempt to equate social Darwinism with eugenics by R. J. Halliday ("Social Darwinism is defined as that discourse arguing for eugenic population control") is historically unconvincing and conceptually unduly restrictive (R. J. Halliday, "Social Darwinism: A Definition," *Victorian Studies* 14 [1971]: 401).

lure of selectionist eugenics, especially in the 1920s. But on the whole, there is no doubting the fact that the concept of evolution played the more prominent role.[64]

Second, a very different set of social Darwinist ideas and concepts found their way into the ideology of Pan-Germanism by 1914. This indeed is how they first came to the attention of general historians. Social Darwinism's place in the ideological synthesis that underpinned the policies of the Pan-German League has been precisely delineated by Roger Chickering, among others. Pan-Germanism, Chickering has remarked, was not a scientific ideology. Some of the men who created it around the turn of the century possessed scientific credentials, "most did not":

> The feat they as a group accomplished required, in any event, the ingenuity of dilettantes. They managed to fuse Gobineau's historical panorama, Wagner's theory of regeneration, antisemitism, and theories of natural selection drawn from Darwin. The infusion of Darwinism, for which most of the credit belongs to the anthropologist Ludwig Woltmann, was the leavening in the synthesis, for it provided these thinkers with a biological metaphor in which to discuss regeneration. Regeneration would take place in the context of interracial struggle, in which the purest race would survive. Darwinism also made it possible to discard Gobineau's fatalism and, with the imprimatur of Schemann himself, to identify racial breeding as the key to arrest race-mixing and the cultural and physical degeneration still associated with it.[65]

Thus the Pan-Germanists' ideology was not simply "social Darwinism," but rather a synthesis that incorporated particular elements of it interpreted in a particular way.[66] Chickering cautions that no complete or systematic statement of this rather eclectic theory appeared before World War I. Yet of the centrality of this version of Darwinian ideas to Pan-Germanism, Chickering is in no doubt. This ideology was tirelessly propagated in the Pan-German League's magazine, in meetings of its local chapters, and in a variety of other racist organizations that the League came to influence. Scientific racists such as Ludwig Woltmann and Otto Schmidt-Gibichenfels lectured at the League's meetings, and the League's publisher, J. F. Lehmann, was also a leading publisher of books on racial hygiene. "Fusing Gobineau and Darwin," as Chickering remarks, "led to the view that the inherent

---

64 Hans-Josef Steinberg, *Sozialismus und deutsche Sozialdemokratie: Zur Ideologie der Partei vor dem Ersten Weltkrieg*, 2d ed. (Bonn, 1972). The most widely read of all Social Democratic texts, August Bebel's *Die Frau und der Sozialismus*, first published in 1878, contained a substantial section on Darwinism, in which he portrayed class struggle as a version of the Darwinian struggle for survival of the fittest and the eventual triumph of socialism as "ein naturgeschichtliches Werden" (60th ed., [Berlin, 1929], 550).

65 Roger Chickering, *We Men Who Feel Most German: A Cultural Study of the Pan-German League, 1886–1914* (London, 1984), 239.

66 See the account of Woltmann's ideas in George L. Mosse, *The Crisis of German Ideology: Intellectual Origins of the Third Reich* (London, 1964), 99–104.

tendency in history was toward cultural degeneration, but that decisive intervention could still reverse, or at least arrest it." From this fusion came not only a campaign to increase the German birth rate (among other things, by providing homes for illegitimate children to improve their survival chances), unite the ethnic Germans across Europe, and find *Lebensraum* for them to live in, but also a vision of international politics as the struggle for the survival of the fittest between Latins, Teutons, and Slavs that could only be resolved by war.[67] Not everyone who supported any of these causes was necessarily a Pan-German, and many people espoused one or the other of them without accepting the whole package. But that there was such an ideological synthesis and that it was held by a significant number of people on the Pan-German far right cannot seriously be doubted.

The Pan-German League was a minority movement in Imperial Germany, but in the approach to World War I it put increasing pressure on the government to adopt a more aggressive foreign policy, and its influence on public opinion was growing. Startling evidence for this influence can be found in the writings of the Reich leadership just before the war. The most famous of these, Bernhardi's book *Germany and the Next War*, published in 1912, although stemming from the pen of a man who had only been head of the historical section of the General Staff and had retired in 1909, was widely debated and undoubtedly expressed the views of many within the military leadership. Bernhardi described war, famously, as a "biological necessity": "Without war, inferior or decaying races would easily choke the growth of healthy budding elements, and a universal decadence would follow."[68] Georg Alexander von Müller, chief of the Imperial Naval Cabinet, saw a prime target of German foreign policy as consisting in "the preservation of the Germanic race against Slavs and Romans."[69] Kurt Riezler, an important adviser of Reich Chancellor Bethmann Hollweg, took the view on the eve of war in 1914 that the major nations of the world were engaged in a ceaseless struggle with one another for the survival of the fittest.[70] The kaiser himself, and even more the crown prince, shared such views of international relations. Erich von Falkenhayn, appointed war minister in 1913 and chief of the General Staff in September 1914, also believed strongly that science had proved nations and races to be engaged in a "struggle for existence" of which military aggression was a necessary part. Recent research, based on

---

67 Chickering, *We Men*, 240–5.
68 Quoted in Crook, *Darwinism, War and History*, 83.
69 Quoted in Imanuel Geiss, ed., *July 1914: The Outbreak of the First World War: Selected Documents* (London, 1967), 22.
70 Hartmut Pogge von Strandmann and Imanuel Geiss, *Die Erforderlichkeit des Unmöglichen: Deutschland am Vorabend des ersten Weltkrieges* (Frankfurt/Main, 1965).

Falkenhayn's newly discovered diaries and letters, shows that he despised the kaiser for failing to bring about war, conspired in July 1914 to create circumstances in which war could be presented to Bethmann Hollweg as a military necessity, looked forward from the start to a war of attrition lasting three or four years rather than the short war so naively expected by many of the troops, and was quite prepared from the beginning to accept that Germany might well lose if that is what the Darwinist logic of world history and racial struggle dictated.[71] The point here is not that all these men were "social Darwinists," nor that they all agreed with everything the Pan-German League said–Hollweg and Riezler, for example, rejected many of the League's more far-reaching demands, and although prepared to risk war in 1914, do not seem on currently available evidence to have deliberately brought it about. Rather, the point is that the Darwinian language of racial struggle had come to infuse many people's thinking abut the relations between states by 1914, above all in Germany. These were not marginal figures on the fringes of academia, nor were they unrepresentative or unimportant. These were the men who led the destinies of Imperial Germany. The view of international relations as interracial struggle for the survival of the fittest according to laws supposedly discovered by Charles Darwin was one of what James Joll described as the "unconscious assumptions" on which statesmen based their conduct of foreign policy at this time. "The linkage of Darwinism with militarism and imperialism," Paul Crook has concluded, "was probably closest in Germany."[72] It was more than merely a confirmation of the existing professional bellicosity of military men. On balance, it made war more rather than less likely to break out.[73]

Linked to these assumptions to a greater or lesser extent was a third major area of public debate in which social Darwinist ideas featured prominently. This was the advocacy of policies of "racial hygiene," which became steadily more influential in the emerging welfare sector before World War I. I have suggested elsewhere how elements of the Pan-German ideological mixture entered the feminist movement before the war, in the defeat of arguments for legalized abortion advanced by many influential women in the movement on the grounds that the international survival of the German race in a future war required a high birth rate.[74] Another illustration of the permeation of welfarist discourse by the language of racial hygiene can be found in the field of criminology and forensic psychiatry. One of the leading criminologists of the

71 Holger Afflerbach, *Falkenhayn: Politisches Denken und Handeln im Kaiserreich* (Munich, 1994).
72 James Joll, *The Origins of the First World War* (London, 1984), 152–3, 184–91.
73 Crook, *Darwinism, War and History*, 30.
74 Evans, *Feminist Movement*, chaps. 5–6.

day, Gustav Aschaffenburg, thought that at least half of all penitentiary inmates were incorrigible, probably on hereditary grounds. The vast majority of criminals, he said, came from "inferior human material." Almost inevitably, they had "physically and spiritually inferior children" who would simply repeat the cycle of crime. It was time, he declared, to prevent them from breeding. Criminals must recognize "that society defends itself with all the means at its disposal."[75] Aschaffenburg considered that the challenges of modern life were too great for the weak human material from which criminals were made:

Life takes its course and crushes the man who cannot cope. Just as the struggle for existence is played out today and will surely be played out through eternity, just as popular morality forces everyone under the yoke of this struggle, so we must all reach an unprejudiced perception and judgment of the dangers to which we are all exposed. And these are far greater than the ability of all these inferior elements in society to withstand them.[76]

Hence the high degree of recidivism observable in the German prison population. Another standard textbook on forensic psychiatry, published in 1901, accepted the argument that criminality could be recognized by physical signs such as malformations of the ear or the size and shape of the forehead. "In general," wrote its editor, Alfred Hoche – later to become notorious as the advocate of the extermination of what he called "life unworthy of life" – "the morbid reduction of a person's capacity to resist his criminal tendencies can be estimated to be the higher, the more he displays physical and mental signs of degeneration under investigation."[77] Even for less dangerous criminals, German criminologists before World War I came increasingly to believe that compulsory sterilization was the remedy. "Individuals of an anti-social disposition" and "moral idiots" had to be stopped from reproducing. They should be removed from society for an indefinite period, irrespective of the nature of their crime, in the interests of an "improvement of social hygiene."[78] Monstrous, inhuman specimens like Jack the Ripper should not be kept alive, with the possibility that they might reproduce: They should be eliminated

75 Dieter Dölling, "Kriminologie im Dritten Reich," in Ralf Dreier and Wolfgang Sellert, eds., *Recht und Justiz im "Dritten Reich"* (Frankfurt/Main, 1989), 222; Gustav Aschaffenburg, *Das Verbrechen und seine Bekämpfung*, 3d ed. (Heidelberg, 1923), 196–201, 220–2, 226–7.
76 Aschaffenburg, *Verbrechen und seine Bekämpfung*, 223. There is a useful brief discussion of this subject in Robert N. Proctor, *Racial Hygiene: Medicine under the Nazis* (Cambridge, Mass., 1988), 202–5.
77 Alfred Hoche, ed., *Handbuch der gerichtlichen Psychiatrie* (Berlin, 1901), 414, 419.
78 Gustav Aschaffenburg, ed., *Bericht über den VII. Internationalen Kongress für Kriminalanthropologie* (Heidelberg, 1912). See also the articles by Graf Gleispach, "Die unbestimmte Verurteilung" (226–43); Prof. Dannemann, "Die Entmündigung chronisch Krimineller als Mittel zur Verbesserug der sozialen Hygiene" (313–21); Hans Maier, "Erfahrungen über die Sterilisation Krimineller in der Schweiz und Nordamerika als Mittel der sozialen Hygiene" (322–31); and H. Klaatsch, "Die Morphologie und Psychologie der niederen Menschenrassen in ihrer Bedeutung für die Probleme der Kriminalistik" (56–73).

from the chain of heredity.[79] Even if criminologists shied away from advocating capital punishment on a large enough scale to be eugenically effective,
some at least were prepared to support it for the most extreme of human
"monsters."[80] The particular branch of criminology that was most vociferous
in advocating such policies – criminal anthropology – was dominated by
Germans and Austrians.[81] But by 1914 such biologistic ways of thinking
about crime had become widespread among forensic psychiatrists as well.
The increasingly professional nature of policing and detective work in the late
nineteenth century also helped spread these ideas and techniques. Policemen
saw them as lending added legitimacy and status to their profession, and soon
textbooks of policing too were filled with pages of photographs detailing the
physiognomical features of various types of criminal, while prison authorities in cities such as Hamburg began to collect the death masks of executed
capital offenders in the hope of applying Cesare Lombroso's techniques to
them as well when they had eventually collected a sufficient number.[82]

To underline the precise significance of these views, it is necessary to recall
that criminologists such as Aschaffenburg actually opposed the death penalty,
because they were unwilling to take the crucial step from arguing that there
was a hereditary element in criminality to proposing that incorrigible criminals should therefore be killed. Another prominent criminologist of the early
twentieth century, Hans von Hentig, declared: "A large proportion of criminals belong to elements in the race which are dying out of themselves."
Investigation showed that they came from families with few children and had
few of their own. From this argument, von Hentig drew the conclusion that
it was not necessary to remove them from the chain of heredity; they would
do it themselves. Eventually he was to be dismissed by the Nazis from his university post because of his protests against their eugenic penal policies in
1933.[83] Clearly, the argument that serious criminality was inherited and therefore serious criminals were incorrigible could be used to justify their biological extermination.[84] Equally clearly, however, such extrapolations were
uncommon before World War I. It took a whole series of historical changes,
including mass slaughter in a world war, military defeat, the overthrow of the
Kaiserreich, and the Revolution of 1918 before criminologists and psychiatrists

---

79 For an account of these views and the controversy they aroused when they were put forward in the
    Archiv für Kriminal-Anthropologie und Kriminalistik, see Peter Gay, *The Bourgeois Experience*, vol. 3: *The
    Cultivation of Hatred* (Oxford, 1994), 165–6.
80 Paul Nacke, cited in ibid., 165.
81 See the list of delegates in Aschaffenburg, ed., *Bericht*.
82 Gustav Roscher, *Grossstadtpolizei* (Hamburg, 1906).
83 Hans von Hentig, *Strafrecht und Auslese* (Berlin, 1914), 216. Aschaffenburg was Jewish, and was also
    dismissed by the Nazis.
84 For a more extended treatment of this topic, see my *Rituals of Retribution*, chaps. 12–16.

could seriously start arguing along these lines. It took a further, massive social and political crisis at the beginning of the 1930s before they could become part of official government ideology. And it took another world war to provide the circumstances in which they could be put into effect.[85]

V

Selectionist social Darwinism – the idea that human society was governed by the struggle, whether between races or between individuals or families, for the survival of the fittest – and the language and concepts that it inserted into welfarist and criminological discourse before World War I had a widespread and growing influence in the discussion of social problems at this time. This was, of course, a language in which a variety of different and often conflicting policies could be articulated. Yet without the emergence of this language, Nazi ideology would not have been able to develop as it did. And its spread during the Weimar Republic helped reconcile those who used it, and for whom it had become an almost automatic way of thinking about society, to accept the policies that the Nazis advocated and in many cases to collaborate willingly in putting them into effect. It may be helpful to conceptualize social Darwinism in these broader historical contexts, indeed, as a language, a collection of words that constituted a discursive framework for debate in these various areas, rather than as a coherent set of ideas or a fully worked-out ideology. It certainly does not help to conflate it with organicist biology or eugenics; the reach of social Darwinist discourses was much wider than that, as we have seen.[86] The history of social Darwinism in Germany goes far beyond the narrow history of science and medicine.

In a similar way, the willing collaboration of the medical profession with Nazi policies in the Third Reich can be explained exclusively neither in terms of its professional interests nor in terms of its scientific ambitions.[87] Doctors were part of the educated middle class, and their social and political attitudes were shaped as much by this fact as by their own specialist training and concerns. They were educated at German universities and were therefore exposed to the conservative, radical-nationalist, and (after 1918) far-right

<hr/>

85 For a balanced treatment of this topic, see Richard F. Wetzell, "Criminal Law Reform in Imperial Germany," Ph.D. diss., Stanford University, 1991; and Wetzell's forthcoming book, which extends coverage through to the 1950s.

86 For the conflation of social Darwinism, organicist biology, and eugenics, see Weindling, *Darwinism*, 303, and Pietro Corsi and Paul Weindling, "Darwinism in Germany, France, and Italy," in David Kohn, ed., *The Darwinian Heritage* (Princeton, N.J., 1985), 683, 698. In the same article, Weindling also confuses social Darwinism with "social factors in the propagation of Darwinism" (697).

87 Benno Müller-Hill, *Murderous Science: Elimination by Scientific Selection of Jews, Gypsies and Others, Germany, 1933–1945* (Oxford, 1988), takes this rather narrow approach; but Müller-Hill is a geneticist, not a historian.

politics that dominated both academic staff and student representation in these institutions.[88] More generally, as Jeremy Noakes has pointed out, the *Bildungsbürgertum*, to which doctors belonged,

was a group which, by the first decade of the twentieth century, was beginning to feel itself threatened by a number of social developments, notably the creation of a "mass" urban society combined with the emergence of a powerful new rival moneyed elite, neither of which shared their values. They both despised and feared the democratizing, levelling aspects of a mass society and what they saw as the crude materialism of the new elite.[89]

The underlying social processes in all this cannot be reduced to the professionalization of biology or the emergence of institutional power bases in the medical field. As Günther Hecht, from the Racial-Political Office of the Nazi Party, once said: "As a political movement, National Socialism rejects any equation with any scholars or researchers or any branches of research within the life sciences. ... National Socialism is a political movement, not a scientific one."[90] Social Darwinist language conferred scientific legitimacy on its exponents, whatever line they took. The rhetoric of science was an important legitimating factor in Nazi imperialism.[91] Hitler took up this rhetoric and used his own version of the language of social Darwinism as a central element in the discursive practice of extermination. By the middle of the war, this discursive practice had been almost entirely cut loose from whatever moorings it might once have had in medicine, science, or social policy. Hitler and the Nazi judicial and police apparatus defined as racially degenerate "anyone whose personality and way of life make it clear that their natural tendency is to commit serious crimes," whether or not the offences in question had actually been committed.[92] The language of social Darwinism in its Nazi variant had come to be a means of legitimizing terror and extermination against deviants, opponents of the regime, and indeed anyone who did not appear to be wholeheartedly devoted to the war effort. The language of social Darwinism helped to remove all restraint from those who directed the terroristic and exterminatory policies of the regime, and it legitimized these policies in the minds of those who practiced them by persuading them that what they were doing was justified by history, science, and nature.

88 Fritz K. Ringer, *The Decline of the German Mandarins* (Princeton, N.J., 1969); Michael H. Steinberg, *Sabers and Brown Shirts: The German Students' Path to National Socialism, 1918–1935* (Princeton, N.J., 1977).
89 Jeremy Noakes, "Nazism and Eugenics: The Background to the Nazi Sterilization Law of 14 July 1933," in Roger J. Bullen et al., eds., *Ideas into Politics: Aspects of European History, 1880–1950* (London, 1984), 78.
90 Quoted in Anne Bäumer, *NS-Biologie* (Stuttgart, 1990), 120.
91 Woodruff D. Smith, *The Ideological Origins of Nazi Imperialism* (Oxford, 1986), 144.
92 Peukert, "Arbeitslager," quoting a draft law of Feb. 1944.

4

Modern German Doctors

A Failure of Professionalization?

CHARLES E. McCLELLAND

This volume of essays would perhaps not have come into being were it not for the nagging and still inadequately answered questions raised by the Nuremberg Tribunal about the "perversion," as Michael Kater has aptly called it, of German medicine. Perhaps the major question still looming over the history of medicine in twentieth-century Germany was succinctly put in the title of Alexander Mitscherlich's 1947 book on the Nuremberg physicians' trials, *Medizin ohne Menschlichkeit*, also translated as *Doctors of Infamy*.[1] How could a modern medical community with a tradition of classical as well as scientific learning, the descendants of Hippocrates and the collective bearers of scientific professionalism, ignore the admonition in the Hippocratic oath to "maintain the utmost respect for human life from the time of its conception?"[2] How could the German medical profession, the peer if not the envy of its colleagues abroad at the outbreak of World War I, have sunk to the level of a colluder in genocide during World War II? Can historical analysis offer anything to answer this question, especially its ethical, legal, and political dimensions? In particular, can the new social history, especially the history of education and professions, add any new hints?

In recent years historians' attention has shifted somewhat from a focus on the tiny minority of German doctors who carried out perverted experiments in death camps or had a direct role in mass murder. It is for the social historian equally interesting to ask about the "normal" people among the nearly 60,000 physicians working in Hitler's Germany. May we justifiably speak, as

---

1 Alexander Mitscherlich with Fred Mielke, *Das Diktat der Menschenverachtung: Medizin ohne Menschlichkeit* (Heidelberg, 1947), translated as *Doctors of Infamy* (New York, 1949).

2 Thus, the phrasing of the 1948 World Medical Association version. (Reprinted with a commentary by Albert Deutsch in *Doctors of Infamy*, xxxviii.) In fact the notion of a particularly grave and binding "Hippocratic oath" (as opposed to the teachings and aphorisms of Hippocrates) appears to be a fairly recent concept, perhaps the result of a twentieth-century Hippocrates revival, because it played little role in modern medical discussions in Germany before 1933 and is not even found in the Oxford English Dictionary.

Michael Kater did in his stimulating *Journal of Contemporary History* article of 1985, of the "failed socialization and professionalization of German medical doctors over previous [to 1933] decades?"[3] Did in fact "elements of their professional development predispose the German physicians to fascistization in the twentieth century and ultimately set many, if not the majority, apart from other doctors of the western world who had once sworn the Hippocratic oath?"[4]

This essay, regretfully, must leave aside such primary questions as that most grievous breach of medical ethics, the misuse of concentration camp inmates and assisting in the Holocaust, because they cannot easily be addressed by analyzing medical professionalization. The number and hierarchical position of the doctors involved was such as to make generalizing from them about the whole medical profession highly dubious. Even camp doctors, as Robert Jay Lifton shows, hardly behaved in a uniform way.[5] Nor does the proclivity of many doctors before 1933 to evince interest in the "eugenics" movement, reproductive sterilization programs, or even euthanasia for the incurably ill constitute a "special case" marking them off from their colleagues elsewhere, including Britain and America.

If the history of professionalization of physicians can shed new light, it is on some other, perhaps less existential questions: Why did *doctors*, especially, find the Nazi party attractive? Even if we can assume that the vast majority of German physicians had nothing to do with medical "perversions," there must have been reasons why so many went along with other aims of the Nazi regime, at least initially. Were they more susceptible than other professional groups? If so, is there indeed something peculiar about their socialization and professionalization?

Michael Kater is not alone in asserting that German doctors suffered from a "legitimation crisis," social insecurity (but at the same time class snobbism), the autocratic tinge to medical training, suspicion of women and Jews as colleagues, and a proclivity toward conservative political views.[6] Yet at the same time, German medical standards, scientific training, and professionalism were admired throughout the world both under and after the Empire, so much so that the Flexner Report on the reform of American medical education in 1910 held it up as *the* model.[7] Were German physicians poorly socialized

3   Michael Kater, "Professionalization and Socialization of Physicians in Wilhelmine and Weimar Germany," *Journal of Contemporary History* 20 (1985): 694.
4   Ibid., 677.
5   Robert Jay Lifton, *The Nazi Doctors: Medical Killing and the Psychology of Genocide* (New York, 1986), esp. chaps. 11–13.
6   Kater, "Professionalization."
7   Abraham Flexner, *Medical Education in the United States and Canada: A Report to the Carnegie Foundation*

or professionalized in comparison to their colleagues abroad or their fellow professionals in Germany? Or, to what extent might the same factors that led to their profession being admired *before* World War I, under the radically changed postwar political, economic and social conditions, have started a process of decline or crisis? Is the antithesis stated in Mitscherlich's title more dramatic than real? Or did highly professionalized modern medicine easily coexist with Nazi barbarism?

To rephrase the looming question into a more manageable one for the purposes of this essay: To what degree can the history of professionalization and professionally organized behavior in an advanced society serve as a useful analytical tool and a key to the tensions that might produce the dramatic reversal in the reputation of German medicine over a mere generation? Although I have little space to explore them here an any depth, I would like to stress the importance of new perspectives of comparative angles of view. How did the other "products" of the German university system, the graduates of the traditional university faculties and later of the technical and other higher educational colleges, evolve in their professional bodies, and did they behave differently from M.D.s? What can one learn by comparisons to the professionalization history of neighboring countries?

Allow me to repeat today a definition of a modern profession I have used elsewhere: "an exclusive, specialized, life-long form of labor which is accessible – in a division-of-labor society – only on the basis of a long, expensive and theoretically-based education."[8] Even in a country where education was relatively inexpensive, the costs of obtaining the necessary qualifications for professions had become high enough by the late nineteenth century to make the "old" professions of medicine and law (the clergy was an exception), as well as such "new" ones as engineering and teaching, into occupations qualitatively much more removed than before from others. It is this process that I mean by "professionalization." University-level education was now the chief watershed and led to a large degree of overlap between the professional class and the *Bildungsbürgertum*. It is therefore hardly surprising to find the attitudes among all German professionals, not just physicians, reflective of the elite values of the university-trained middle class.

It is important to note that learned professions (including medicine) did not enjoy in previous centuries the consistently high public esteem they came

for the Advancement of Teaching (New York, 1910); see also Abraham Flexner's *Medical Education in Europe* (New York, 1912).

8 Charles E. McClelland, "Zur Professionalisierung der akademischen Berufe in Deutschland," in Werner Conze and Jürgen Kocka, eds., *Bildungsbürgertum im 19. Jahrhundert*, vol. 1: *Bildungssystem und Professionalisierung in internationalen Vergleichen* (Stuttgart, 1985), 237.

to have by 1900 (and still, according to public opinion surveys, tend to retain today).[9] It is perhaps not exaggerating too much to point out that the medical butchers of Auschwitz had only to fall back to the level of the medical pioneers of a century before, if that far, to find their technical (if not moral) peers. From the inception of their organization into modern national associations, all German professions aimed at *die Hebung des Standes* – the raising of the collective professional "estate." German physicians followed some of the same paths toward this as their counterparts in other fields in Germany, as well as some shared with physicians abroad; they also, however, pursued professionalization under some unusual and even unique conditions.

Perhaps no other modern or modernizing profession had come to depend so heavily for its legitimation on swift advances in science as was the case of medicine and relatively less on strategies of market control. The degree to which the German medical profession was "scientified" under the Empire was probably the highest in the world. (British and even French physicians could also scoff at the relative German neglect of hospital or clinical training and "bedside manner.") Pride in "scientific" achievement could nevertheless be shared by the leadership groups in the medical profession itself and the leadership of the German higher educational system, backed by the German states with sensible policies and lavish financial resources. As I have argued elsewhere, barring artificial restrictions on admission to medical training (which neither government higher-education policy nor a majority of German physicians favored), the path for limiting ruinous competition in the profession lay exactly in the promotion by the profession of ever-higher educational qualifications for new physicians.[10]

9 Even one of the founders of the prestigious University of Göttingen referred contemptuously to the necessity of creating a medical faculty in order to produce a few *Würgengel* (angels of death), "so that the dead can be conveyed to the cemetery in an orderly fashion"; just as the King of Prussia decreed that lawyers should wear distinctive robes so that the people could "see the scoundrels coming." See J. G. von Meiern, as cited in Götz von Selle, *Die Georg-August-Universität zu Göttingen, 1737–1937* (Göttingen, 1937), 27; Adolf Weissler, *Geschichte der Rechtswissenschaft* (Leipzig, 1905), 310. By contrast, doctors have enjoyed increasing esteem over the last century, demonstrable among other things by public opinion polls. The Institut für Demoskopie in Allensbach in a survey of German professions' public esteem in the fall of 1993 showed that 81 percent of surveyed Germans had high respect for doctors. The next most respected occupational group was pastors (40 percent), followed by lawyers (36 percent), and, as a poor fourth, university professors (33 percent). Politicians, journalists, and schoolteachers did significantly worse (9 percent, 17 percent, and 15 percent, respectively). Of course the road from eighteenth-century *Würgengel* to 1990s public hero was littered with many public complaints, justified skepticism, and outright mistrust, just as in any other country. Yet many documented public criticisms of the medical care system were often heartily shared by the professionals themselves.

10 At various times since the foundation of the DÄVB in 1873, some doctors expressed the wish that a *numerus clausus* be adopted by German universities to limit the number of professionals being turned out. Articles and letters in medical journals sometimes made such calls; occasionally, resolutions were unsuccessfully proposed to the national medical conventions (*Ärztetage*). Yet even in the

One can only speculate about the resulting proclivity of many German doctors to seek status reinforcement from the outside. Recourse to "authority" such as science was certainly one strategy. When this appeared to fail, as during the Great Depression, a turn to the "strong state" had its appeal (even though the *Nationalsozialistische Deutsche Arbeiterpartei*, or NSDAP, was basically more in sympathy with "alternative" than "school" medicine, as German M.D.s discovered to their horror in 1939 with the passage of the Lay Healer's Law). Perhaps the question to be raised – and it certainly cannot be answered here – is not so much why German doctors were "authoritarian" as why French and British doctors did not get an opportunity to throw in their lot with an initially successful fascist regime.

The *process* of professionalization is an almost universal phenomenon accompanying modernization, urbanization, and industrial as well as post-industrial change. It should not, however, be thought of as an absolute condition (either there is professionalization or there is not), or as irreversible, or as linearly continuous, or "progressive." It is almost impossible to conceive of something called "perfect professionalization," because the very term designates a process that is far from uniform in time, geography, or even among different occupations. Should such perfection ever be momentarily achieved, however, it could hardly be maintained, at least in a changing and relatively free market society.

A look at the historical vicissitudes of the professionalization process in Germany, and particularly with regard to German medicine, might show us this most dramatically.

One could reasonably argue that German medicine was professionalizing well down to 1900, even to the start of World War I, although under conditions different from those in many foreign countries.

The professionalization of modern German medicine began well before the creation of a German national state. Even under the Empire, the education and certification of doctors remained a prerogative of the federal states, as did the administration of medical ethics (in the course of time increasingly through *Ärztekammer*, or medical chambers). The medical profession continued to be organized locally and regionally, with the National Medical Association (*Deutscher Ärztevereinsverbund*, or DÄVB, founded in 1873) as a league of regional medical societies rather than an association of individual

depths of the Great Depression, the German Medical Association was never willing to endorse much more than restrictions on the number of physicians that could be admitted to panel practice, which it negotiated with the sickness funds. The DÄVB represented 95 percent of German licensed physicians by the 1920s. For more detailed discussion, see Charles E. McClelland, *The German Experience of Professionalization: Modern Learned Professions and Their Organizations from the Early Nineteenth Century to the Hitler Era* (Cambridge, 1991), 142, 183.

members. Membership in medical societies was voluntary; but in most states membership in the medical chambers was or became compulsory, and the leadership of both types of professional organization tended to overlap.

The DÄVB was concerned chiefly with the status of the profession, including issues of training and certification. The local and state medical chambers dealt mostly with policing medical ethics, but these were defined in practice more by questions of unfair competition than malpractice involving patients. It is worth noting that certain categories of physicians, for example, military and state medical officers, were not required to belong to the chambers on the argument that their bureaucratic superiors would supervise their activities. Finally, although sickness insurance funds to some degree predated the founding of the German Reich, they remained local and diversified in administration and structure even after the creation of a national health insurance system in the 1880s. Their counterpart was the nationally organized Hartmann-Bund (to which doctors *did* belong as individual members), which in turn affiliated with the DÄVB before World War I.

German medical leaders had boldly struck a bargain with the new national government in 1869. Despite the localized and heterogenous nature of the medical profession and its working conditions, medicine was one of the two major traditional professions (along with attorneys) to be affected by a national "framework law." The medical profession, just then organizing on a national scale, even conceded the lifting of laws against *unlicensed* practice, or "quackery," in order that the *Reichsgewerbeordnung* declare medicine a "free profession." This meant that medicine would no longer be tightly controlled by state bureaucracies but be left to the free play of the market, within certain limits. The chief spokesperson and negotiator for the medical profession in striking this deal was the Berlin Medical Society, itself heavily influenced by liberal ideology and a professorial faith in the obvious superiority of "school" medicine.

Not all members of the DÄVB were entirely happy with this national legislation. The practice of medicine as covered by the *Reichsgewerbeordnung* was treated as a "trade." Not only did this seem demeaning to many physicians, it rankled even more that nonlicensed health-care providers, such as herbalists, wise women, shepherds and others dismissed by the M.D.s as "quacks," were allowed to practice freely also. Many in the medical profession, as well as the DÄVB, persisted in demanding a national physicians' code (*Reichsärzteordnung*) that would, inter alia, suppress competition from these so-called *Kurpfuscher*. Such an aim was quite consistent with "power" theories of professionalization, which posit the drive to monopoly over the market as the only real goal of professional organizations, as well as with the attitudes of doctors in other countries (e.g., America).

Failing to convince the state to criminalize "quack" practice, however, the medical profession fell back on arguments that only school medicine, with its ever-higher educational and scientific requirements, provided real therapy. Ironically, the expansion of the sickness fund system, although having an unwelcome effect on the complete freedom of doctors in matters of treatment and fees, at least helped in the marginalization of quacks. (The funds nevertheless continued to hire paramedically trained people such as medical students and nurses for tasks the profession believed should be carried out by fully licensed physicians.)

The practical effect of continued endorsement of the most open access to medical training consistent with completion of secondary school was a flood of new doctors, with especially high crests in years of slow economic growth. A minority of doctors began raising calls for a *numerus clausus*, or restriction on the number of students admitted to the study of medicine, as the least painful form of professional market control. Yet all such calls were resisted by the majority of the rapidly growing German medical profession and its major organization, the DÄVB. Its persistent answer for overcrowding came from another angle – that of *Verwissenschaftlichung*. Raising the cost of medical education in terms of time and difficulty of study and examinations was the route chosen consistently by the DÄVB (and, beginning a generation later, also of the American medical profession). Yet there was also a limit to manipulation of such standards of knowledge: They could not arbitrarily be increased or decreased over short time periods, because the arguments for *increasing* them were linked to the progress of knowledge. A countervailing "interest of state" also led in the direction of easy access to medical training for various reasons – whether wartime emergency (as in 1914–18), need to fill panel physicians' slots in an expanding health insurance scheme, or even meritocratic and democratic ideology.

As in other fields of study, medicine changed its traditional student recruiting base, especially in the early twentieth century. Traditionally a field for ambitious young men of commercial and lower-middle-class families (compared to law, which drew heavily on the *Bildungsbürgertum* and administrative elites), medicine had also offered a haven to scions of Jewish families in the German Empire – precisely because it was a "free" profession. The expansion of student bodies in the early twentieth century, and especially in the 1920s, meant a far larger number of future physicians facing stiff competition; for many, financial exigency during student years and worry about the future; and a sense of desperation about the need to change the system if they were to survive. The Nazi promise to rid universities of Jews and women – in effect a *numerus clausus* affecting some 36 percent of medical students in 1933 – thus had a certain attraction, especially among students whose social and economic backgrounds made their future professional existence precarious in the extreme.[11]

Thus the German path to increased professionalization paralleled the path of ever-higher scientific and educational qualifications *precisely for the younger aspirants to the profession*. There were already numerous complaints about overproduction of doctors, ruinous competition, sinking average incomes, and the like by the beginning of the twentieth century. The progressive inclusion of more and more citizens in the mandatory health insurance scheme, although providing more patients, also limited the fees and working conditions of panel physicians.

One must also consider the unique set of conditions of the German medical market caused by sickness insurance. It undoubtedly facilitated, inter alia, the support of many more doctors than would have been possible without it. At first a mere cloud on the horizon in the 1880s, it was greeted with indifference, or even positively by doctors. Even later it never upset German physicians in any way remotely comparable to the tantrums of American doctors against "socialized medicine" over the past seventy years. No majorities of German physicians ever called for the abolition of the sickness funds, which were a rational substitute for the old obligation (also abolished in 1869) of any doctor to treat any indigent patient gratis. Further, until the Insurance Reform of 1911, mandatory coverage had been extended to citizens in the lower-income classes, which opened up a new market in services, even if the regulated fees were low.

Even when the medical profession began to collide with other social and political institutions, it showed both power and responsibility. One might cite the widespread strikes of 1913 against the provisions of the new insurance law, which forced a compromise on the insurance funds. In these steps toward greater professional solidarity and organization, German doctors pushed through many long-standing demands, such as the insurance patients' right to choose their physician.

If power over the market in services is the best indicator of "successful" professionalization, as the current fashionable theory holds (with "perfection" equaling "monopoly"), German medicine probably could not be said to compete equally with British or American equivalents in 1914. But by many other traditional measures of professionalization, such as the existence

11   Ibid., 183.

of self-regulating ethics bodies (*Ärztekammer*), prestige and public trust, economic security, a high degree of inclusiveness in professional organizations and of effectiveness of the same, and autonomy in the exercise of one's professional practice, one can see on the whole marked advances in 1914 over the previous half century.

Instead, some historians have referred to the phenomena of interwar Germany in terms of "deprofessionalization," with characteristic massive overcrowding, economic insecurity and ruthless competition, and the entry or expansion of recruits from heretofore little-included strata of the population. What made the economic crisis of Weimar Germany even more wrenching for young medical professionals, however, was that the scientific standards set already before 1914 were not relaxed (except during World War I). Thus professional standards remained nominally high, whereas professional prospects became very dim for a generation.

Can professionalization and deprofessionalization take place at the same time? Ironically, both tendencies appeared present in the tumultuous years of the Weimar Republic.

The results of World War I greatly exacerbated the conditions under which all doctors worked, but they were especially dire for young people. If the universities of Imperial Germany were producing too many physicians, as was argued in 1913, then those of the Weimar Republic went into hyperinflation. Competition for clients was made even more acute by the economic crises of the Weimar era, during some of which even the medical insurance coverage had to be curtailed.

These conditions were not unique to Germany. The successor states to Austria-Hungary experienced similar phenomena of deprofessionalization. Well before and more vehemently than in the German Reich, for example, Hungarian doctors and lawyers developed a strong affinity for fascist doctrines and anti-Semitic jargon, of which they had been remarkably free before 1914. As in Germany, Hungary had a very large number of physicians who happened to be Jewish. The proportion of Jewish physicians in the lands of the former Austro-Hungarian empire was even higher than in Germany, where it was quite high by standards further west.

Trends of deprofessionalization (in terms of income, status, occupational security, and even social esteem) appear to have had the greatest impact on the young, the economically less well-off, and the nonspecialist. Not surprisingly, the leadership of the DÄVB and other medical associations tended to belong to the senior generation and to be cushioned by success against many of the effects of deprofessionalization. One could thus legitimately hypothesize a "professionalization crisis" as a major cause for the support found among

German doctors–particularly among younger ones–for Nazi promises to make not only the German race but the medical profession "healthy" again.[12]

One should not, of course, conclude either that the DÄVB and the German medical profession generally were inclined to enthusiasm for democracy, liberalism, or leftist causes. Physicians were by necessity members of the *Bildungsbürgertum*, and most were operating small businesses, in economic terms. The political left constituted the enemy, in the eyes of most doctors, if only because of the structure and functioning of the national health insurance system. Germany's *Krankenkassen* negotiated contracts with the country's panel physicians that determined their working conditions and fees. Even when these contracts were negotiated with the powerful DÄVB/Hartmann-Bund, German doctors viewed the sickness insurance funds as dominated by representatives of the workers that they covered, in other words, by socialist, union, or communist influences. At the very least, German physicians regarded the labor-dominated sickness funds as threats to their autonomy and livelihood; at worst, they viewed the funds–with their single-minded concern for cheap, mass treatment under very restricted bureaucratic direction–as the enemy of good medical practice.

Considering that the anti-Marxist rage of the NSDAP was at least as strong a lure to German voters as anti-Semitism, one would think a shared antipathy toward the left would have attracted doctors more than many other professional groups to the "brown" ranks. And it no doubt did serve as an attraction for those who joined the Nazi Federation of German Doctors (*Nationalsozialistischer Deutscher Ärztebund*, or NSDÄB). But the DÄVB (like most professional organizations at the time) adopted a position above the parties and attempted, with varying but considerable success, to couch its lobbying and arguments in nonpartisan terms.

The German medical profession, and its organizations, were disproportionately influenced by German doctors who happened to have Jewish backgrounds. The open and cooperative attitudes of an older generation of German doctors had become a thorn in the side of younger aspirants by the late 1920s. The fact that younger German doctors and medical students founded the NS Ärztebund already in 1929 is not so much an index of the virulence of the brown disease among German doctors: It is rather a sign that fascist resentments could not get very far in the major national medical organizations, including the most important one, the DÄVB.

---

12 Michael Kater has written that the "bulk of Nazi supporters among the physicians ... before 1933 were young rather than old, insecure rather than established, desperately casting about for chances of gainful self-employment and economic stability rather than opportunities for self-sacrifice to augment the fortunes of some political party." *Doctors under Hitler* (Chapel Hill, N.C., 1989), 64.

The virulent anti-Semitism of the NSDAP would logically have had more appeal to members of the medical profession than most others, simply because it had been one of the few to be completely open to Jews under the Empire. Thus young, frustrated aspirants to a secure medical practice and income often found (particularly in big cities) that they had to compete with older, well-established Jewish physicians. According to one contemporary study, Jews made up 16 percent of all Prussian doctors on the eve of the Nazi seizure of power (as opposed to about 1 percent of the population).[13] The professional organizations and their directors reflected also the high percentage of Jews in medicine. Ironically, too, the very permeation of professional organizations by doctors of Jewish background posed a formidable barrier for a Nazi takeover from within – undoubtedly one of the reasons for the early founding of the NSDÄB as a separate organization. In other words, the existence of the NSDÄB, often cited as an indicator of the strength of Nazi sentiment in the German medical profession, may more correctly be seen as an indicator of the failure of Nazi physicians' influence in the DÄVB.

Let us finally review our considerations of how the dynamics of professionalization and the specifics of the German environment for professionals interacted, especially in view of the relationship of the medical profession to Nazism.

I have argued that German medicine was indeed highly professionalized by the end of the Hohenzollern empire, with a number of important qualifications. Less than in some countries, the monopoly status of German physicians as dominators of the market in health services was only uncertainly protected. Strong competition and specialization were other signs that the medical profession was far from unified in solidarity. A state-mandated medical insurance system disrupted the traditional doctor-patient relationship even as it brought expanded, if not usually highly lucrative, practice.

Yet the path chosen by the medical profession to strengthen its position – including ever-higher educational and certification requirements – was effective in many ways, if not as arbitrary and immediate as the imposition of a *numerus clausus*. The effective resistance of the Hartmann League and its ally, the DÄVB, to encroachments by sickness funds in 1913 showed the power of professional solidarity, and repeated "doctors' strikes" in the 1920s also made an impact.

13 Comité des délégations juives, ed., *Das Schwarzbuch: Tatsachen und Dokumente: Die Lage der Juden in Deutschland* (Paris, 1934), 81, 84. Jews comprised 27 percent of the Prussian attorneys and about 15 percent of the dentists. By contrast, the percentage of Jews in the higher civil service in all Germany was less than 0.3 percent.

Had Germany not frittered away much of its newfound prosperity and political stability in World War I, one could easily imagine a continuing expansion of the medical profession (which occurred anyway) along with the maintenance of satisfactory professional working conditions (which did not happen). The disruptions of the war and the socioeconomic turmoil of the early and late phases of the Weimar Republic, however, exacerbated the real and perceived problems of the German medical profession. Especially the younger aspirants witnessed a trend toward proletarianization of their incomes, insecurity in their practice, increasing competition, and even the crumbling of the medical insurance system, all worse in 1932 than ten years earlier. Despite these threats to professional status, despite what some have termed "deprofessionalization," doctors, not even young ones, in Germany then or since then have seldom considered the option of changing careers. Far more, if not a majority, appeared to prefer to change the "system."

The last Weimar governments attempted feebly to relieve some of the crisis phenomena by facilitating admission of panel practitioners who had been waiting years, but this typical effort merely reduced the number of patients (and thereby fees) per physician. The Nazi government, starting in 1933, pursued its typical carrot-and-stick tactic of dissolving autonomous professional organizations (such as the DÄVB and Hartmann League) and replacing them with brown ones, while simultaneously offering the appearance of long-standing concessions, as with the creation of the *Kassenäzteliche Vereinigung* to assure smoother relations between sickness funds and panel physicians, the *Reichsärztekammer* and the *Reichsärzteordnung* (hollow concessions, as it turned out). Despite reduction of competition, by throttling medical enrollments, purging Jewish and leftist physicians, and so forth, any promises of "normalization" and reprofessionalization that National Socialism dangled before the German medical profession in the early 1930s were later made a mockery by the most serious assault on professional standards seen in modern times, accelerating through the peacetime years and intensifying during World War II.[14]

These crisis phenomena have been cited for clues to the undoubtedly high rate of membership by doctors in Nazi organizations *after* January 1933. Low

---

14 The introduction of the *Reichsärzteordnung* (Physicians' Ordinance) and a *Reichsärztekammer* (Reich Physicians' Chamber) in 1935 and 1936, respectively, delivered the token but not the substance of reforms German doctors had been requesting for decades. Like most other National Socialist legislation on the professions, both these measures reduced rather than enhanced physicians' autonomy. The chief objective "gain" in the mid-1930s, partly because of the purges to eliminate leftist and Jewish physicians from competition and partly by raiding the health-insurance funds, was a certain increase in doctors' average incomes. These rose from a low of RM 9,300 in 1933 to RM 15,000 by 1938, incidentally making doctors the best-paid professional group for the first time in history. See Walter Wuttke-Gronberg, ed., *Medizin im Nationalsozialismus* (Tübingen, 1980), 347.

rates of participation *before* that date, the relative lack of success of the NSDÄB, and the autonomy to the bitter end of the DÄVB provide evidence sustaining the interpretation that many doctors (like even more civil servants) opportunistically shifted their bets.[15] (Just as many did again in 1945.) The goal still presumably remained the growth of their professional autonomy, power, income, and status – just as it did after 1945 again.

The professionalization stories of other groups, from attorneys (the learned profession with the highest percentage of Jews) to schoolteachers, vary in detail, but not in dramatic substance.[16] Whereas the Nazis' League of National Socialist Jurists had been able to attract only a meager 1,500 lawyers to the end of 1932, it found another 78,500 members the year following January 30.[17] Purges, restrictions on admission, the Nazi takeover under the disguise of a new national lawyers' code and national lawyers' chamber also improved the economic lot of the remaining (and far fewer) attorneys, but only until the beginning of the war.[18]

Perhaps what we can hypothesize from the history of modern professionalization is that highly organized and well-educated professionals behave in roughly similar ways in the face of overweening social and political crises. These include attempts to improve their own position – *den Stand zu heben* – and rarely include a component of "civic courage." Opportunism and, at best, resignation in the face of force majeur has been more the rule than the exception with all major professional groups in societies taken over by dictatorships of whatever ideology.

German doctors did not behave differently from lawyers, professors, engineers, chemists, schoolteachers, or other "professionals." The statistical variant that is obvious – more German doctors joined the National Socialist Party or its organizations after 1933 than other professional groups – is interesting only if one holds medical professionals to a higher standard of moral responsibility than other professionals. Even if one makes this assumption, one must look carefully at motives and conflicted aims. (It is not, for example,

15 Civil servants, who had not joined the NSDAP in any higher percentage than was found in the general population through 1932, made up 81 percent of the new members joining between Jan. 30 and May 1, 1933. See McClelland, *Experience*, 221.
16 See in particular the complicated account in Konrad H. Jarausch, *The Unfree Professions: German Lawyers, Teachers and Engineers, 1900-1950* (New York, 1990), chap. 6: "The Illusion of Reprofessionalization." Although admitting that opportunism, economic motives, and resignation played major roles in the lack of loud resistance to totalitarian regimes in Europe (including bolshevik and fascist ones), Jarausch nevertheless insists on locating the root of the corrosion of German professionalism in the turn away from nineteenth-century liberal values (*The Unfree Professions*, 226–7), a reductive fallacy based on the semantic identification of modern "professions" with "free" or "liberal" occupations.
17 Bernd Wunder, *Geschichte der Bürokratie in Deutschland* (Frankfurt/Main, 1986), 140.
18 McClelland, *Experience*, 223.

fashionable today to point out that the Hippocratic Oath forbids abortion or that Nazi medical directives at least partly upheld this aspect of the doctors' supposed creed.) Enthusiasm for a greater state-sanctioned medical control over society was not necessarily "Nazi," unless one wants anachronistically to color Rudolf Virchow and other nineteenth-century medical "liberals" brown. Given the lavish Nazi promises to "reprofessionalize" medicine, offered by no other political party in such unqualified sweep, one might almost be surprised how *few* M.D.s snapped at the lure in 1933 and subsequent years.

One can easily read the recent literature on university professors of history and other fields[19] to find a certain "continuity of values" spanning at least the years from 1910 through 1960, and beyond. According to this literature, German professors did not *need* to join the NSDAP because they were already halfway in it, mentally. If this reasoning holds up, why did doctors egregiously rush to the swastika flag in such numbers?

The NSDAP had reasons for wanting to recruit medical doctors to its ranks that simply transcended its reasons for wanting lawyers, professors, teachers, and other professionals. These reasons went along with the Nazis' desire to recruit engineers, while also subverting any vestigial sense of professional independence on their part. Jeffrey Herf has given a label to this: reactionary modernism.[20] As Michael Kater and others have argued, public *Gesundheitspflege* was to be transformed into *Volksgesundheitspflege* with a brown stamp.

Yet it does not mean that concern about the "national health" or right-wing ideas before 1933 automatically made M.D.s more susceptible to specifically Nazi ideas. A close reading of the publications of Rudolf Virchow, an unimpeachably "liberal" leader and influence in German and world medicine in the second half of the nineteenth century and beyond, clearly indicates an acceptance of an etatist, interventionist philosophy of care "for the people." It is by no means clear to this researcher how many of the M.D.s who joined the NSDAP or its organizations might have seen the *promise* of the self-styled "Government of German Renewal" of 1933 as one that gave a green light to Virchow's frustrated demands for a "national health policy" beyond Bismarck's social insurance system.

We cannot imagine what German doctors thought in 1932 without also looking at what American, British, French, and Polish doctors also accepted

---

19 Karen Schönwälder, *Historiker und Politik: Geschichtswissenschaft im Nationalsozialismus* (Frankfurt/Main, 1992); and Helmut Heiber, *Universität unterm Hakenkreuz* (Munich, 1991–).
20 Jeffrey Herf, *Reactionary Modernism: Technology, Culture and Politics in Weimar and the Third Reich* (Cambridge, 1984).

as "up-to-date" and "scientifically founded" orthodoxy. This orthodoxy included eugenics, euthanasia, sterilization, and experimentation on human subjects without much regard to their "consent." One of the reasons so few German doctors were put on trial in Nuremberg (let alone thousands of others who perhaps should have been in the dock) was a lack of consensus among the Allies' advisors about what the minimal standards of medical ethics really were.

To return to Michael Kater's charge, which has thankfully provoked this essay, it seems to me dubious if German doctors were especially badly socialized and professionalized. If we wish to understand why so many doctors (a statistically obvious variant among the professions) joined the NSDAP, we might as well ask why so many of them cooled to it, even before the onset of World War II and the Holocaust. We might as well also ask why, in a world dominated by "experts," as today, doctors feel utterly frustrated in their "profession" – why they feel blocked from doing what they were trained and sworn to do, to preserve and improve human life.

Maintaining the profession at a high moral cost has also been defended under other dictatorships with the classic argument of "preventing worse" or, in the case of the medical profession, combating the deterioration of the national health in the wake of deprofessionalization.

Two world wars and Hitler did more to undermine Germany's national health than any imaginable plague. In the light of post-1945 experience, the German medical profession (and not it alone) appears to have absorbed the lesson that war and racism are not "healthy." The fact that the German medical profession survived Nazism and went on to adapt again to world standards of health care for the "clientele" is often ruled out as evidence about "Nazi medicine." All statements about professions, however, must be placed on a chronological continuum. It is just as valid today to ask the uncomfortable question "Why were GDR judges unacceptable to West German lawyers and politicians?" as to ask "Why did the Allies accuse so few German physicians in the trials at Nuremberg?"

We must also not restrict our field of inquiry solely to German doctors. A "professionalization crisis" and an "illiberal" backlash is also easy to find in other Continental countries not yet dominated by Hitler Germany. The history of Hungarian doctors and lawyers presents a sad but accurate mirror image of German events, even though the Hungarian dictator Horthy personally (and with some public and even professional backing) resisted the Nazi Holocaust.[21]

---

21 See Maria Kovács, *The Politics of the Legal Profession in Interwar Hungary* (New York, 1987); Victor Karady, "Antisémitisme universitaire et concourrence de classe: La loi de numerus clausus en

The answers we get from the history of professions will depend on the questions we ask. If we ask if German M.D.s were especially susceptible to Nazi allures, the answer is yes. If we could ask the same questions, under the same historical circumstances, of M.D.s elsewhere, the answer might be more alarming and often positive. (The anti-Semitism of American doctors in the face of pre-Holocaust European refugees is now a sad but little-publicized fact.) If we ask whether German doctors were attracted to the NSDAP because of their socialization and professionalization, the answer is not so clear. An authoritarian political regime and historical tradition is not entirely necessary to explain authoritarian and haughty thinking in doctors (leave alone other professions).

The history of professionalization can and should raise questions about the gap between ideals and realities in the minds of professionals. This gap has always yawned. It has become more and more gaping as professionals organize in highly sectoralized modern societies. If the altruistic ethos claimed by most modern professions may seem weak compared to self-serving rhetoric, anxiety about survival, fears of competition, and opportunism, it is nevertheless an ethos, the obligation that binds expert to client and justifies professional privilege. The special difficulties and threats to the German medical profession were both real and perceived under the Weimar Republic. With the political eclipse of traditional "middle class" political parties under the weight of the Depression, coupled with the opportunistic targeting of professional groups by the NSDAP, it is not hard to understand the way a professionalization crisis could translate into a sense of having no serious political options.

The history of German medicine in the twentieth century shows us the consequences of interrupted professionalization. It does not deliver us the paradigmatic example of evil consequences of professionalization as such, which so many historians of German professions are inclined to seek out. There are enough evil consequences of professionalization, just as there are those of industrialization and the "iron cage" described by Max Weber. Examining the interrupted professionalization of German doctors in an international and comparative framework may help us better to understand the fragility of the "professionalizing project" and the dangers posed to professional autonomy by the powerful forces of modern societies. The temptation to secure elusive aims of the profession by resorting to authoritarian rule – because democratic, parliamentary government seemed unable to meet

Hongrie d'ancien régime," *Actes de la recherche en sciences sociales* 34 (1980); and the essays by both authors in Charles E. McClelland, Stephan Merl, and Hannes Siegrist, eds., *Professions in Modern Eastern Central Europe* (Berlin, 1995).

those aims – was strong in many European countries in 1933. The falseness of the NSDAP's reprofessionalization promises only became apparent when it was too late to climb down from the tiger's back. That experience, in turn, must go a long way toward explaining the relatively successful alliance between professions and parliamentary democracy after 1945.

5

The Mentally Ill Patient Caught between the State's Demands and the Professional Interests of Psychiatrists

HEINZ–PETER SCHMIEDEBACH

In comparison to other natural and medical sciences, German psychiatry in the nineteenth century was characterized by its particularly close relationship to the state and society, its late establishment as an academic discipline, and its precarious relationship to the principles of scientific methods. In 1805 Prussia agreed to reform the system of caring for the mentally ill along the lines suggested by Johann Gottfried Langermann (1768–1832).[1] With this decision, the largest and most important German state accepted responsibility for this group of people. In contrast to other medical disciplines, psychiatry had to respond to special pressures from interest groups as well: the attempt by doctors interested in psychiatry to establish a new discipline and to receive the full recognition of their medical colleagues; the state's demands to get the mentally ill off the streets, perhaps forcing them to work and thereby making them productive members of society; and last but not least, the interests of the patients and asylum inmates, interests that unfortunately counted little.

To trace and understand the development of psychiatry in Germany, the historian must inquire into the forces behind these interactions, as they played themselves out within this field of varied interests. The changing role of psychiatrists and the newly emerging tasks of psychiatry were, and are, related to the social construction of what is called "mental illness." Mental illness can best be described as an interpretation of social behavior by means of pathological terms derived from medical concepts, in other words, as a transformation of social abnormality into pathological normalcy.

Defining "mental illness" inevitably involves making value judgments about individual behavior with regard to social rules of society and applying

* I would like to thank Rebecca Ripple and Paul Lerner for their suggestions.

1 For information on Langermann and his concept, see Hans Laehr, "Johann Gottfried Langermann (1768-1832)," in Theodor Kirchhoff, ed., *Deutsche Irrenärzte: Einzelbilder ihres Lebens und Wirkens* (Berlin, 1921), 1:42–51. Klaus Dörner, *Bürger und Irre: Zur Sozialgeschichte und Wissenschaftssoziologie der Psychiatrie* (Frankfurt/Main, 1969), 275–9.

medical concepts to social phenomena. Although all diseases are to some extent socially constructed, nowhere is this clearer than in the case of mental illness. The medical concepts of mental illness developed by the academic physicians since the early nineteenth century emerged within a framework of conflicting interests pursued by psychiatrists, on the one hand, and by society and the state, on the other hand. Psychiatrists were slowly attaining the recognition they sought and expanding their professional competence concerning social issues. Meanwhile, society and the state searched for an authority with academic legitimation, one that could work with patients according to the principles of a modern society that was based on a division of labor and services. This meant that every kind of medical, social, and juridical contact with mentally ill people should avoid any trace of arbitrariness and unrestrained brutality. In this field of interwoven interests, psychiatrists gained room to define various tasks by referring to the wishes and expectations of society and the state. Perhaps it is fair to say that psychiatrists and the state were the two parties involved in negotiations in which the patient was the subject about which they were negotiating. Late in the nineteenth century, we find an attempt of the patients to enter into these discussions themselves and to have their needs taken into account. The growth of an anti-psychiatric movement is clear evidence of their efforts.

The emergence of this movement was to a large extent due to new regulations of the 1890s that concerned when and how individuals were to be committed to an asylum.[2] These reforms produced two results. First, the mental health care system was made more uniform. The division between the urban community responsible for poor, mentally ill residents and the county boards was abolished. As a result of this measure, the state gained better control and therefore had more power over the mentally ill patient. Second, police and administrative authorities became the crucial institutions with the right to make decisions about mental illness and internment.

In 1892, 111 people, including members of the aristocracy, the scientific community, elected representative assemblies, the print media, the church, and the legal system published an announcement demanding a uniform law concerning the mental health care system.[3] This law was intended to guarantee individual rights of freedom and establish a control of the asylums by laymen. During the next fifteen years the movement founded some

---

2 See Dirk Blasius, *Der verwaltete Wahnsinn: Eine Sozialgeschichte des Irrenhauses* (Frankfurt/Main, 1980), 93–7.
3 For an international comparative survey of the laws and a recent history of legislation, see Ernst Rittershaus, *Die Irrengesetzgebung in Deutschland nebst einer vergleichenden Darstellung des Irrenwesens in Europa* (Berlin, 1927), 4–115.

organizations, such as the *Bund für Irrenrechtsreform* (Federation for the reform of laws concerning the mentally ill) and published their own journals. Most of the members belonged to the liberal bourgeoisie; only a few doctors and psychiatrists joined the movement.

Forced by the spirit of the 1918–19 revolution, the *Bund für Irrenrechtsreform* struggled in the following period to obtain the freedom of inmates thought to be victims of the old regime, which had stigmatized them as "mentally ill querulous persons."[4] Despite the fact that some members of the newly established parliament supported the aims of the movement and wanted to use the ideas of the federation for the intended draft of a new law, the movement failed and disappeared during the second half of the 1920s. The result was due to the reluctance of psychiatrists and the refusal of some German states to relinquish an area of their competence and to collaborate with the central government in agreeing on a uniform mental health law.[5] But the activities of these organized laypersons and patients provoked a discussion about the individual rights of inmates and the practice of internment. This discussion yielded approximately 170 publications, which forced psychiatrists to come to terms with these important issues.[6]

In this chapter, I trace the history of psychiatry from the beginning of the nineteenth century to the end of the Weimar Republic. During this period psychiatrists attempted to attain the recognition they wanted as a fully acknowledged medical discipline. Thus medicine, in general, was fast becoming the most important academic discipline, charged with the task of evaluating social behavior on the basis of a scientific legitimacy.

At the beginning of the nineteenth century, psychiatry was outlined as a distinct medical discipline by Johann Christian Reil (1759–1813).[7] From this point forward, it took almost one hundred years for psychiatry to become fully recognized as a medical discipline and fully established within the curriculum of a university medical education.

Despite the fact that psychiatry eventually succeeded in becoming integrated into the medical scientific society, the newly established discipline

4 See anon., "Revolution im Irrenwesen," *Die Irrenrechts-Reform: Zeitschrift des Bundes für Irrenrecht und Irrenfürsorge* 11 (1919): 160–3.
5 For more information on the so-called antipsychiatric movement, see Gabriele Feger, "Die Geschichte des 'Psychiatrischen Vereins zu Berlin' 1889–1920," Med. diss., Freie Universität Berlin, 1982, 220–47. Blasius, *Der verwaltete Wahnsinn*, 124–42. Andreas Dahm, "Zum Phänomen der Antipsychiatrie seit dem 19. Jahrhundert," Med. diss., Universität Bonn, 1983.
6 The number 170 was given by one of the psychiatrists who sought to analyze this movement; see Bernhard Beyer, *Die Bestrebungen zur Reform des Irrenwesens: Material zu einem Reichsirrengesetz: Für Laien und Ärzte* (Halle, 1912), 649–59.
7 See Johann Christian Reil, *Rhapsodieen über die Anwendung der psychischen Curmethode auf Geisteszerrüttungen* (Halle, 1803), 478–80.

differed from other medical disciplines in two important ways. First, in the early asylums founded at the beginning of the nineteenth century, about one third of the inmates consisted of patients suffering from chronic mental disturbances. These patients had already had a long period of hospitalization and had virtually no chance of being rehabilitated. Instead of providing a process of healing and thus performing the "natural" and original task of physicians, psychiatrists were confronted with the question of what they should do with this large number of patients. This unique task set psychiatrists apart from the majority of physicians. This problem of chronic, or so-called incurable, inmates provided a social challenge. At the end of the century, important groups of politicians and psychiatrists began to look increasingly at the cost of caring for these incurable inmates. They also began to consider the worth of these human beings in a rational, economic sense. Their work led to the creation of a professional attitude that regarded the money invested into the mental health care system as an unnecessary expense, an expense that should be reduced to the disadvantage of the incurable inmates.

Second, some asylum inmates were regarded as dangerous to themselves and to society. The security interests and fears of the general public, especially at the end of the nineteenth century, were closely connected to the institutions of psychiatry. Providing for public health and combating epidemic diseases were among the traditional tasks performed by physicians. But the demands of providing public security cast psychiatrists in a role akin to that of prison guards. A considerable number of psychiatrists – making efforts to demonstrate evidence of the social usefulness of their discipline – were ready to accept this challenge, especially when failures concerning the scientific explanation and treatment of mental illness could not yet be overlooked. But by accepting this role, the psychiatrists became part of a security system, and the patient was pushed to be a foe of society, comparable to a thief or a murderer.

It is important to consider the historical context when tracing the development of psychiatry during the nineteenth century. I want to emphasize three main issues. First, during the first half of the nineteenth century, some vastly different concepts of mental illness and its treatment stood in opposition to each another. Second, the integration of psychiatry into scientific medicine was accompanied by a new concept of asylum organization and treatment. It was also characterized by both an extraordinary optimism concerning future psychiatric-scientific findings and the demands of equating the mentally ill person with the somatically ill patient. Third, the jeopardizing of this hopeful and optimistic progress at the end of the century compelled psychiatrists to delineate new tasks, while at the same time social Darwinism was integrated into psychiatry. Another important consideration was the overall cost of the growing number of asylum inmates. The emergence of this financial problem was connected to the fundamental questioning of the social worth of the human beings who suffered from chronic mental illness and who were regarded as unable to contribute to the social and economic welfare of society. It is obvious how psychiatry and psychiatrists were tied up in a network of different discourses dealing with such dissimilar issues as medical research techniques and the social worth of human beings.

In this context the following questions are important: What were the aims of psychiatric activity concerning both the mentally ill individual and the organization of asylums? Which steps were taken toward integration into university medicine and how did psychiatrists strive to overcome any difficulties that arose? Which new fields of psychiatric activity were defined in order to enlarge professional competence? What were the changing connotations of the label "mental illness"?

EDUCATIONAL CONCEPTS OF SELF–DISCIPLINE AND THE ROLE OF PUBLIC ASYLUMS

Based on the acknowledgment of the state's obligation to provide for mentally ill patients, the first half of the nineteenth century witnessed a wave of asylum building, financed by the various German states. The foundation of such institutions was linked to the states' expectation of increasing the number of inmates able to work or to live in society. At this time, medical views of mental illness were strongly influenced by contemporary philosophical currents.

As Otto M. Marx has pointed out, early nineteenth-century German psychiatry is typically presented as a dispute between those who saw the origins of mental illness in the mind – the mentalists or psychicists – and those who interpreted it in purely biological terms – the somaticists.[8] But this simple notion applies to only one aspect of a complicated admixture of psychiatric contexts. Klaus Dörner has emphasized that the psychicists were concerned with issues of ethics, law, and morality in society, especially when

8 Otto M. Marx, "German Romantic Psychiatry, Part 1," *History of Psychiatry* 1 (1990): 351; and Otto M. Marx, "German Romantic Psychiatry, Part 2," *History of Psychiatry* 2 (1991): 1–25. Marx points out that this simple notion applies only to the contest between the early representatives of the period, J. C. A. Heinroth and Maximilian Jacobi. For a survey about the German psychiatry in the first half of the nineteenth century and its roots, see Udo Benzenhöfer, *Psychiatrie und Anthropologie in der ersten Hälfte des 19. Jahrhunderts* (Hürtgenwald, 1993).

they stressed the questions of the insanity defense and the role of forensic psychiatry. As members of university faculties, they felt obliged, as civil servants, to devote their efforts to serving the conservative state. Accordingly, they considered the connection between mental disorders and the ethical and moral conditions needed to stabilize a functioning conservative state. With moral and educational concepts, they aimed to create diligent, pious, and obedient subjects. Thus, psychicists provided psychiatry with a "sociological approach," certainly along conservative lines.[9]

Some of the so-called mentalists attempted to base psychiatry on psychology, as an independent field without a physical basis.[10] One of the representatives of this group, Carl Wilhelm Ideler (1795-1860), who received the first special appointment (*Extraordinariat*) for psychiatry at the Berlin medical faculty in 1839, was a leading figure in that field.[11] In his scientific work, he tried to embrace the anthropological dualism between instincts (*Triebe*) – which were the natural power of the mind – and a morally or ethically based self-control or self-discipline (*Selbstbeherrschung*).[12] This self-discipline prevented the instincts from becoming passions. In a harmonious and balanced state of mind, the individual attained circumspection (*Besonnenheit*), which provided a high level of moral and ethical freedom. But if mental discipline became disturbed, instincts could transform into passions, which would then dominate the mind and infect the soul. The individual, by losing his self-confinement and self-consciousness, would thus become mad. Only by applying bodily restraint and coercive means could the passion be subdued and the patient's circumspection be restored.

Carl Wilhelm Ideler developed a psychiatric scheme grounded in psychology and anthropology with an inherent moral and ethical code; it was to be applicable to all persons as well as all social, political, and religious institutions.[13] Ideler used this scheme on individuals as well as on the public, which gave his scientific reflections a strong political subtext. When he stated that the mad individual tends to destroy social order and act as if he were freed from all social rules – a behavior Ideler considered typical of revolutionaries – he depicted a horrible political scenario that evoked the anxieties shared by all conservative groups.[14] Based on his psychiatry, he drew a paral-

---

9   Klaus Dörner, *Bürger und Irre*, 318–43.
10 Ibid., 324–5.
11 On Ideler, see ibid., 326-34. See also Gesa Wunderlich, *Krankheits- und Therapiekonzepte am Anfang der deutschen Psychiatrie (Haindorf, Heinroth, Ideler)* (Husum, 1981), 57–81.
12 Carl Wilhelm Ideler, *Grundriss der Seelenheilkunde* (Berlin, 1835), 1:238.
13 Carl Wilhem Ideler, "Über das Verhältniss der Seelenheilkunde zu ihren Hülfswissenschaften," *Allgemeine Zeitschrift für Psychiatrie* 3 (1846): 399–401.
14 Carl Wilhelm Ideler, *Grundriss der Seelenheilkunde* (Berlin, 1838), 2:248, 205.

lel between the unfolding of society's liberal economic and social forces and the unrestrained passions of the individual.[15]

The somaticists were more varied and included directors of asylums, forensic physicians, and university professors interested in psychiatric issues. They attempted to diminish religious-ethical speculation and to establish psychiatry on an exact scientific somatological foundation. Despite the fact that some of them were sympathetic to liberalism, they cannot be regarded as a unified group of liberal progressives. Some of them, such as Christian Friedrich Wilhelm Roller (1802–78), who founded the public asylum at Illenau in 1842, were politically conservative.[16] But convinced of the somatic basis of mental illness, they stopped seeking moral guilt or innocence in the mentally disturbed patient; instead of making moral assessments, they superseded these judgments by performing only "help and compassion." Driven by a patriarchal philanthropism, they sought treatments that were as mild as possible, treatments that consisted of both mental guidance and medical assistance.

The acceptance of the mentally ill person and his alienating behavior was certainly augmented by doctors with a somatic orientation. Clinical observation of the patient's behavior – sometimes combined with the postmortem assessment of the pathological alteration of brain and nerve tissue – became a more common method of obtaining information about the material basis of mental illness. The directors of the newly founded asylums tended to consider themselves benevolent rulers of their own little realm. They tried to construct a social entity that was ruled by the psychiatrist who acted much like a good monarch. They saw themselves as considerate pater familias who lived within the asylum in close contact with "their" patients, sharing leisure-time activities, excursions, and other amenities with the patients. Paradoxically, this was an obvious attempt to create a small intact world of insanity within a changing and challenging social environment and in a civilization that was said to cause mental illness by its accelerated rhythm of life and by the tremendous demands of the modern world. Legitimized by their philanthropism, some directors used or abused the inmates to build up a walled-in retreat and to repulse the influences of modern society, particularly the negative consequences of industrialization and urbanization. Both groups' efforts led to the creation of obedient patients – the psychicists through moral and ethical conditioning and the somaticists by means of paternalistic philanthropism.

15 See Dörner, *Bürger und Irre*, 327–8.
16 On Roller and his asylum, see Clemens Beck, "Die Geschichte der 'Heil- und Pflegeanstalt Illenau' unter Chr. Fr. W. Roller (1802–1878)," Med. diss., Universität Freiburg, 1984.

INTEGRATION INTO SCIENCE AND JURIDICAL CHALLENGES

It is important to take note of this kind of appropriation of the asylums by the directors in order to understand the vehement rejection of Wilhelm Griesinger's (1817–68) reform proposals of the 1860s.[17] In 1865 Griesinger was appointed to the newly created chair of psychiatry at the University of Berlin. His idea of an integrated system of asylums was regarded as a threat because he seemed bent on destroying the intact little world of the patriarchal director. Some might have seen an expropriation of the social and daily environment in which they were rooted.[18] Griesinger subdivided the mentally ill patients according to the duration of their illness and differentiated between chronically and acutely ill patients. He claimed there should be two kinds of asylums: the urban asylums for the acutely ill and the rural asylums for the chronically ill patients. In the case of a change in status, a patient was discharged from one institution and handed over to the other.[19] Thus, it was no longer considered a necessity that the director should live within the asylum.

Griesinger's differentiation between chronic and acute patients superseded the old, traditional separation into curable and noncurable patients. By doing so his picture of the mentally ill person was closer to that of the somatic patient. According to Dörner, Griesinger was the first German psychiatrist to formulate a complete paradigm of psychiatry as an academic discipline.[20] With his phrase "mental illness is rooted in a failure of the brain," Griesinger clearly linked the somatic approach to other medical science disciplines. He drew scholarly attention not only to anatomical ideas but also to physiological and psychological ones[21] and to the social environment needed to assess the mental disturbance.[22] This branch of brain psychiatry, introduced by

17 Recent biographies on Griesinger include Bettina Wahrig-Schmidt, *Der junge Griesinger im Spannungsfeld zwischen Philosophie und Physiologie: Anmerkungen zu den philosophischen Wurzeln seiner frühen Psychiatrie* (Tübingen, 1985); Ulf Jacobsen, "Wissenschaftsbegriff und Menschenbild bei Wilhem Griesinger: Ein Beitrag zur Geschichte des ärztlichen Selbstverständnisses im 19. Jahrhundert," Med. diss., Universität Heidelberg, 1986; Bettina Wahrig-Schmidt, "Wilhelm Griesinger (1817–1868)," in Dietrich von Engelhardt and Fritz Hartmann, eds., *Klassiker der Medizin* (Munich, 1991), 2:172–89; see also Alexander Mette, *Wilhelm Griesinger*, Biographien hervorragender Naturwissenschaftler, Techniker und Mediziner, vol. 26 (Leipzig, 1976).

18 See Heinz-Peter Schmiedebach, "Wilhelm Griesinger," in Wilhelm Treue and Rolf Winau, eds., *Berlinische Lebensbilder: Mediziner*, Einzelveröffentlichungen der Historischen Kommission zu Berlin, vol. 60 (Berlin, 1987), 129.

19 Wilhelm Griesinger, *Gesammelte Abhandlungen: Psychiatrische und nervenpathologische Abhandlungen* (Berlin, 1872), 1:294–304.

20 See Klaus Dörner, *Bürger und Irre*, 378.

21 Wilhelm Griesinger, "Über psychische Reflexaktionen: Mit einem Blick auf das Wesen der psychischen Krankheiten," *Archiv für physiologische Heilkunde* 2 (1843): 76–113. Wilhelm Griesinger, "Neue Beiträge zur Physiologie und Pathologie des Gehirns," *Archiv für physiologische Heilkunde* 3 (1844): 69–98.

22 See Martin Schrenk, "Griesingers neuropsychiatrische Thesen und ihre sozialpsychiatrischen Konsequenzen," *Nervenarzt* 39 (1968): 441–50.

Griesinger, became an important field of psychiatric research during the last quarter of the nineteenth century and paved the way for the growth of neurological research. Outstanding academics belonging to this field include Theodor Meynert (1833–92) and Carl Wernicke (1848–1905), who distinguished the various forms of aphasia.

At the same time, Griesinger demanded human rights for the mentally ill, which meant equating those patients with the somatically ill,[23] performing therapy without the use of physical restraints or brutality, and avoiding moral and religious attitudes in therapy.[24] Griesinger's psychiatry was influenced by John Conolly (1794–1866), who introduced the idea of a nonrestraint system, originally proposed by Robert Gardiner Hill (1811–78). Griesinger made great strides in integrating the new discipline of psychiatry into the existing curriculum of scientific medicine. Griesinger's approach already reflected economic considerations, an issue that was increasing in importance at the end of the nineteenth century. Griesinger complained about the high costs of the construction of new asylum buildings and wanted patients to work for two reasons. First, work was a good antidote to idleness, which was thought to lead directly to mental deterioration. Thus, work activity produced a preventative and therapeutical effect. Second, Griesinger recognized the possibility of recovering a portion of the costs needed for running asylums by letting the inmates work. He also quantified the working abilities of the mentally ill and estimated their capacities to be as high as a fifth of the working capacity of a healthy individual.[25]

Griesinger's endeavor to integrate psychiatry as a scientifically based medical discipline into the medical curriculum was now legitimized by the authority of science. This attempt to enlarge their competence concerned forensic medicine, civil law, and penal law. Beginning in 1867, some psychiatric societies engaged the problem of life insurance. Many insurance companies refused to pay benefits to the bereaved family in cases of suicide. In 1868 the Society of German Psychiatrists (*Verein deutscher Irrenärzte*) wrote sixteen insurance companies, claiming that these companies were responsible for all such cases in which a psychiatrist's expertise could have been acquired to show that the policyholder had committed suicide because of proven mental illness. Psychiatrists attempted to link the business of life

---

23 Wilhem Griesinger, *Die Pathologie und Therapie der psychischen Krankheiten*, 2d ed. (Stuttgart, 1861), 470.

24 See Heinz-Peter Schmiedebach, "Mensch, Gehirn und wissenschaftliche Psychiatrie: Zur therapeutischen Vielfalt bei Wilhelm Griesinger," in Johann Glatzel, Steffen Haas, and Hein Schott, eds., *Vom Umgang mit Irren: Beiträge zur Geschichte psychiatrischer Therapeutik* (Regensburg, 1990), 83–105.

25 Wilhelm Griesinger, *Gesammelte Abhandlungen*, 300.

insurance with their professional competence.[26] Apart from this attempt to attain professional influence, psychiatrists exerted themselves to take on new responsibilities in areas that had heretofore been the province of judges. Carl Westphal's effort to evaluate homosexual behavior within a medical and psychiatric framework is one such example. In 1868 Westphal described what he called "contrary sexual perception" (*conträre Sexualempfindung*) as a symptom of a neuropathic state of hereditary genesis, at times linked with other "perverse inclinations." Therefore, this "abnormality" should be discussed in a medical and not in a juridical context.[27] This example clearly demonstrates how the psychiatrists identified socially striking behavior as a product of mental disturbance and transformed it into a normal pathological category.

But psychiatrists went further and inserted opinions into the discussion of penal law reform in the North German Confederation (*Norddeutscher Bund*) during the late 1860s. The debate dealt with the soundness of mind and the freedom of will concerning a punishable offense and insanity as a defense. The psychiatrists intervened, saying that in addition to the paragraph concerning feeblemindedness, there was a need to integrate a new paragraph into the law that would regulate reduced soundness of mind. This provided the necessary differentiation between a real mental illness and other disturbed psychic states.

But the government's advisory commission was quite skeptical and rejected the psychiatrists' proposals. The commission feared that medical expert witnesses could be found who, by neglecting their original task of supporting the law, would protect defendants against the law with reference to what the commission called "alleged medical arguments taken from psychiatry."[28] In the late 1860s, state authorities obviously did not acknowledge psychiatry to be a fully legitimate scientific medical discipline. Psychiatry was labeled an alleged medical discipline that endangered the safety interests of both society and the state.

At the time, important psychiatrists were allied with the liberal part of the bourgeoisie. But by rejecting proposals made by the state's commission, they endangered their professional interests, and thus during the following years, they increasingly aligned themselves with the state's interests.

During the next few years, psychiatry gained new responsibilities and developed a scientific conception of criminal control. Prompted by the

26   Heinz-Peter Schmiedebach, *Psychiatrie und Psychologie im Widerstreit: Die Auseinandersetzung in der Berliner medicinisch-psychologischen Gesellschaft, 1867–1899* (Husum, 1986), 242–3.

27   Carl Westphal, "Die conträre Sexualempfindung, Symptom eines neuropathischen (psychopathischen) Zustandes," *Archiv für Psychiatrie* 2 (1870): 73–108.

28   See Heinz-Peter Schmiedebach, *Psychiatrie und Psychologie*, 68.

writings of Cesare Lombroso (1835–1909), who painted a refined portrait of the natural "born criminal" in the last quarter of the nineteenth century, international debates centered on a reassessment of classical penal codes. Lombroso, who worked as a professor of psychiatry in Pavia and Turin, claimed to have identified significant anatomical and physiological characteristics that distinguished the criminal from his or her normal counterpart.[29] With this delineation of the "criminal type," which he described as an atavistic remnant of an ancestral type, Lombroso sought to construct a scientific system in which diagnostic signs could provide the basis for a preventative model of criminal control: "Once the characteristics of innate criminality were identified, it was possible to know in advance those predestined toward antisocial behavior and eliminate or treat them before they became a danger to society."[30]

Lombroso wanted to provide for the safety of society. He did not investigate crime, but inquired into the mind and body of the criminal. He emphasized somatic signs of a person, which he thought yielded evidence of inborn and hereditary "moral insanity." His concept of "moral insanity" transformed criminal behavior into somatically induced pathological phenomena, the domain of medicine and psychiatry.

Apart from the shift from criminal to pathological content, Lombroso's work embraced two important approaches. First, security of society is one of the highest values that had to be supported by the psychiatrists; second, the thesis of an inborn "inferiority" (*Minderwertigkeit*) of the nervous system and the brain leading to insanity and crime referred to the theory of degeneration, which had previously been elaborated by Benoit-Augustin Morel (1809–73).[31] In this way an alleged breakdown of nervous tissue and/or of the brain was used to explain criminality as well as insanity. Similarly, an unchangeable somatic constitution of individuals seemed to justify social hierarchy and aggressive means, such as castration, to solve social problems.

Lombroso's concept could be used to consider social problems only with regard to individual constitutional patterns. The state and society were liberated from having to bear the responsibility for worsening social conditions. The way to solve social problems, such as crime, alcoholism, and so forth, was strongly related to the individual "pathological" constitution of

29 For more information on Lombroso and the perception of his ideas by German psychiatrists, see Carla Maria Gadebusch Bondio, "Die Rezeption der kriminalanthropologischen Theorien von Cesare Lombroso in Deutschland von 1880–1914," Ph.D. diss., Freie Universität Berlin, 1994, 100–91, 239–371. Daniel Pick, *Faces of Degeneration: A European Disorder c. 1848 to c. 1918* (New York, 1989).
30 Ruth Harris, *Murders and Madness: Medicine, Law, and Society in the 'fin de siècle'* (Oxford, 1991), 81.
31 For more information on Morel's theory, see ibid., 51–6.

the socially and politically conspicuous person. At the end of the nineteenth century, a large number of German psychiatrists discussed Lombroso's theories. Although they did not always accept his notions, many of his basic ideas were integrated into German psychiatric thinking.

PUBLIC HEALTH, RATIONAL DISPOSABILITY OF HUMAN BEINGS, AND WAR

Despite the fact that by no means all psychiatrists agreed with Lombroso's main thesis (atavistic signs as somatic evidence of insanity and criminality), the idea of a social and individual pathology became conceptualized in terms of scientific anthropology and hereditary psychiatry. According to historian Paul Weindling, this reflected the emerging "professionalism of psychiatrists, as well as the growing bourgeois 'angst' of the criminal, disease, and riotous masses."[32] At the end of the nineteenth century, the general ideology that integrated these very different factors was Darwinism, especially social Darwinism.

Weindling's definition of Darwinism embraces the general conviction of the truth of evolution that includes such diverse mechanisms as "Lamarckian" adaptation and psychic factors, such as will and learning powers. "Social Darwinism gave legitimacy to a variety of interests in an expanding industrial society, and cannot be identified as an exclusively right-wing ideology."[33] Additionally, Weindling points out that Darwinism was both a scientific and a social movement. In this way, it boosted the authority of scientific experts who, by the early twentieth century, came to stress the values of hierarchy, order, and historical traditions, thus rejecting the liberal attitudes of the mid-nineteenth century.[34]

Based on this general assessment, Weindling argues persuasively for the differentiation of social Darwinians that includes politicians and literary figures as well as scientists and physicians.[35] Focusing on German psychiatrists, this broad spectrum becomes less differentiated. Darwinism could be used to support theories of mental and physical degeneration, and from the 1880s on, psychiatry began to adopt eugenic theories. But the readiness and the graduation of using social Darwinistic patterns to explain mental illness or to construct eugenic models of coping with behavior of socially abnormal persons was dependent on other attitudes. First, the dimension

---

32 Paul Weindling, *Health, Race and German Politics between National Unification and Nazism, 1870–1945* (Cambridge, 1989), 81.
33 Ibid., 28.
34 Ibid., 40.
35 Ibid., 40–154.

of being afraid of degeneration was a crucial item in this context. Some psychiatrists, such as Adolf Schott (1870–1937), Friedrich Rohde (1857–1919), and prior to World War I, Oswald Bumke (1877–1950), who later joined the eugenic movement, did not support ideas of racial hygiene. They argued against overestimating the degeneration process. Despite the fact that they were influenced by social Darwinistic ideology, they rejected all compulsory eugenic measures.[36] Second, another group of psychiatrists tried to maintain the viewpoint of strict scientificity. This group was divided in two subgroups. The first argued that hereditary components of most of the mental diseases were not yet known. Thus eugenic intervention should not be allowed. The second subgroup pursued a somatic biochemical or pathophysiological approach and tried to explain psychic phenomena by molecular movements or similar models. Most neurologists, who gained organizational autonomy in the first decade of the twentieth century by founding their own organization in 1906, belonged to this group.[37] All of the psychiatrists associated with one group or the other were more or less influenced by Darwinistic or social Darwinistic ideas. Of course, it was possible – dependent on the process of enlarging scientific knowledge – to change one's mind and to associate with another group, so that this differentiation, which is based on psychiatric and medical items not on political opinions, does not give a consistently fixed delineation.

The public health campaigns against degeneration, venereal diseases, and alcoholism – campaigns that were joined and supported by psychiatrists – furthered the idea of prevention. To a great extent, these campaigns were dedicated to the welfare of the society and the nation, if one takes into consideration the costs of caring for the mentally ill as well as the perceived deterioration of national health. Thus the views of physicians and psychiatrists coincided with the politics of Imperial Germany and were an attempt to strengthen national power.

Within the section of neurology and psychiatry of the Society of German Scientists and Physicians, 75 percent of the speakers dealing with degeneration between 1886 and 1913 supported the "racial hygienic movement."[38] They used well-known aggressive and brutal terms, such as "weeding out

36   See Gerd Udo Jerns, "Die neurologisch-psychiatrischen Vorträge in der Abteilung für Neurologie und Psychiatrie der Gesellschaft Deutscher Naturforscher und Ärzte von 1886 bis 1913," Med. diss., Freie Universität Berlin, 1991, 398–9.
37   See ibid., 29–30. For more information on the development of German neurology, see Hans-Heinz Eulner, *Die Entwicklung der medizinischen Spezialfächer an den Universitäten des deutschen Sprachgebietes* (Stuttgart, 1970), 257–82.
38   Jerns, *Die neurologisch-psychiatrischen Vorträge*, 397.

psychopathic persons of inferior value," and integrated those terms into scientific terminology. By propagating castration, prohibiting marriage of the mentally ill, and secluding alcoholics and prostitutes, these psychiatrists attempted to fight the perceived decline of culture. Pretending to support high cultural values, psychiatry went to great lengths to present itself as the defender of the national and social welfare.

Beginning in the 1870s, the number of asylums and the number of inmates increased dramatically. Despite the fact that a similar development occurred in other European countries, the number of inmates in Prussia, by comparison, grew markedly. In 1880 there were 27,000 cases treated in all Prussian asylums; by 1910 the number had increased to 143,000. During the 1890s the transition from public care to governmental control was most evident.[39] This process reflected the changing relationship between state and society during the last quarter of the nineteenth century. The economic crisis of the 1870s revealed the vulnerability of the social and political system in Germany. Governmental administration could aspire to provide for the safety of society and provide the solution to what it labeled the "problem of the mentally ill."

Three governmental prescriptions, those of 1894, 1896, and 1904, displayed the growing interest of the police in the affairs of the mentally ill. In 1894 the state tried to attain control over those patients outside the asylums, many of whom were in the so-called family care system. The government estimated that 50 percent of the total number of mentally ill patients belonged to this noninstitutionalized group.[40] It took steps to bring such individuals into the asylums, thus guaranteeing public safety. The emancipatory and liberal approach of the mid-nineteenth century, which considered the mentally ill individual a human being who should be integrated into society and who should have the same rights as all other citizens, was replaced by a system of control linked to a more pessimistic outlook. Psychiatry submitted to a system of control to which we can also ascribe laws aimed at suppressing the political left, such as the *Sozialistengesetze* (anti-Socialist laws forbidding political activity, 1878–90).

The psychiatrist Emil Kraepelin (1856–1926) gained influence in this changing situation.[41] Like Lombroso, Kraepelin, the first director of the German Research Institute for Psychiatry founded in 1917, considered crime

39 Blasius, *Der verwaltete Wahnsinn*, 94.
40 Ibid., 95.
41 For biographical information on Kraepelin, see Kurt Kolle, "Emil Kraepelin 1856–1926," in Kurt Kolle, ed., *Grosse Nervenärzte*, vol. 1 (Stuttgart, 1956): 175–86; Emil Kraepelin, *Lebenserinnerungen* (Berlin, 1983). On his concept, see Hans-Georg Güse and Norbert Schmacke, *Psychiatrie zwischen bürgerlicher Revolution und Faschismus* (Kronberg, 1976), 101–84.

a social disease.[42] He defined the social consequences for society, not dependence on social environment, as the crucial issue of mental illness. Practical psychiatry, he argued, should focus on the insecurity produced by the mentally ill patient and on the "unlimited misery" in society that could be traced to mental disturbances.[43] Kraepelin was also involved in the German temperance movement and fought against the alleged explanations for degeneration of future generations. His psychiatric work was influenced by the therapeutic pessimism of the late nineteenth and early twentieth centuries. The meager therapeutic results and the insufficient explanations of madness based on material or somatic concepts, inevitably led to the rise of prevention, improvement of society, and neutralization of deviants. According to Eric J. Engstrom, public education and internment of the mentally ill were pushed to the forefront.[44] But Kraepelin did not confine himself to these issues. Apart from focusing on serology – at the University of Munich he established a serological laboratory in 1907 – he created an accessible classification system of mental illnesses, which distinguished between psychoses of exogenous and endogenous origins. In defining this differentiation, he did not refer to pathological, etiological, or symptomatic foundations but rather to perturbations of perception and disturbed functions of the mind, as well as to the whole course of the disease's development. Moreover, Kraepelin defined a new field of psychiatric competence. In doing so he opened the door for the participation of psychiatry in the process of constructing a society based on the rational utilization of human resources.

Kraepelin was concerned with practical aspects of medicine and avoided reflections on illness in a general sense. He stated that illness is a notion of value that, in its general form, does not interest the physician. He wanted to assess concrete situations and to make decisions of practical importance. But being aware of the fact that standards are required for this purpose, he emphasized a notion of illness in a practical sense and defined it as an unacceptable deviation from the norm.[45]

The psychiatrist was supposed to have the responsibility for defining the standards of mental and physical abilities needed for social and professional tasks in society. Only after having defined these standards could the doctors evaluate the whole population with reference to these standards. These

42 See Eric J. Engstrom, "Emil Kraepelin: Psychiatry and Public Affairs in Wilhelmine Germany," *History of Psychiatry* 2 (1991): 111–32.
43 Emil Kraepelin, *Einführung in die psychiatrische Klinik*, 3d ed. (Leipzig, 1916), 3.
44 Engstrom, "Emil Kraepelin," 114.
45 Kraepelin, *Einführung in die psychiatrische Klinik*, 243; see also Emil Kraepelin, "Ziele und Wege der psychiatrischen Forschung," *Zeitschrift für die gesamte Neurologie und Psychiatrie* 38 (1918): 192.

evaluations could, for example, be applied to the following topics: suitability for military services, aptness for school requirements, soundness of mind, and legal capacity. With this new task, the psychiatrist became a crucial control system able to assess the rational sharing of resources of human beings. By making such assessments, the individual would have been deployed with reference to social and industrial efficiency but not according to individual preference.

This tendency to declare that the interests of the general public have a higher value than those of individuals became most obvious during World War I. Wartime conditions also underscored the view that human beings could be considered "material" to be used according to the needs of the nation. In 1872 a military physician clearly described the role of military medicine as "economic administration" of the "most valuable war material," the individual soldier. The physician wrote that "the individual is not to be taken in consideration when the existence of the whole is in question."[46] A large number of physicians shared the viewpoint of reducing human beings to material, even when aspects other than the victorious survival of the "holy whole" were concerned. Especially with regard to what was called "scientific progress," they carelessly legitimized war, which was said to make human scientific material available. In this context, the pathologist Ludwig Aschoff (1866–1942) explicitly stressed the relevance of dissecting fallen soldiers because it could give the broadest possible statistical basis of the somatic constitution of the healthy male portion of the population between twenty and forty years of age.[47] Thus, the war provided scientific material and readied the human body for further medical research.

It is not surprising then that such an attitude influenced the therapeutic relationship between the doctor and the patient. If a patient's individual interests and needs did not count for much, then it would not be possible to establish a respectful and careful intimacy between the doctor and the patient. The war conditions encouraged increased aggressiveness and brutality in the relationship between doctors and patients, often legitimized by the doctors alluding to the extreme war situation and the struggle for survival

---

46 F. Kratz, *Recrutirung und Invalidisirung: Eine militärärztliche Studie* (Erlangen, 1872), 2: "Das Individuum darf nicht berücksichtigt werden, sobald es sich um die Existenz des Ganzen handelt," quoted in Johanna Bleker, "Medizin im Dienste des Krieges – Krieg im Dienste der Medizin: Zur Frage der Kontinuität des ärztlichen Auftrages und ärztlicher Werthaltungen im Angesicht des Krieges," in Johanna Bleker and Heinz-Peter Schmiedebach, eds., *Medizin und Krieg: Vom Dilemma der Heilberufe 1865 bis 1985* (Frankfurt/Main, 1987), 16.

47 See Heinz-Peter Schmiedebach, "Sozialdarwinismus, Biologismus, Pazifismus – Ärztestimmen zum Ersten Weltkrieg," in Bleker and Schmiedebach, eds., *Medizin und Krieg*, 103–4.

that demanded sacrifice from everyone. According to Peter Riedesser and Axel Verderber, the majority of German psychiatrists and neurologists were engaged in the development and application of therapies, absolutely aware of the extremely brutal character of these intrusive measures.[48]

War provided psychiatry with the opportunity to support the widespread national and patriotic aim of victory, and psychiatrists were eager to demonstrate that they were indispensable. Professional interests, the desire to strengthen the discipline, and nationalist convictions were all interrelated.

The transition of values perpetuated by the war not only reduced the worth of a single human being, but also led to a differentiation and selection of human beings into more or less valuable individuals. Only those who were strong enough and able to contribute to the survival of the nation were regarded as valuable. A large number of psychiatrists shared this thinking, which became relevant with regard to the treatment of "war neurosis."[49] The aim of this often violent treatment, as mentioned previously, was to get the soldier back to the front as rapidly as possible. Sigmund Freud described the function of the doctors as something "like machine guns behind the front."[50] Psychiatry integrated itself into the military machinery by submitting completely to the conditions and aims of warfare. By neglecting the interests of the individual patient, psychiatrists supported the process of turning human beings into disposable resources.

The alleged inferiority of mentally ill individuals led to reduced care and rationed food supplies in numerous asylums during the war. According to Igor Weimann, who has studied this topic concerning the public asylums of Saxony, the number of rooms available for the mentally ill persons was also reduced. Especially after 1917 the funds for nutrition were reduced dramatically, while at the same time the facilities that were swept clean of the mentally ill inmates were used to treat injured soldiers coming from the front. Whereas the mentally ill patients suffered from hunger, the military patients received outstandingly large food portions.[51] As a result of this conscious neglect and mistreatment, about 70,000 people died of malnutrition in German asylums between 1914 and 1918.[52] Physicians did not produce this

48 See Peter Riedesser and Axel Verderber, *Aufrüstung der Seelen: Militärpsychologie und Militärpsychiatrie in Deutschland und Amerika* (Freiburg, 1985), 12.

49 See Paul Lerner's chapter on war neurosis in this book.

50 See K. R. Eissler, *Freud und Wagner-Jauregg: Vor der Kommission zur Erhebung militärischer Pflichtverletzungen*, (Vienna, 1979), 53.

51 Igor Weimann, "Die Auswirkungen des ersten Weltkrieges auf die psychiatrische Betreuung in den sächsichen Landes-, Heil- und Pflegeanstalten in der Zeit von 1914 bis zum Beginn der zwanziger Jahre," Med. diss., Universität Leipzig, 1992, 59–62, 72.

52 During World War I, 140,234 inmates died in German asylums. Compared with the average mortality of prewar times, this means a surplus of 71,786 persons. See Hans Ludwig Siemen, *Menschen*

development; the decisions were made by the governments and parliaments of the individual states. But at least in the case of Saxony, nobody, neither the doctors nor the politicians, supported the interests of the helpless asylum inmates.[53]

The very aggressive attitude toward the patients, especially toward soldiers with "war neurosis," was caused by the physicians' interests in unmasking war-shy individuals. The point was to ensure and strengthen the pugnacity of the German army and to serve the aims of the whole. This attitude persisted after the war and was applied to the so-called pension fraud, meaning a patient who tried to obtain a legal, legitimate pension after being injured in a traumatic accident. But one can find these efforts already at the end of the nineteenth century.[54] However, the experience of war, with the inevitable changing of human relations, had an impact on the increasingly aggressive attitude of medical experts. This can be likened to a continuation of fighting after the war had ended. The well-known booklet of Karl Binding and Alfred Hoche on the extermination of lives not worth living continued this aggressive attitude evoked during the war but now disguised as academic reflections.[55]

During the Weimar era, psychiatry was characterized by the following tendencies. The field of theoretical and scientific psychiatry was characterized by multiple psychiatric discourses due to the newly gained freedom that undermined traditional academic forms of thinking. The then recent results of neuroendocrinology were discussed, and some newly developed methods of brain surgery influenced psychiatry. Film, a new medium, was used to

---

blieben auf der Strecke: Psychiatrie zwischen Reform und Nationalsozialismus (Gütersloh, 1987), 29–30; see also Weimann, "Die Auswirkungen," 56–7. Weimann carefully studied the situation in Saxony during the war and points out that between 1914 and 1917 the mortality of the inmates in the asylums reached a fourfold rate, whereas the mortality of the population in Saxony only increased by a factor of 1:2.

53 Weimann, *Die Auswirkungen,* 94–5.

54 See Esther Fischer-Homberger, *Die traumatische Neurose: Vom somatischen zum sozialen Leiden* (Bern, 1975), 56–73; see also Heinz-Peter Schmiedebach, "Die 'Traumatische Neurose' – Soziale Versicherung und der Griff der Psychiatrie nach dem Unfallpatienten," in Susanne Hahn and Achim Thom, eds., *Kolloquium zum 100. Geburtstag von Henry Ernest Siegrist (1891–1957)* (Leipzig, 1991), 154–9.

55 Karl Binding and Alfred Hoche, *Die Freigabe der Vernichtung lebensunwerten Lebens: Ihr Mass und ihre Form* (Leipzig, 1920). For more information on this issue, see Karl Heinz Hafner and Rolf Winau, "'Die Freigabe der Vernichtung lebensunwerten Lebens': Eine Untersuchung zu der Schrift von Karl Binding und Alfred Hoche," *Medizinhistorisches Journal* 9 (1974): 227–54. Gerhard Baader, "Die Medizin im Nationalsozialismus: Ihre Wurzeln und die erste Periode ihrer Realisierung, 1933–1938," in Christian Pross and Rolf Winau, eds., *"nicht misshandeln": Das Krankenhaus Moabit, 1920–1933: Ein Zentrum jüdischer Ärzte in Berlin: 1933–1945 Verfolgung, Widerstand, Zerstörung* (Berlin, 1984), 79–81. Hans-Walter Schmuhl, *Rassenhygiene, Nationalsozialismus, Euthanasie* (Göttingen, 1987), 115–25. Rolf Winau, "Die Freigabe der Vernichtung 'lebensunwerten Lebens,'" in Johanna Bleker and Norbert Jachertz, eds., *Medizin im "Dritten Reich,"* 2d ed. (Cologne, 1993), 162–74.

document psychomotoric reactions in order to differentiate various kinds of illness.[56] Some psychiatrists, such as Alfred Guttmann and Arthur Kronfeld, performed self-trials by means of the application of mescaline, hoping to produce artificial hallucinations in order to perceive the feelings of their patients.[57] In contrast to prewar times, psychoanalysis received little psychiatric attention.[58] All these different items, which were by no means accepted universally by the psychiatric community, induced vivid and frank discussions over controversial and innovative approaches.

In the area of practical health care for mentally ill patients, some new reforms took place. Between 1924 and 1929, the large majority of German asylums tried to establish a therapeutical system that was characterized by the attempt to keep the highest possible number of inmates busy and to make the interior circumstances of life similar to those outside of the asylums. Most of the large asylums established an outdoor care system for follow-up-treatment. In this period of consolidation, visits to psychiatric asylums rose dramatically; for example, in 1929 about 300,000 patients received treatment in 415 asylums with 168,000 beds.[59] But in the following years, forced by the world economic crisis and attempts to reduce the costs of the mentally ill patients, the shift toward radical eugenic solutions occurred. The willingness to solve social problems by applying biological means was on the increase. In this context, some of the German states, such as Prussia and Saxony, drafted laws on sterilization. These laws were not regarded as means to regulate individual, freely chosen birth control, but rather as necessary means to overcome social problems.

According to historian Hans-Ludwig Siemen, these concepts of cutting down expenses improved on the wishes of practically oriented psychiatry to become an efficiently working institution whose purpose was to separate out

---

56 Wilhelm Liepmann, "Psychomotorische Studie zur Konstitutionsforschung," *Deutsche Zeitschrift für Nervenheilkunde* 106 (1928): 146–9.

57 Alfred Guttmann, "Halluzinationen und andere Folgeerscheinungen nach experimenteller Vergiftung mit Anhalonium Lewini (Mescal)," *Neurologisches Zentralblatt* 40 (1921): suppl., 384–5.

58 Yet before World War I there were only a few discussions on psychoanalysis. In 1909 Karl Abraham gave a lecture on psychoanalysis and hysterical dreams at a meeting of the *Berliner Gesellschaft für Psychiatrie und Nervenheilkunde*, but was not successful. Theodor Ziehen especially rejected all psychoanalytic ideas; see Karl Abraham, "Psychoanalyse hysterischer Traumzustände," as well as Theodor Ziehen, "Remarks about Abraham's Paper on Psychoanalysis," both in *Neurologisches Zentralblatt* 28 (1909): 1291. In 1913 the *Deutsche Verein für Psychiatrie* discussed this issue. Eugen Bleuler supported psychoanalysis in his paper, whereas Alfred Hoche did just the opposite. See Thomas-Peter Schindler, "Psychiatrie im Wilhelminischen Deutschland im Spiegel der Verhandlungen des 'Vereins der deutschen Irrenärzte' (ab 1903: 'Deutscher Verein für Psychiatrie') von, 1891–1914," Med. diss., Universität Berlin, 1990, 120–2.

59 See Hans-Ludwig Siemen, "Reform und Radikalisierung: Veränderung der Psychiatrie in der Weltwirtschaftskrise," in Norbert Frei, ed., *Medizin und Gesundheitspolitik in der NS-Zeit* (Munich, 1991), 193.

human beings with socially divergent behavior. Additionally, the readiness to identify curable patients from incurable ones and to restrict dramatically the life conditions of the incurable increased sharply.[60]

The history of practically oriented psychiatry was governed by three crucial elements at the end of the Weimar period. First, there were the claims for preservation and development of achievements concerning differentiated forms of care systems and modern treatment. Psychiatric asylums and hospitals should become more like hospitals by having high access rates, short treatment durations, and high discharge rates. Second, experts wanted to establish low-budget institutions for incurable and particularly troublesome individuals. Third, the demands for repressive eugenic measures, such as sterilization, were to give psychiatry a new task. Thus, psychiatrists believed they could now control socially abnormal behavior.[61] Psychiatry could use these elements for presenting itself as an indispensable discipline, one that provided for the very special interests of society, the nation, and the state. In a reciprocal way, the general public could refer to the psychiatrists for scientifically legitimized proposals.

CONCLUSIONS

During the period between 1815 and 1933 the interests of German psychiatry – or important groups of psychiatrists – became closely aligned with those of the state and society. We find exceptions to this general tendency, however, after 1848, when a large group of psychiatrists espoused the political contents of liberalism (e.g., human rights for the mentally ill), and during the Weimar period, when psychiatry engaged in a vital and broadly based discourse with many innovative approaches.

By aligning their interests so closely with the state's, psychiatrists tried to make their discipline indispensable and to integrate the field into the medical curriculum at the universities. Whereas psychiatrists used the state and society for the establishment of their discipline, society and the state used psychiatry to derive scientifically valid schemes and concepts for managing social abnormality.

The main issues of psychiatric activity changed in concert with the state's and society's needs. During the first half of the nineteenth century, Germany was characterized by the first wave of industrialization. The creation of a patient with self-discipline became the primary concern of psychiatry. At the end of the century, in contrast, psychiatry exerted itself to fulfill the function

60 Ibid., 196.
61 Ibid., 199.

of police control and tried to become a crucial element in the control system and in the rational apportionment of human resources. These tendencies grew more pronounced during World War I, when psychiatry integrated itself into the military by submitting to the conditions of warfare.

Wartime meant radical change in two ways. First, the transformation of ethical values. The worth of a single human being diminished, the welfare of the entire community was declared to be of higher value. At the same time, those who suffered from mental disturbances were regarded as having inferior value. Second, an aggressive brutality concerning the relationship between doctors and patients was initiated and continued into the years of the Weimar Republic.

During the whole period, mental illness described a behavior that was atypical and thus conspicuous. A person gained medical attention only through behavior that violated social or religious norms. But the connotations of the notion "mentally ill" changed. During the first half of the nineteenth century, a mad person was characterized as someone who felt little or no connection to society's rules and as someone who was without self-control, thus endangering social order. At the end of the century, mentally ill persons were seen primarily in terms of their capacity for economic performance. Because of their inability to work like healthy persons, the mentally ill were seen as a burden on society.

6

Rationalizing the Therapeutic Arsenal

German Neuropsychiatry in World War I

PAUL LERNER

The doctors hold the sieve into which male humanity is poured, in order to separate out the fit from the unfit. The netting of this sieve is getting wider and wider. Eventually so wide that almost nothing will be left above. Everything falls through into the bins which have to be kept full for the ravenous war.

Alfred Polgar, 1917

The worst thing is not that many hysterics who remain uncured must be compensated with high pensions, but that they are lost to the army in our hour of greatest need, and what's more, that these people mostly young, physically healthy individuals become worthless parasites on human society, self-pitying hypochondriacs and spineless weaklings.

Dr. Robert Gaupp, Tübingen, May 1917

As the celebrations of the beginning of World War I faded and the belligerent armies dug trenches across the western front, a puzzling epidemic that would debilitate as many as several hundred thousand German soldiers began to appear.[1] The most common symptoms included sleeplessness, uncontrollable shaking, and disorders of speech, sight, hearing, or gait, all without detectable organic basis. Soon the individuals who came to be called "war neurotics" began to fill up army hospitals; their symptoms often deemed incurable, many were discharged with pensions or sent to their hometowns

---

1 The official *Reichswehr* statistics list the number of soldiers who were hospitalized for nervous illness as 313,399. The war neuroses in a narrower sense include hysteria, neurasthenia, and nervous shock, and several subdiagnoses, which amount to roughly 62 percent of those cases, hence 194,300. See *Sanitätsbericht über das Deutsche Heer im Weltkriege, 1914–1918*, vol. 3: "Die Krankenbewegung bei dem Deutschen Feld- und Besatzungsheer" (Berlin, 1934), 145-9. This number, I would argue, can only be used as a very rough estimate. It is actually a record of the number of hospital admissions, and not actual patients, so it overlooks the possibility of multiple admissions. It also fails to take into account those who were never treated.

for treatment. Yet, by 1916 German psychiatrists and neurologists had begun to make progress against this national emergency, and soon afterwards an elaborate system for diagnosing, treating, pensioning, and reassigning the war neurotics was put in place.

Accounts of war neurosis in Germany have focused above all on its ethical dimensions.[2] The zealous collaboration of doctors in military aims, widespread application of brutal and dangerous methods of treatment; and shifting pension policies in times of economic crisis have all been cited as medical-ethical transgressions that set the precedent for the role of doctors in National Socialism. Cliché depictions of army psychiatrists forcing shell-shocked soldiers back into combat and the high mortality rates in mental institutions during the blockade constitute, for some historians, the prehistory of psychiatric participation in the Nazi euthanasia program.[3]

This chapter parts from such perspectives by placing the treatment of the war neuroses into the medical-historical context of the war.[4] It calls attention to the central, but often overlooked fact that wartime psychiatrists and neurologists acknowledged the "legitimacy" of psychogenic illness. Thus, rather than declaring all neurotics simulators or malingerers and simply forcing them back to their divisions, doctors medicalized the condition and constructed an intricate system for its diagnosis and treatment.[5] The medicalization process meant radically increased control of individual lives by doctors; but as we will see, doctors had phenomenal success at abolishing debilitating symptoms and restoring individuals' ability to function and work.

2   See Hans Ludwig Siemen, *Das Grauen ist vorprogrammiert: Psychiatrie zwischen Faschismus und Atomkrieg* (Giessen, 1982), 7–51; Peter Riedesser and Axel Verderber, *Aufrüstung der Seelen: Militärpsychiatrie und Militärpsychologie in Deutschland und Amerika* (Freiburg, 1985); Karl-Heinz Roth, "Die Modernisierung der Folter in den beiden Weltkriegen," *1999: Zeitschrift für Sozialgeschichte des 20. und 21. Jahrhunderts* 2 (July 1987): 8–75; and Esther Fischer-Homburger, "Der Erste Weltkrieg und die Krise der ärztlichen Ethik," in Johanna Bleker and Heinz-Peter Schmiedebach, eds., *Medizin und Krieg: Vom Dilemma der Heilberufe 1865 bis 1985* (Frankfurt/Main, 1987), 122–34.
3   Siemen, *Das Grauen ist vorprogrammiert.*
4   Much of the excellent work on "shell shock" in the British army emphasizes issues of professionalization, the gendering of diagnoses, and the place of psychiatry in the modern welfare state. See Elaine Showalter, *The Female Malady: Women, Madness, and English Culture, 1830–1980* (New York, 1985), 167–95; Elaine Showalter, "Rivers and Sassoon: The Inscription of Male Gender Anxieties," in Margaret Randolph Higonnet et al., eds., *Behind the Lines: Gender and the Two World Wars* (New Haven, Conn., 1987), 61–9; Martin Stone, "Shell Shock and the Psychologist," in W. F. Bynum, Roy Porter, and Michael Shepard, eds., *The Anatomy of Madness* (London, 1985), 2:242–71; Eric T. Dean Jr., "War and Psychiatry: Examining the Diffusion Theory in Light of the Insanity Defense in Post-World War I Britain," *History of Psychiatry* 4 (1993): 61–82; Ted Bogacz, "War Neurosis and Cultural Change in England, 1914–1922: The Work of the War Office Committee of Enquiry into 'Shell-Shock,'" *Journal of Contemporary History* 24 (April 1989): 227–56; and Tom Brown, "Shell-Shock in the Canadian Expeditionary Force, 1914–1918: Canadian Psychiatry in the Great War," in Charles Roland, ed., *Health, Disease and Medicine: Essays in Canadian History, Proceedings of the First Hannah Conference on the History of Medicine, McMaster University, 1982* (Toronto, 1984), 308–32.
5   See Eric J. Leed, *No Man's Land: Combat and Identity in World War I* (Cambridge, 1979), 163–92.

The complexity of medicalization, that is the co-occurrence of healing and controlling, dictates the need for a new approach to the war neurosis issue. Here conventional notions of psychiatric continuity in German history will be challenged through the paradigm of rationalization, the principles of wartime, and postwar industrial reconstruction, which emphasized efficiency, standardization, and the full utilization of human resources. Rationalization was embraced across the social spectrum and was applied by Weimar era social reformers to the organization of daily life.[6] This chapter argues that these same principles governed wartime psychiatric practice. Its discussions of hypnosis, electrotherapy, and the reorganization of military psychiatry show how the priorities of speed, efficiency, and the needs of the national economy redefined the perception and treatment of the mental health of Germany's men.

GERMAN PSYCHIATRY GOES TO WAR

Germany's medical professionals greeted the war with nearly unanimous support. Most doctors mobilized quickly and enthusiastically, and by the war's end, some 26,000 would serve in the war effort.[7] Many saw the war as a means of improving their professional status, which had been threatened in the preceding decades by the institution of social insurance, whereas others viewed it as an opportunity to gain influence over state health policy.[8] For a generation of neurologists and psychiatrists, the war represented a chance to demonstrate their patriotism and indispensability to the nation. Those born in the 1860s had reached the peak of their professional productivity and, in many cases, attained university chairs in the decade before the war; afterward they would achieve the height of their prominence.[9] Members of this

6   For discussions of rationalization as a feature of wartime and Weimar industry and as a principle of social organization, see Annemarie Tröger, "The Creation of a Female Assembly-Line Proletariat," in Renate Bridenthal, Atina Grossmann, and Marion Kaplan, eds., *When Biology became Destiny: Women in Weimar and Nazi Germany* (New York, 1984), 237–69; Atina Grossmann, "The New Woman and the Rationalization of Sexuality in Weimar Germany," in Ann Snitow, Christine Stansell, and Sharon Thompson, eds., *Powers of Desire: The Politics of Sexuality* (New York, 1983), 159–71; and Mary Nolan, "The Infatuation with Fordism: Social Democracy and Economic Rationalization in Weimar Germany," in W. Maderthauer and H. Gruber, eds., *Chance and Illusion: Labor in Retreat* (Vienna, 1988), 151–84.
7   Paul Weindling, "Social Hygiene and the Birth Rate in Wartime Germany," in Richard Wall and Jay Winter, eds., *The Upheaval of War: Family, Work and Welfare in Europe, 1914–1918* (Cambridge, 1988), 417–39; Heinz-Peter Schmiedebach, "Sozialdarwinismus, Biologismus, Pazifismus: Ärztestimmen zum Ersten Weltkrieg," in Bleker and Schmiedebach, eds., *Medizin und Krieg*, 93–121; and Johanna Bleker, "Medizin im Dienst des Krieges, Krieg im Dienst der Medizin: Zur Frage der Kontinuität des ärztlichen Auftrages und ärztlicher Werthaltung im Angesicht des Krieges," in Bleker and Schmiedebach, eds., *Medizin und Krieg*, 13–28.
8   Schmiedebach, "Ärztestimmen zum Ersten Weltkrieg."
9   A striking number of the leading German authorities on war neurosis were born in the same decade,

generation had matured during an era of intense scientific rivalry between Germany and France; as a consequence of German advances in pathology and hygiene and the new preeminent status of Central European universities, they were particularly prone to a chauvinistic brand of medical nationalism.

This war enthusiasm was, of course, shared by others of the same class and social standing, but doctors often added uniquely medical justifications. Numerous doctors looked forward to the war as an experiment that would answer pressing questions about the relationship of culture and environment to mental and nervous health. Many psychiatrists depicted war as a premodern antidote to the deteriorating conditions of industrial modernity and believed that exposure to fresh air and nature would heal soldiers' psyches. Oblivious to the realities of modern warfare, they idealized the upcoming conflict as the solution to a perceived crisis of mental health and lauded the healthful psychological consequences of the mobilization of the national community. Among these doctors were some of the leaders of German university psychiatry, including Karl Bonhoeffer from Berlin, who observed the decreasing incidence of alcoholism during mobilization; Freiburg psychiatrist Alfred Hoche, who credited mobilization with emptying out the "luxury sanatoria"; and Robert Sommer of Giessen, who linked war with times of great human achievement and progress.[10] The Swiss-born Otto Binswanger, professor of psychiatry at Jena, explained the positive effects of war, "the great purifier" (*grosse Reiniger*), on the health of the nervously ill as follows:

I had a whole series of weak-nerved youths in treatment over the course of the last year and up to the time of the war's outbreak: anxious, cowardly, irresolute, weak-willed creatures, whose consciousness and feelings were determined only by their own egos and who amounted to nothing more than whiners, complaining of physical and mental pain. Then came the war. The illnesses fell away as though beaten out of them. They reported to their divisions, and what seems even more remarkable to me, every single one of them, with only one exception, has held up to this day. ... Thus, even among those with sickly natures ... the war has done its job.[11]

With the exception of cases of so-called mobilization psychosis, the beginning of the war produced relatively few instances of psychiatric illness. This

became the leaders of German university psychiatry and neurology immediately after the war, and retired in the 1930s. A partial list with wartime university affiliation follows: Gustav Aschaffenburg, Cologne (b. 1866); Karl Bonhoeffer, Berlin (b. 1868); Robert Gaupp, Tübingen (b. 1870); Alfred Hoche, Freiburg (b. 1865); Max Nonne, Hamburg (b. 1861); Robert Sommer, Giessen (b. 1864); Robert Wollenberg, Strassbourg (b. 1862).

10 See, e.g., Karl Bonhoeffer, "Über die Abnahme des Alkoholismus während des Krieges," *Monatsschrift für Psychiatrie und Neurologie* 41 (1917): 382–5; Alfred Hoche, *Krieg und Seelenleben* (Freiburg, 1914); Robert Sommer, "Zur Psychologie des Krieges und deren Erfindungen," unpublished MS, Sommer papers, vol. 14, Handschriftenabteilung der Universitätsbibliothek, Justus-Liebig-Universität, Giessen.

11 Otto Binswanger, *Die Seelischen Wirkungen des Krieges* (Leipzig, 1914), 21–2.

confirmed German medicine's assumption of the superior health of German men. Furthermore, most doctors shared the view that neuroses were essentially selfish complaints; the appeal of the war was that it reoriented concern away from the individual and toward the good of the whole nation. But, as the German advance bogged down during the fall and winter of 1914–15, the psychological strain of modern, mechanized war made itself felt, and military hospitals began to fill up with puzzling cases of hysterical and functional disorders.

Data from prior wars had, in fact, alerted German psychiatrists that they would have a role to play in the upcoming conflict. This was especially true of the Russo–Japanese War, in which dozens of cases of neurasthenia or nervous exhaustion among Russian troops had been reported.[12] Furthermore, concern with degeneration in Germany's urban and industrial centers had spread among doctors, hygienists, and social reformers; many feared that Germany's men did not possess the nervous strength necessary to endure a prolonged war.[13] Psychiatrists in particular expressed concern over the nation's deteriorating mental health as indicated by the flooding of asylums and increasing suicide rates.[14] Connections between deviant behavior and the influence of the big city milieu were the subject of numerous empirical studies, including, among others, Karl Bonhoeffer's examinations of Breslau prisoners for alcoholism and vagabondage and Robert Gaupp's work on mental illness in Munich.[15] But despite the medical and popular discourse on the crisis of mental health, the first reports of epidemic male hysteria caught German doctors wholly unprepared.

THE RISE AND FALL OF "TRAUMATIC NEUROSIS"

The onset of the war neurosis problem reignited debates over the relationship between traumatic experiences and post-traumatic neuroses. Beginning with the alleged discovery of "railway spine" in Great Britain, the right of

12 See P. M. Awtokratow, "Die Geisteskranken im Russischen Heere im Russisch-japanischen Kriege," *Allgemeine Zeitschrift für Psychiatrie* 64 (1907): 286–319; and Robert Wollenberg, "Nervöse Erkrankungen bei Kriegsteilnehmern," *Münchener Medizinische Wochenschrift, Feldärztliche Beilage* 61 (1914): 2181–3.

13 See Bernd Ulrich, "Nerven und Krieg- Skizzierung einer Beziehung," in Bedrich Loewenstein, ed., *Geschichte und Psychologie: Annäherungsversuche* (Pfaffenweiler, 1992), 163–91.

14 In Prussia, e.g., between 1880 and 1910, the number of asylum inmates increased more than fivefold, from 27,000 to 143,000; during this period the population increase was less than 1.5-fold, from 27 million to 40 million. Thomas-Peter Schindler, "Psychiatrie im Wilhelminischen Deutschland," Med. diss., Freie Universität Berlin, 1990, 92.

15 Robert Gaupp, "Die klinischen Besonderheiten der Seelenstörungen unserer Grossstadtbevölkerung," *Münchener Medizinische Wochenschrift* 53 (1906): 1250–2, 1310–13; and Karl Bonhoeffer, "Ein Beitrag zur Kenntnis des grossstädtischen Bettel- und Vagabondentums: Eine Psychiatrische Untersuchung," *Zeitschrift für die gesamte Strafrechtswissenschaft* 21 (1901): 5.

victims of railroad or factory accidents to financial compensation for loss of their ability to work had spawned disagreement over how to deal with sufferers of the ailment psychiatrists now call posttraumatic stress disorder.[16] The Berlin neurologist Hermann Oppenheim theorized that these conditions constituted a distinct disease entity that he named "traumatic neurosis"; the core of the condition, he wrote, lay in undetectable microscopic changes in the brain or central nervous system caused by the physically jarring accident experience. But, what Oppenheim's detractors seldom acknowledged, was his belief that the psychological consequences of trauma also played a significant role.[17] Oppenheim's opponents, in contrast, often viewed sufferers of psychic trauma as pension seekers and advocated cutting off compensation to restore their ability to function productively. Crucial to the latter position, however, was that it acknowledged the "legitimacy" of the illness; that is, sufferers from traumatic or "pension neurosis" were not seen simply as simulators, but as genuinely ill. Their malady was termed a sickness of will (*Willenskrankheit*). Alfred Hoche well represented the psychogenic position in 1910 when he wrote:

Still an unknown concept thirty years ago, today an illness, a cancer on the organism of our whole working class, and justifiably the cause for serious concern. This peoples' epidemic [*Volksseuche*] arose not only chronologically after the enactment of the accident insurance legislation, but also in direct causal relationship. The law has, without doubt, produced the illness. ... It is not the case, as was assumed at the beginning, that it is a matter of simulation, of intentional faking of symptoms that are not there. The individuals are in fact sick, but they would be well, strangely enough, if the law did not exist.[18]

Indeed, if the laws did not exist, to extrapolate Hoche's statement, these individuals would not be collecting pensions; instead they would be working. The psychogenic position thus valorized work and equated neurotic illness with the desire to escape working. During the war, as the nation was gripped by labor and manpower shortages, these assumptions took on explicit moral

16 For detailed discussions, see Esther Fischer-Homburger, *Die Traumatische Neurose: Vom Somatischen zum Sozialen Leiden* (Bern, 1975); Greg Eghigian, "Die Bürokratie und das Entstehen von Krankheit: Die Politik und die Rentenneurosen, 1890–1926," in Jürgen Reulecke and Adelheit Gräfin zu Castell-Rüdenhausen, eds., *Stadt und Gesundheit: Zum Wandel von Volksgesundheit und kommunaler Gesundheitspolitik im 19. und frühen 20. Jahrhundert* (Stuttgart, 1991), 203–23; Gabriele Moser, "Der Arzt im Kampf gegen 'Begehrlichkeit und Rentensucht' im Deutschen Kaiserreich und in der Weimarer Republik," *Jahrbuch für Kritische Medizin* 16 (1992): 161–83; and Eric Caplan, "Medicalizing the Mind: The Invention of American Psychotherapy, 1800–1920," Ph.D. diss., University of Michigan, 1994, esp. chap. 1.
17 Hermann Oppenheim, *Die traumatischen Neurosen, nach den in der Nervenklinik der Charité in den 5 Jahren 1883-1889 gesammelten Beobachtungen* (Berlin, 1889).
18 Alfred E. Hoche, "Geisteskrankheit und Kultur," in Alfred E. Hoche, *Aus der Werkstatt* (Munich, 1935), 16.

and political dimensions, with the result that pension collection was at times cast as unpatriotic and even sick behavior.

After the turn of the century, as a new generation of psychiatrists and neurologists began to weigh in on the issue, general medical opinion turned against the traumatic neurosis theory, blaming it for a perceived epidemic of pension neurosis.[19] Meanwhile, Oppenheim, having been denied a professorship at the university, opened a private clinic in northern Berlin and devoted his attention primarily to other issues. The urgency of the war neurosis problem brought the two positions into direct and open conflict. Proponents of traumatic neurosis viewed the war neurotics as confirmation of their theory, citing perceived connections between munitions explosions and the incidence of neurosis. Oppenheim, for one, presented evidence that many cases of traumatic neurosis arose during sleep, hence for him a psychogenic etiology was ruled out. Oppenheim's detractors, however, were ultimately able to produce significant evidence to the contrary. Studies on prisoners of war and those with serious injuries showed that neuroses seldom occurred among these groups, suggesting that only those in need of an excuse to get away from the war were likely to "flee into illness" through neurosis.[20] Other studies produced evidence that soldiers well behind the front lines were more likely to become hysterics or neurasthenics than those actually in combat, suggesting that fear of the front and desire to escape service were responsible.

The two approaches came into direct conflict at a now infamous 1916 congress, when the German Psychiatric Association convened in Munich to discuss wartime nervous and mental illnesses; there the traumatic neurosis issue was hotly debated, and Oppenheim found himself attacked by a group of psychiatrists and neurologists, including most vociferously, Max Nonne and Robert Gaupp.[21]

Oppenheim's defeat could perhaps best be explained with recourse to the fact that the traumatic neurosis diagnosis would have been far more expensive for the state; deemed organically ill and incurable, all war neurotics would have had to be discharged with pensions. But ultimately decisive in the debate

---

19 Historians have generally failed to recognize the influence of psychogenicism among German psychiatrists and neurologists of this time; too often and perhaps owing to the lingering influence of Freud's own accounts, psychoanalysis and somaticism are posed as the only alternatives. My research reveals that many well-established psychiatrists occupied a middle ground simultaneously dismissive of psychoanalysis yet adherent to a form of psychogenicism. For an early, yet very persuasive, statement of this position, see Hannah Decker, *Freud in Germany: Revolution and Reaction in Science* (New York, 1977).

20 See Friedrich Mörchen, "Traumatische Neurose und Kriegsgefangene," *Münchener Medizinische Wochenschrift* 63 (1916): 1188–90.

21 See "Verhandlungen des Deutschen Vereins für Psychiatrie zu München am 21. und 22. September 1916," *Allgemeine Zeitschrift für Psychiatrie* 73 (1917): 162–233.

were the successes in treatment that backers of psychogenicism could claim for methods derived from suggestion or crude forms of psychotherapy. Nonne, about whom much will be said below, pointed to his success through hypnosis and suggestion as proof that these disorders were products of the mind and not the body. As he recalled years later:

> I've never experienced before or since so much participation in a debate. Thirty-six men spoke in the discussion and thirty of them declared that they agreed with my presentation. Professor Oppenheim, who at that time was the generally recognized, authoritative leader of German neurologists, saw himself totally isolated in his conception of the "traumatic neurosis" which he attributed to the anatomical consequences of trauma. ... This most accomplished man, who had been the teacher of many neurologists, and who had swallowed hard the fact that he never had received an official chair, who was hypersensitive to attack, could not overcome this defeat – he had fought for years for his concept, the traumatic neurosis, and the topic was "loaded with *Affekt*." A year later he suffered a heart attack for which he, a long time sufferer from hypertension, was predisposed.[22]

The widespread acceptance of psychogenicism, however, did not mean complete psychiatric unanimity.[23] One unresolved issue, the role of the so-called psychopathic constitution, or disposition, in neuroses and psychoses, remained a point of contention.[24] Nonne and Hoche argued that any individual, when exposed to the conditions of battle, could develop neurotic symptoms. Gaupp, Binswanger, and Bonhoeffer represented the majority opinion, which held that functional psychogenic disorders were possible only in the presence of a preexistent psychopathology. Hence, for the latter group, neurotics were essentially considered psychopathic. But the importance of manpower to the war meant that these psychopaths had to be treated, a function foreign to both university psychiatrists and asylum doctors. The latter had, before the war, played a role best described as warehousing those deemed unfit for life in society. The former, mostly engaged in research

22 Max Nonne, *Anfang und Ziel Meines Lebens* (Hamburg, 1971), 179–80.
23 Space limitations prevent this essay from dealing with the complicated position of psychoanalysis in this story. But it should be stressed that, though psychogenicism represented a degree of convergence between mainstream psychiatry and psychoanalysis, it did not alter the marginal status of psychoanalysis. A sizable and useful literature on this topic exists, including Geoffrey Cocks, *Psychotherapy in the Third Reich* (New York, 1985), chap. 2; Johannes Reichmayr, "Psychoanalyse im Krieg," in P. Passet and E. Modena, eds., *Krieg und Frieden aus Psychoanalytischer Sicht* (Frankfurt/Main, 1983), 36–58; Peter Büttner, "Freud und der Erste Weltkrieg: Eine Untersuchung über die Beziehung von Medizinischer Theorie und gesellschaftlicher Praxis der Psychoanalyse," Ph.D. diss., Ruprecht-Karls-Universität, Heidelberg, 1975; Kurt Eissler, *Freud as Expert Witness: The Discussion of War Neurosis between Freud and Wagner-Jauregg*, trans. Christine Trollope (Madison, Wis., 1986).
24 See Fritz Fränkel, "Über die psychopathische Konstitution bei Kriegsneurosen," *Monatschrift für Psychiatrie und Neurologie* (1920): 287–309; Karl Pönitz, *Die klinische Neuorientierung zum Hysterieproblem unter dem Einflusse der Kriegserfahrungen* (Berlin, 1921).

and observation in new university facilities, returned to the act of treatment only under the conditions of the war.[25]

DEPLOYING ACTIVE TREATMENT

> The therapy of the hysterical disorders of war has gradually developed into a neurological specialty, which governs the whole military organization all the way through discharging and pension setting.[26]
>
> Dr. Karl Birnbaum

The year 1916 witnessed unprecedented loss of life in the battles of Verdun and the Somme. The surprising resilience of the French army and the nature of that year's fighting meant greater and greater manpower needs. At the same time, paralyzing labor shortages gripped industries crucial to Germany's war economy.[27] The year 1916 also saw the first widespread therapeutic successes against war neurosis and the development of new approaches to the administration of neuropsychiatric treatment. Cases once dismissed as incurable were subjected to programs designed to reclaim simultaneously potential labor power, trim burdensome pension obligations, and free up overcrowded hospital facilities. These measures were put into place as part of a new, rationalized system for dealing with war neurotics. The result was an "assembly line" approach to classifying patients and a system that redefined individual health in terms of the collective needs of the German war effort.

The early practice of sending neurotic soldiers home from the beginning of the war was soon overturned and deemed the worst possible solution — having attained the fulfillment of his wish in his return home and enjoying the "damaging pity" of his neighbors, the soldier, it was argued, would never get better. Thus, special sections for neurotics were added to hospitals near the front.[28] Untreated neurotics were rarely sent back into action for fear of risking relapse; furthermore, the presence of neurotics was believed damaging to troop morale as it could encourage others to simulate neurotic symptoms.[29] Instead, and by acknowledging the "legitimacy" of the neuroses, psychiatrists and neurologists supervised the construction of a complete

25 See Siemen, *Das Grauen ist vorprogrammiert*; Bogacz, "War Neurosis"; and Brown, "Shell-Shock."
26 Karl Birnbaum, "Ergebnisse der Neurologie und Psychiatrie: Kriegsneurosen und -psychosen auf Grund der gegenwärtigen Kriegsbeobachtungen: Sammbelbericht V," *Zeitschrift für die Gesamte Neurologie und Psychiatrie: Referate und Ergebnisse* 14 (1917): 241.
27 In the words of one historian, "The problem was how to reconcile the military's insatiable manpower-requirements with industry's desperate need for skilled labour ... the only way adequately to supply the soldiers needed at the front was to call them back to Germany!" (Richard Bessel, *Germany After the First World War* [Oxford, 1993], 13–14).
28 See G. Ronald Hargraves, Eric Wittkower, and A. T. M. Wilson, "Psychiatric Organisation in the Services," in Emanuel Miller, ed., *The Neuroses in War* (New York, 1940), 163–80.
29 Karl Bonhoeffer, "Psychiatrie und Krieg," *Deutsche Medizinische Wochenschrift* 40 (1914): 1777–9.

system for screening, treating, and rehabilitating war neurotics. As stated by the Berlin neurologist Max Lewandowsky, they aimed to "systematically construct a net, through whose meshing no neurotic not rid of his symptoms can slip."[30] These measures meant that, in the words of Dr. Karl Pönitz, "there was no possibility for slipping away.... [It was] a sealed system, a closed front against the war hysterics."[31]

The fighting of 1916 rendered conditions in military hospitals unmanageable. One solution to the overcrowding and shortages of staff and resources came through the development of a new, aggressive approach to the treatment of the neuroses. Starting in 1916 a series of methods called "active treatment" came into widespread use and replaced the milder rest and bath cures that had been fruitlessly practiced earlier in the war. These new methods were all derived from psychogenicism; all relied on suggestion to coax or force the patient out of his illness. To accommodate these methods and to prevent neurotic patients from influencing organically ill patients, the construction of new hospital stations especially designed for nervously ill patients was ordered.[32]

Doctors applied the principles of suggestion as they saw fit, and several individuals achieved great fame in promoting their own variations. "The war neuroses are in their essence curable, and these days the great majority of cases are in fact cured. There are numerous ways to do this, and to swear by one method alone is foolish. The doctor cures through his personality, not through his method," wrote Gaupp.[33] Military medical authorities did not prescribe treatment methods, deferring to the experiences and preferences of practicing doctors and the particularities of individual cases.[34] Nonne echoed this when he summed up his therapeutic observations from the war in 1922. "Each person should use the method which he has mastered, for which he has the talent and the faith and with which he has had success, and each method is successful when it is practiced by the right doctor in the proper manner."[35]

30 Max Lewandowsky, "Was kann in der Behandlung und Beurteilung der Kriegsneurosen erreicht werden?" *Münchner Medizinische Wochenschrift: Feldärztliche Beilage* 63 (1917): 1028.
31 Pönitz, *Klinische Neuorientierung*, 32.
32 See the memorandum from Generalarzt Georg Friedrich Wilhelm Schultzen, Sanitätsdepartement des Kriegsministeriums, "Behandlung und Beurteilung von Kriegsneurotikern," Berlin, Sept. 7, 1917, Archiv der Eberhard-Karls-Universität Tübingen, Akte Nr. 308/42.
33 "Gaupp spricht über die Neurosen und Psychosen des Krieges," Archiv der Eberhard-Karls-Universität, Tübingen, Akte Nr. 308/42, "Gaupp."
34 Bayerisches Kriegsministerium, "Behandlung von Kriegsneurotiker," Feb. 19, 1917, Bayerisches Hauptstaatsarchiv Munich (hereafter cited as BayHStA), Abt. Kriegsarchiv, Stellv. Gen. Kom. des II. Armee Korps, Sanitätsamt, Bd. 14, Akte 1.
35 Max Nonne, "Therapeutische Erfahrungen an den Kriegsneurosen in den Jahren, 1914–1918," in Karl Bonhoeffer, ed., "Geistes- und Nervenkrankheiten," vol. 4 of *Handbuch der ärztlichen Erfahrungen im Weltkrieg, 1914–1918*, ed. Otto von Schjerning (Leipzig, 1922), 106.

The adoption of active therapy meant that methods that had been previously eschewed or condemned by established medicine were brought back into the psychiatric repertoire. Prewar psychiatry had been characterized primarily by the search for scientific legitimacy and for long-term solutions to the perceived crisis in mental health. Methods of treatment for mental and nervous illnesses had received little professional attention in the years immediately preceding the war.[36] Precisely during the war German psychiatry was attaining the heights of "modernity" and "scientificity" with the 1917 establishment of Emil Kraepelin's long-awaited institute for research into the biological basis of mental illness.[37] But at the same time, leading neuropsychiatrists began reaching back to early nineteenth-century forms of treatment that depended upon the subjective role of the doctor's personality and outdated notions of the doctor-patient relationship. These subjective treatments lay paradoxically at the core of the highly schematized, objective system for processing neurotic soldiers.

Active treatment consisted of methods that sought to cure through force or discipline, those based upon deception, and those aimed to enlighten the patient by uncovering the roots and causes of his illness. Although methods based upon force have almost exclusively captured the attention of historians, most doctors experimented with all three kinds of treatment. The most well-known methods of active treatment were suggestive hypnosis, which Nonne contributed to the therapeutic arsenal, and Fritz Kaufmann's so-called overpowering method (*Überrumpelungsmethode*), which applied electric current with a regimen of exercises and military commands.

Other methods were based upon non-hypnotic suggestion (*Wachsuggestion*), such as Kurt Goldstein's method of phony operations, which played upon the patient's belief that his illness was somatic and surgically curable; Rothmann's and Hirschfeld's practice of using narcotics to stupefy their patients before attempting to talk them out of their symptoms; and Otto Binswanger's isolation technique, which was based on the soothing "rest-cure" developed by Silas Weir Mitchell for neurasthenia, but as practiced by Binswanger, attempted to bore the patient out of his illness through deprivation of food, light, and human contact. Raphael Weichbrodt, among others, promoted suggestion through long baths (*Dauerbäder*); the patient would be instructed that he could leave the bath only after he was cured. Particular methods were also used for localized hysterical symptoms. The

36 See Schindler, "Psychiatrie."
37 See Matthias M. Weber, "'Ein Forschungsinstitut für Psychiatrie…' Die Entwicklung der deutschen Forschungsanstalt für Psychiatrie in München zwischen 1917 und 1945," *Sudhoffs Archiv für Geschichte der Medizin* 75 (1991): 74–89.

laryngologist Otto Muck developed a technique that terrified psycho-genically mute patients in order to evoke a scream (*Angstschrei*); Robert Sommer similarly tricked functionally deaf patients into acknowledging that they heard an audible stimulus by ringing a bell behind their heads and measuring their reaction. Psychotherapy as we know it scarcely existed, but some doctors did treat patients by having them reenact traumatic battle scenarios until they were freed of their symptoms. Even a modified form of psychoanalysis was practiced during the war, most notably by Ernst Simmel in a station for nervous disorders in Poznan.[38]

Many of these methods were touted as cures for long-standing cases where the symptoms had "hardened" because of the early policy of sending neuro-tics home. All represented a new aggressiveness in dealing with neurotic illness, and doctors boasted of their efficiency, affordability, and speed. Methods based on suggestion recognized the importance of the hospital atmosphere to psychic therapy. This involved maintaining strict military discipline and preventing the hospital from being too pleasant, hence making certain that the "flight into illness" was a less attractive alternative than "the flight into health" through military or industrial service.

But what did the flight into health actually mean? The claims of individ-ual doctors such as Nonne and Fritz Kaufmann of cure rates above 90 per-cent were well publicized. These phenomenal results were not unique to those doctors with near celebrity status. In preparation for a 1918 meeting at the medical department of the Prussian Ministry of War in Berlin, neurolo-gists and psychiatrists, on order from the deputy general commands of the different armies, posed the following questions to neurosis stations through-out Germany: (1). How many sufferers of the so-called war neurosis have been treated since the creation of the neurosis section? (2). In how many cases was the ability to work or a high ability to serve reached? (3). How many officers have been there?[39] Kaufmann himself reported that in the two years since the establishment of the Ludwigshafen neurosis station, at least 90 percent of the 1,500 patients treated had been released with at least the ability to work. Approximately 95 percent, he added, were freed from their symptoms.[40]

38 Nonne, "Therapeutische Erfahrungen"; Kurt Singer, "Prinzipien und Erfolge der aktiven Therapie bei Neurosen," *Zeitschrift für Physikalische und Diätetische Therapie* 9 (1918): 275–85; R. Weichbrodt, "Zur Behandlung hysterischer Störungen," *Archiv für Psychiatrie* 57 (1917): 519–25; Kurt Goldstein, "Über die Behandlung der Kriegshysteriker," *Medizinische Klinik* 13 (1917): 751–8.
39 Letter from Seydel, Kriegsministerium, Medizinalabteilung to Sanitätsämter, May 31, 1918, BayHStA, Stellv. Gen. Kom. des II. Armee Korps, Bd. 14, Akte 2.
40 BayHStA, Stellv. Gen. Kom. des II. Armee Korps, Sanitätsamt, Bd. 14, Akte 2.

A report from the second Bavarian Army Corps in Würzburg claimed that almost 94 percent of the 3,000 neurotics who had been treated in its three neurosis stations had been released as able to work.[41] The records of dozens of stations throughout Bavaria and Württemberg reveal that rates in the low 90s were common. A station in Speyer reported a curing rate of 92 percent and boasted of its speed and efficiency:

The patients on average had been through 183 days of unsuccessful treatment in different hospitals before being sent here. ... [T]here are cases which had been in treatment for two or more years. ... Here the treatment time through the disappearance of the hysterical symptoms was twenty-two days in a private room; after which came fourteen days for confirming the results in a three-bed room; then work therapy followed whereby patients worked in agriculture or in their professions for on the average thirty-one days before being discharged.[42]

These results judged treatment success on a scale that equated curing with the restoration of the ability to serve in the military or at least to work without danger of relapse. A highly differentiated system was used whereby patients were judged capable of long- or short-term work or service on the front, in the *Etappe* (rear areas), at a garrison, or in home territory. Officers were always treated and counted separately from enlisted men and were usually diagnosed differently. More likely to be called neurasthenic or simply exhausted, officers were spared the methods of active treatment and were usually sent to pleasant rustic settings for recuperation.[43]

But for common soldiers, active treatment consisted of aggressive attempts to abolish the symptoms that prevented them from working. Healing was thus reconceptualized as enabling the patient to work productively and disqualifying him from a pension. As stated by Berlin neurologist Kurt Singer, "[C]urrent experience after thousands of cases has taught us that every ... neurotic can be freed of his symptoms. For his peace-time occupation, for service through working [*Arbeitsverwendung*], hence for the question of compensation and pension, removing the symptoms has the same significance as curing."[44]

As Germany's labor and manpower shortages reached crisis proportions, work became not only the goal of treatment but also an integral part of the therapeutic process. Desperate conditions saw the conflation of the alleged good of the patient with Germany's military and economic needs. Work

41 Ibid.
42 Ibid.
43 See the material by the Bund deutscher Offiziersfrauen in Sächsisches Hauptstaatsarchiv, Dresden, Gen. Kom. des XII. Res. Korps, Akte 19540, "Schriftwechsel, Sanitätsdienst Allgemeines." For a discussion of neurasthenia among English officers, see Showalter, *The Female Malady*, 167–95.
44 Singer, "Prinzipien und Erfolge der aktiven Therapie."

became emblematic for health, morality, and patriotism; it also created an atmosphere deemed desirable for recovering patients. Working battalions for neurotic soldiers were formed, and the acts of healing and recuperation were relocated from crowded hospitals to factories or farms.[45] The hospital, because it was filled with other patients lying around and living off state resources, was portrayed as an unfavorable environment for a neurotic. Pity was also condemned as having a destructive influence on morale, and neurotics were to be kept away from lay people who would indulge their woes. The two alternatives of prolonged hospital stays and pension collection were thus believed equally damaging, and the doctor's task was redefined as delivering nervously ill soldiers as quickly as possible from overcrowded and understaffed hospitals into the war economy's labor force.

Throughout Germany workshops were added to military hospitals, and new hospitals were constructed in agricultural settings and adjacent to factories. A variety of occupational retraining programs were developed for those no longer able to practice their prewar jobs and to redirect individuals into agricultural and industrial jobs essential for the war effort; continuing education courses and lectures were organized to prevent idleness, and whenever possible, hospital inmates were sent out to work during the day. Letting patients remain unoccupied was, in the words of an official from the Saxon Ministry of War medical department, "a serious moral danger for the individual and economically damaging to the general public. It also works against the patient's speedy and complete recovery."[46]

Many of these measures originated in the state of Baden and were known as the Baden system. In 1916 in the Black Forest town of Hornberg, the army's medical office first called for the cooperation of a munitions factory with a nearby neurosis station. Heidelberg psychiatry professor Karl Wilmanns reported, "[I]t is due to the sympathetic cooperation of these gentlemen that the goal of turning great numbers of the nervously ill into capable workers in the war economy has been reached. Since then neurotics, who for years had been moved from hospital to hospital without ever being cured, have been cured under the favorable influence of cured comrades, often immediately after their admission."[47]

As the advantages of this system became clear, similar policies were enacted throughout Germany and Austria-Hungary. According to Wilmanns:

45 Pönitz, *Klinische Neuorientierung*, 32.
46 SHStA, Dresden, Stellv. Gen. Kom. des XII. Armee Korps, Akte Nr. 12708, "Beschäftigung der Verwundeten," 12.
47 Karl Wilmanns, in Badischer Heimatdank, "Bericht über die Sitzung des bad. Landesausschusses der Kriegsbeschädigtenfürsorge, 26. Oktober 1917," 43–4, Bundesarchiv, Abt. Potsdam, Reichsarbeitsministerium, film no. 36069.

"For hospital stations, large, empty inns were preferred; these facilities were wonderfully suited for the nervously ill, and at the same time they strongly supported the innkeepers, who were suffering terribly from the war. The hospitals also enable factory owners to overcome labor shortages, to release the female workers who are so necessary for agricultural work, and to free children and youth from occupations that are dangerous to their health."[48] These sites also kept neurotics away from the unfavorable influence of big cities.

Successes in the treatment of neurotics led to new programs designed to lessen the enormous burden of pension payments on the state treasury. Patients originally discharged and pensioned early in the war were required to appear before so-called invalid inspection boards (*Invaliden-Prüfungs-Geschäfte*). Although the initial pensioning policy had established a five-year period before reexamination would be necessary, starting in 1917, reexaminations organized by the deputy general commands occurred annually, and many of the neurotics who had been previously discharged as incurable were subjected to the new methods of active therapy.

The Prussian Ministry of War in Berlin established the following principle for neuropsychiatric care: "[T]he main approach to dealing with war neurotics [is] to help them to a full utilization of their mostly psychologically inhibited ability to work."[49] Health officials also called for the establishment of central observation centers, where neurotics were to be sorted out based on ability to work and treatment needs. A Bavarian doctor proposed establishing six or seven observation centers in the territory of each army corps, each with 150 beds. "All men with unclear diagnoses are to be sent to the observation stations; there they are not to be treated, rather only their illnesses are to be ascertained. Fourteen days should be sufficient. ... Company doctors and hospitals must hold to the diagnoses from the observation station under all circumstances and must treat in accordance with them."[50] The result was a rationalized system for regulating the flow of neurotic soldiers. The acts of diagnosis and treatment were to be conducted separately, and in a manner akin to an assembly line, "genuine" neurotics were first separated from simulators and the chronically mentally ill (*geisteskrank*). Neither group was considered treatable, and both were thought to exercise a negative influence on the other patients. Particularly excitable neurotics were often sent to mental

48 Ibid., 44.
49 Kriegsministerium, "Nachprüfung beim Prüfungsgeschäft," BayHStA, Stellv. Gen. Kom. des I. Armee Korps, Bd. 156, "Invaliden Prüfungsgeschäft."
50 Letter from Dr. Kimmel, BayHStA, Stellv. Gen. Kom. des II. Armee Korps, Sanitätsamt, Bd. 15, Akte 3: "Kriegsinvalidenfürsorge."

institutions.[51] Only neurotics whose pensions had been set at 65 percent or higher were to be reexamined if treatment were deemed worthwhile by the examining board; these individuals were then sent to a specialized station where they were likely to be hypnotized or exposed to electric current.[52]

Thus, during the war the goal of neuropsychiatric treatment was reoriented around work. Wartime measures separated the acts of diagnosing, treating, and rehabilitating, and hospital stays were kept as short as possible. Treating war neurotics was endowed with particular significance for the economy and the war effort. Gaupp declared war neurotics "the most important category of patients in our army. ... the neurosis stations are the only ones in the whole land which are always full."[53] Whereas some doctors viewed their task as analogous to that of the preacher, others stressed the pedagogical or the disciplinary dimensions of treating neurotics. But common to these perspectives was the elevation of the doctor's role and the frequent depiction of treatment sessions as struggles or battles of will between doctor and patient. The doctor, armed with superior rank and the convictions of patriotism and morality, had to exert his strength of will to bring the patient back into health. Doctors' descriptions constantly emphasized the importance and difficulty of their task. In the words of Gaupp, "[T]he stronger the patriotism and social conscience of a doctor today, all the more self-sacrificing and energetic he will be in curing hysterics and in the battle against the obsession with pensions, which makes social parasites and miserable hypochondriacs out of physically healthy young men."[54]

Kaufmann acknowledged, "[I]t cannot be denied that the overpowering method places great demands on the nerves of the treating doctor. But the success makes all the effort worthwhile."[55] According to Nonne, the treatment of war neurotics was too important to be even discussed by lay people. "Concerning the treatment of war neurotics, only those who themselves have treated may write and talk about it, since only then can one give proper

51 R. Gerz, "Bericht über die vom preuss. Kriegsministerium (Sanitätsdepartment) nach Berlin einberufene Versammlung der Neurotikerärzte." BayHStA, Stellv. Gen. Kom. des II. Armee Korps, Sanitätsamt, Bd. 14, Akte 1.
52 That is, if their ability to earn had been diminished to 65 percent or more of its prewar value. "Nachprüfung beim Prüfungsgeschäft," BayHStA, Stellv. Gen. Kom. des I. Armee Korps, Bd. 156, "Invaliden Prüfungsgeschäft."
53 Robert Gaupp, *Die Nervenkranken des Krieges, Ihre Beurteilung und Behandlung: Ein Wort zur Aufklärung und Mahnung unseres Volkes* (Stuttgart, 1917).
54 Robert Gaupp, letter to Königliches Württemberg Gericht der stellvertr. 53. Infantriebrigade, Ulm, May 24, 1917, Archiv der Eberhard-Karls-Universität, Tübingen, Akte Nr. 308/42, "Gaupp."
55 Fritz Kaufmann, "Die Planmässige Heilung komplizierter psychogener Bewegungsstörungen bei Soldaten in einer Sitzung," *Münchener Medizinische Wochenschrift, Feldärztliche Beilage* 63 (1916): 802–4; Nonne wrote that only his occasional angry outbursts saved him from becoming nervous himself after working with nervous patients for fifty years. See Nonne, *Anfang und Ziel*, 179.

dignity to the sum of physical and mental labor it takes to bring a neurotic through physical-psychological pedagogy to flight into health from flight into illness."[56]

MAX NONNE AND THE REVIVAL OF HYPNOTHERAPY

At that time [1889], I had no idea that twenty-five years later I would give hypnosis honor and fame through the treatment of war neuroses.

The war brought us immense work in Eppendorf... already after several months we saw a condition that had before only very rarely been seen, the condition of Hysteria virilis, "male hysteria." This condition had been shown before by Charcot in Paris. At that time we had said, "such a thing only occurs among the French, in Germany there is no male hysteria."[57]

Dr. Max Nonne

Hypnosis was one of the most common forms of active treatment used during the war. Its rediscovery by mainstream medicine as a treatment for war neurosis was owed above all to the neurologist Nonne. A closer analysis of Nonne's life and his role in the treatment of war neuroses throws light on the convergence of medical nationalism and professional development that framed the wartime rediscovery of hypnosis.[58]

Nonne's career trajectory mirrors the development of neurology as a medical specialization in Germany.[59] His path at the Eppendorf hospital in Hamburg, from his 1887 beginning as a neurologically trained assistant in internal medicine to his directorship of the section for nerves (*Nervenabteilung*) in 1896 (which he ultimately renamed the neurological clinic) chronologically corresponds with neurology's progression out of internal medicine and its development of near disciplinary autonomy and the ability to set its own research agendas and administer distinct clinical facilities. Typical for members of his generation, Nonne had reached professional maturity before the war, and as evidenced by his participation in an elite team

---

56 Nonne, "Therapeutische Erfahrungen," 105.
57 Nonne, *Anfang und Ziel*, 177–9.
58 There is very little historical literature on Nonne. Despite his role during the war, he does not appear in most histories of hypnotism. For biographical details the best sources remain his autobiographical reflections and an unreliable essay that portrays him, I think unjustifiably, as decidedly anti-Semitic and intractably opposed to psychoanalysis. Georg Schaltenbrand, "Max Nonne," in Kurt Kolle, ed., *Grosse Nervenärzte* (Stuttgart, 1963), 3:164–73.
59 Albrecht Hirschmüller, *Freud's Begegnung mit der Psychiatrie: Von der Himmythologie zur Neurosenlehre* (Tübingen, 1991), 38. See also Hans-Heinz Eulner, *Die Entwicklung der medizinischen Spezialfächer an den Universitäten des deutschen Sprachgebietes* (Stuttgart, 1970).

of German and Swedish doctors called to attend to Lenin on his sick bed, he achieved national and international fame in the 1920s.

When Nonne was a young assistant doctor, German neurology and psychiatry were still overshadowed by French achievements in the field. As many of his German-speaking contemporaries, most famously in the case of Sigmund Freud, Nonne journeyed to France in 1889 to learn from the master, Jean-Martin Charcot.[60] At that time Charcot dominated France's medical-intellectual community. His typological studies of hysteria had turned the Salpetrière clinic into an international center for the study of the neuroses. Charcot had turned to hypnotism in the late 1870s; the interest of a doctor so respected and admired legitimated the controversial art as a subject of research, if not as a therapeutic method. For Charcot, hypnosis was a way of understanding the mind of the hysteric; it provided a view of the psychopathological states proximate to hysteria. In the words of one historian, it represented a kind of psychophysiological vivisection.[61]

Nonne stayed at Salpetrière for only six weeks; he was indeed impressed by Charcot's charisma, but remained skeptical of the authenticity of his therapeutic demonstrations and was put off by the Frenchman's purported arrogance and distance. "As a German – it was only eighteen years after the peace of Versailles – I could not expect more affability from Charcot with his strongly chauvinistic attitude, nor did I."[62] However, Nonne did remain in Paris long enough to enjoy the sights, in particular the Louvre, Notre Dame, and Versailles where, inspired by the events of eighteen years before, he swelled with pride at the founding of the German Empire.[63] His travels next took him to Nancy where he observed Charcot's rival Hippolyte Bernheim. Bernheim had challenged Charcot's belief in the proximity of the hypnotic state to hysteria; he and his Nancy followers emphasized the therapeutic applications of hypnosis. They also criticized Charcot's somatic view of hysteria and stressed the role of suggestion. In their view the charismatic Charcot had influenced his obedient patients to conform to his ideas of the illness and hence to physically recapitulate the hysterical states that he had documented. Bernheim and the other members of the Nancy school were thus posing a form of psychogenic mechanism in opposition to Charcot's

60 See Mark Micale, "Charcot and the Idea of Hysteria in the Male: Gender, Mental Science, and Medical Diagnosis in Late Nineteenth-Century France," *Medical History* 34 (Oct. 1990): 363–411; and Jan Goldstein, *Console and Classify: The French Psychiatric Profession in the Nineteenth Century* (Cambridge, 1987).
61 Ruth Harris, *Murders and Madness: Medicine, Law, and Society in the Fin de Siècle* (Oxford, 1989), chap. 5.
62 Nonne, *Anfang und Ziel*, 76.
63 Ibid., 78.

somaticism. They argued that suggestibility was not a sign of mental pathology; in fact, their work showed that ordinary persons accustomed to obedience, such as soldiers, were easily suggestible.[64]

In Nancy, Nonne enjoyed Bernheim's demonstrations of the bankruptcy of Charcot's ideas. Afterward, he journeyed to Switzerland to the eccentric Auguste Forel, then director of the Burghölzi Sanatorium. Forel was also experimenting with hypnosis and therapy and had a major impact on the young Nonne. "Here it became clear to me how correct Bernheim had been when he attributed Charcot's influence to suggestion and not to his '*passes*.'"[65] But after returning to Hamburg, Nonne seems to have turned his back on what he experienced in France. His research interests over the next two decades chiefly involved the study of organic diseases of the nervous system; his growing reputation in the first decade of the twentieth century owed mostly to work on syphilis and multiple sclerosis.[66]

Nonne reported that he saw his first neurotic patient, a case of psychogenic mutism in a young lieutenant who had participated in the Belgium campaign, already in October 1914. "Then I remembered what I had seen with Forel in Zurich and what I had practiced as an assistant to [Karl] Eisenlohr at Eppendorf. The hypnosis succeeded easily in this case and the lieutenant was suddenly cured." Nonne's skills with hypnosis improved, and his successes were soon recognized, "I gained great confidence in my method and in my ability to carry it out. The clinic became convinced of my special abilities and 'calling'. ... Several assistants helped me; particularly talented was a doctor named Wachsner. Our reputation grew and with it the stream of patients who were sent to us from other hospital stations, where no one had any idea what to do with these people."[67]

Nonne's particular method of hypnosis functioned through suggestion. With hypnosis Nonne could more easily exert his own will over that of the patient; he could convince hypnotized patients that their maladies were not real and lodge that fact in their consciousness. "We use hypnosis," he explained, "so that through the altered state of consciousness we can gain influence over that positive strength of will that enables the symptoms to be overcome."[68] Nonne's suggestive hypnosis constrasts significantly with the more familiar form of hypnotherapy, known as cathartic, which several other doctors, influenced by Freud and Breuer's 1895 theory of hysteria, practiced during the war. The goal of cathartic hypnosis is for the patient to recover

64 See Harris, *Murders and Madness*; and Alan Gauld, *A History of Hypnotism* (Cambridge, 1992), chap. 16.
65 Nonne, *Anfang und Ziel*, 79.
66 Schaltenbrand, "Max Nonne," 43.
67 Ibid., 178.
68 Nonne, "Therapeutische Erfahrungen," 109.

repressed memories (or fantasies) and through abreaction to be cured of neurotic symptoms. In suggestive hypnosis, the patient is treated as the object or recipient of therapy.[69] In the latter method, the doctor retains full control of the therapeutic process, as would a surgeon, and the results occur quickly and predictably, but the condition is not actually cured.

Nonne listed three necessary conditions for success with hypnosis: absolute self-confidence on the doctor's part, complete subordination of the patient, and the creation of an atmosphere in which being cured was, for the patient, a foregone conclusion. He confessed that, when not in the proper mood, he lacked the resolve and concentration to successfully perform hypnotism. "On days with good reports from the front, I was able with the first stroke to almost effortlessly put the man into the desired hypnotic sleep; on gray, unhappy days on the front, my ability to get started was lacking or completely absent."[70] Nonne did acknowledge that he could not cure every case. "A perceptive neuropsychiatrist – and neuropsychiatrists must be perceptive – can tell very soon if there is a 'fluid' [*Fluidum*] between him and the patient. If the fluid isn't there, then all efforts are in vain."[71]

After Nonne demonstrated his technique at the 1915 gathering of the Southwest German Association for Psychiatry and Neurology in Baden-Baden, his method gained national and soon international attention. That same year he had a silent film made about patients with functional psychogenic disorders. The nine-minute film, which is curiously reminiscent of Charcot's photographic depictions of the hysterical states, consists of roughly a dozen before-and-after scenes of patients. First Nonne, clad in his long white coat, presents each patient, wearing only underwear. He demonstrates the patients' symptoms, which include disorders of gait, inability to stand, speech disorders, and "clown-like" hysterical convulsions similar to Charcot's *grande hystérie*. Then follows a cut, after which the patient is seen in his post-treatment condition – after hypnosis or suggestion we are to assume – in almost every case, fully cured.[72]

As his fame grew, Nonne traveled around Germany, lecturing and performing hypnosis before private circles, psychological associations, and groups of military doctors in such cities as Munich, Constance, Koblenz, Berlin, and Metz. He described a Dresden appearance as follows:

69 Ruth Leys, "Traumatic Cures: Shell Shock and the Question of Memory," *Critical Inquiry* 20 (Summer 1994): 623–62.
70 Ibid., 179.
71 Ibid., 183.
72 Max Nonne, *Funktionell-motorische Reiz und Lähmungs Zustände bei Kriegsteilnehmern und deren Heilung durch Suggestion und Hypnose* (Hamburg, 1916). I would like to thank Alfons Labisch for generously allowing me to view this film.

I've almost never experienced a more tense situation as that when Dr. Wachsner and I were led into a great room in which more than seventy war neurotics sat and lay about, surrounded by more than fifty military doctors, who were waiting impatiently and perhaps silently hoping that I too wouldn't get anywhere with these patients. If you know that I always performed my hypnosis alone, that I would find myself alone with the patient in a small room, then it should be clear how difficult this situation was for me, to perform my art before more than 100 eyes, and that this was really not conducive to lifting my self confidence. The first case was only half successful. However I received such applause to my utter amazement that I gained self-confidence and could go after the patients who were brought to me full speed ahead.[73]

During a second visit to Dresden, Nonne appeared before the reserve medical corps of the Saxon army. The king of Saxony was even scheduled to attend, but according to Nonne, lacked the attention span to endure the hour-long lecture and hence changed his mind. Ultimately, Nonne traveled to such distant cities as Riga, Rio de Janeiro, Montevideo, and Buenos Aires to perform his method before enthusiastic audiences.[74]

Nonne's hypnotic therapy did, however, have its share of critics. Detractors condemned it as a step back into prescientific medicine. When Nonne presented his findings before the Association of Hamburg Doctors (*Ärztlicher Verein zu Hamburg*), he was criticized by Kurt Böttiger, who charged that hypnosis degraded both doctors and patients.[75] Through hypnosis, the doctor suppresses the patient's feelings and imagination, but at the same time, degrades himself by pretending to believe in medieval nonsense in order to achieve the full effect. Böttiger claimed that he preferred to appeal to the patient's sense of reason, in short to heal the patient by enlightening him about the virtues of serving the fatherland, rather than forcing or tricking his symptoms away.

An even harsher attack came from the Leipzig doctor, Erwin Niessl von Maiendorf. Niessl wrote that hypnotism actually worsened the condition of neurosis sufferers; he doubted the authenticity of Nonne's public appearances:

But where the shaking disappears suddenly upon waking up out of hypnosis, it is a question only of successful theater for the self-aggrandizement of the performing doctor, but it is never really a cure. It is convenient for the hypnotist to say, "the man is now capable of field duty," he gets rid of him as quickly as possible and sends him away from his field of vision. But if one were to follow up such alleged cures with

73   Nonne, *Anfang und Ziel*, 180–1.
74   Ibid., 179, 181.
75   Kurt Böttiger, "Diskussion zum Vortrag Nonne: Zur therapeutischen Verwendung der Hypnose bei Fällen von Kriegshysterie," *Neurologisches Zentralblatt* 35 (1916): 261–2.

objective examinations, one would find the well known fact that *hysteria is never cured through suggestion* [emphasis his].[76]

This critique echoes the general disapproval of hypnosis among established physicians in Germany before the war. Even as Nonne was dazzling medical and military authorities with his traveling hypnosis show, many German states were cracking down on the proliferating incidence of nonlicensed *hypnotiseurs*. Immediately after the war attempts were made to revive a 1910 bill that would have made hypnosis, when performed by an unlicensed practitioner, harshly punishable.[77] The increased presence of so-called quacks was attributed by Prussian authorities to both the war-induced shortage of doctors at home and the hysterical and nervous civilian population.[78] In such volatile times, hypnosis was considered particularly dangerous; even its representation in film was censored.[79]

Nonne's revival of hypnosis can be made clearer when reexamined in light of his confrontation with Hermann Oppenheim and his sojourn in France. Nonne's attack on Oppenheim and Bernheim's challenge of Charcot have striking parallels. In both cases a younger man, early in his career, championed psychogenicism and the therapeutic potential of suggestion against a dominant neurologist whose career was associated with the materialist explanation of neurosis. In Nonne's case his belief in suggestion and psychogenicism put him on the side of a growing number of German university neurologists and psychiatrists, whereas Oppenheim's views were typical of marginal doctors, many of whom were Jewish and in private practice.[80] By humiliating Oppenheim, Nonne may have been enjoying his belated revenge against Charcot. At the same time he was certainly aiding his own professional ascent and contributing to the triumph of German university science over the threat of a costly "pension neurosis" epidemic.

76 E. Niessl von Maiendorf, "Über pathologische Tremorformen zur Kriegszeit," *Monatschrift für Psychiatrie und Neurologie* 23 (1916): 221–36.
77 "Entwurf eines Gesetzes gegen Missstände im Heilgewerbe." *Verhandlungen des Reichstages* XII Legislative Periode, 2. Session, 1909–11, Bd. 277 (1909–10), 2759.
78 See, e.g., a letter from the Ministerium des Innern to the Berlin Polizeipräsidium, Oct. 6, 1919, Geheimes Staatsarchiv Preussischer Kulturbesitz, Berlin-Dahlem, I. HA Rep. 76, Kultusministerium, VIII B Akte Nr. 1325, Bl. 258, "Anwendung des Hypnotismus und des Magnetismus zu Heilzwecken."
79 See Harris, *Murders and Madness*; letters between Karl Bonhoeffer and a Dr. Bulcke of the Film Censorship Office, Reichs Ministry of the Interior, Archiv der Humboldt-Universität zu Berlin, Charité, Nervenklinik, Akte Nr. 37, "Gesetzte u. Gesetzesentwürfe Reichsgesundheitsamt (Erbgesetz), 1922–1934."
80 Whether Oppenheim's Jewishness played a role is a question that demands more research. For an interesting evocation of the observation that Jewish doctors were more likely to tend toward somaticism, see Edward Shorter, *From Paralysis to Fatigue: A History of Psychosomatic Illness* (New York, 1992), 219–20.

FRITZ KAUFMANN AND CONTROVERSY OVER ELECTROTHERAPY

It is the great contribution of a Mannheimer, a very humane neuropsychiatrist [*Nervenarzt*] whom I know well, Dr. Fritz Kaufmann, that he has devoted all of his strength and energy to treating and curing these shakers and stutterers, as well as other hysterical conditions. By reaching back to well-known methods that have been proven over decades, he has succeeded, through the application of electric current… in completely curing stubborn cases and in rendering the patients, even if as occasionally, unable to serve in the war, completely capable of working. This treatment was quickly taken up all over Germany (in France, Austria and Hungary as well) and the most glowing reports of success have been coming from all sides.

Dr. Robert Gaupp[81]

Without doubt, electrotherapy was the most controversial method of treatment employed during the war; the deaths and injuries it caused epitomize the worst wartime breeches of medical ethics. Freud's testimony in Werner Wagner-Jauregg's trial over the usage of electrotherapy is one of the most dramatic and well-known episodes in medicine during this period.[82] Less known are the proceedings against several other doctors and popular protests against brutality and severe pension policies. Here Kaufmann's method will be discussed as a second example of the revival of old therapeutic methods into the neuropsychiatric repertoire.

As popularized by Fritz Kaufmann, electric current was one component in a therapeutic regimen that included strict military discipline and suggestive preparation. In his initial presentation of the so-called overpowering method in 1916, Kaufmann lamented that, with the exception of Nonne's work with hypnosis, most treatments were ineffective or of short duration.[83] He proposed instead an active method that "forced" patients to be cured, and hence addressed the pension problem and the labor shortage simultaneously.

The first step in Kaufmann's four-step method involved preparing the patient psychologically for the upcoming treatment session. The patient had to be informed that the session would be painful and most importantly that he would be cured in it. The second step involved the application of

---

81 Robert Gaupp, "Die Behandlung der nervösen Schüttellähmung durch starke elektrische Ströme," Archiv der Eberhard-Karls-Universität, Tübingen, Akte Nr. 308/89, "Kriegsneurose."

82 Eissler, *Freud as Expert Witness.*

83 See Fritz Kaufmann, "Die planmässige Heilung komplizierter psychogener Bewegungsstörungen bei Soldaten in einer Sitzung," *Münchener Medizinische Wochenschrift, Feldärztliche Beilage* 63 (1916): 802–4.

alternating current in cycles of two- to five-minute bursts, followed by exercises. All the while, the third component, military subordination and discipline, was to be followed. That is, during the cycles of current and exercise, military orders were to be given and the patient's subordinate rank to the doctor would be constantly emphasized. Kaufmann's fourth requirement was the doctor's conviction that once the treatment began, it could not be stopped before complete curing. That is, if the doctor relented, then the condition would become "fixed" and thus nearly impossible to remove.

Kaufmann claimed that his method was superior to Nonne's hypnosis for two reasons. It required less skill and training to not do harm to the patient with electricity than with the far more dangerous hypnosis, and with hypnosis there was, according to Kaufmann, always the danger that the treatment could actually strengthen the patient's resistance to being cured.[84]

Kaufmann of course did not invent treatment with electric current; its history purportedly stretches back to ancient times when Galen used the shocks from electric eels to treat gout.[85] Around the beginning of the nineteenth century, electrotherapy was first used to treat hysterical disorders, but only in the late nineteenth century did it become a common therapeutic method among psychiatrists. However, by the turn of the century, its usage began to wane as doctors lost faith in its uniquely curative powers and saw that ordinary suggestion could achieve equivalent results.[86]

In a manner similar to Nonne, who had witnessed hypnosis during his early training, Kaufmann recalled having observed electrotherapy at Wilhelm Erb's neurological clinic in Heidelberg where he had worked as an assistant at the beginning of the century; Nonne and Gaupp, too, had served as assistants at the prestigious clinic.[87] The symptoms exhibited by war neurotics reminded Kaufmann of a young female hysteric who had been cured there through a combination of verbal suggestion and painful alternating current. But there was a crucial difference between earlier forms of electric treatment and its application in the treatment of war neuroses. Previously pain had been considered an undesirable but necessary side effect of electrotherapy, which was used for the healing properties attributed to electric current. In particular after the discovery of the electric properties of the brain and nervous system and in consequence of the enormous hopes pinned on electricity as an agent

---

84 The advantages of nonverbal suggestion in Austria-Hungary were clear because doctors often faced patients with whom they shared no common language. Eissler, *Freud as Expert Witness*, 52.

85 Edward Stainbrook, "The Use of Electricity in Psychiatric Treatment during the Nineteenth Century," *Bulletin of the History of Medicine* 22 (1948): 156. See also Michael Hubenstorf, "Elektrizität und Medizin," in Rolf Winau, ed., *Technik und Medizin* (Düsseldorf, 1993): 241–57.

86 Stainbrook, "Electricity," 175.

87 Kaufmann, "Planmässige Heilung."

of modernization, miraculous healing powers were ascribed to electric current. But in the treatment of war neurotics, it was precisely the pain and the shock and not other qualities of the electricity that were considered the curative agents. Most wartime practitioners of electrotherapy credited its remarkable healing powers to its suggestive effect, which was generally believed to be strengthened by hierarchical military relationships.[88]

The appeal of electrotherapy lay in its speed and reliability; curing rates of 97 percent were not uncommon.[89] Furthermore, its usage of the trappings of technology made it appear more modern and thus less offensive than hypnosis and other "old-fashioned" techniques to modern research psychiatrists. Gaupp was a staunch defender of the method and intervened to protect several of its practitioners, but it is doubtful that he used it himself. "Recently a document was published in which an author reports that he cured 270 hysterical shakers, each in one electrotherapeutic session ... what would it lead to if we gave up active treatment just to avoid the self-pitying complaints of hysterics?"[90] Robert Sommer proposed a method of electrotherapy that required only a source of electricity and a rheostat for resistance. It was not only inexpensive but also viable even outside of the special neurosis hospitals.[91] Others praised the power of electrotherapy to cure instantly longstanding cases. As stated by Wilmanns,

[A] very significant step forward in the treatment of hysterical neuroses is the introduction of electric current as a suggestive method of curing and its adaptation to the particular military relations. ... Patients who were stuck in bed for months and years with paralyzed limbs, who needed wheelchairs and had become dependent on those around for help were freed from their symptoms in a few minutes with the impressive procedure.[92]

But electric treatment met with growing opposition in medical as well as lay spheres; several doctors, alarmed by reported instances of death and serious injury in late 1916 and 1917, warned of its abuse.[93] However, ethical criticism of the method was rare among doctors; they generally lauded its therapeutic efficacy while urging more cautious applications of the method,

88 I am indebted to Heinz-Peter Schmiedebach for this observation.
89 Birnbaum, "Ergebnisse."
90 Robert Gaupp, letter to K. Württemberg Gericht der stellv. 53. Infantriebrigade, Ulm, May 24, 1917, Archiv der Eberhard-Karls-Universität, Tübingen, Akte Nr. 308/42, "Gaupp."
91 Rossbach, "Kurzer Bericht über den Kurs über Elektrodiagnostik und Elektrotherapie in Giessen am 2. und 3. April 1917, BayHStA, Stellv. Gen. Kom. des I. Armee Korps, Akte Nr. 189, "Besondere Heilverfahren."
92 Wilmanns, "Bericht," 43.
93 T. Christen, "Schädigung durch Sinusströme," *Deutsche Medizinische Wochenschrift* 43 (1917): 1536–7; M. Lewandowsky, "Über den Tod durch Sinusströme," *Deutsche Medizinische Wochenschrift* 43 (1917): 1169. For the opinion of an early critic of Kaufmann who changed his mind, see Kurt Mendel, "Die Kaufmannsche Methode," *Neurologisches Zentralblatt* 36 (1917): 181–93.

more thorough screening out of patients with weak hearts, and application of current only to insensitive body parts.[94]

Patients took their complaints against particularly brutal doctors to their political representatives and to local welfare offices.[95] Medical brutality in general was discussed in the Bavarian *Landtag*, and in several cases *Landtag* deputies called upon state officials to monitor particular doctors.[96] At least two Württemberg physicians, Martin Freund and Gustav Liebermeister, were singled out for allegedly brutal electrotherapy. In both cases Gaupp came to their defense. "It may be that advancing experience will succeed in making painful electric current superfluous; but it can be said with certainty that at the time when Liebermeister took up the strong faradisation of hysterics, which brought on him the court's accusations, what he practiced was the best and most successful procedure."[97] Gaupp also lamented that popular intrusions into medical affairs made it more difficult for doctors to do their jobs. For suggestive methods to be effective, unquestioning faith in the doctor was necessary. Kaufmann himself does not seem to have been subjected to such attacks. In 1917 he claimed that other doctors were more "Kaufmannish" than he and that his method had become milder with time.[98] Kaufmann continually stressed that current only be applied in short bursts and by highly qualified doctors.

Yet, complaints against brutal electrotherapy increased. Due to the perception of a deepening public mistrust in doctors, the Ministry of War launched a public relations campaign. It called for doctors to avoid any actions and utterances that might give the impression of brutality and encouraged the usage of hypnosis and other, milder treatments instead of electric current.[99] But at the same time, communications from the Ministry of War stressed its support of and faith in its doctors and its reluctance to interfere in their affairs.[100]

94 H. Boruttau, "Todesfälle durch Sinusströme," *Deutsche Medizinische Wochenschrift* 43 (1917): 808–9.
95 See "Beschwerde über Begutachtung und Gutachter," Bundesarchiv, Abteilung Potsdam, Reichsarbeitsministerium, film no. 36027.
96 See Archiv der Eberhard-Karls-Universität, Tübingen, Akte Nr. 308/42, "Gaupp."
97 Robert Gaupp, letter to Königliches Württemberg Gericht der stellv. 53. Infantriebrigade, Ulm, May 24, 1917, Archiv der Eberhard-Karls-Universität, Tübingen, Akte Nr. 308/42, "Gaupp."
98 See Fritz Kaufmann's comments in "Verhandlungen des Deutschen Vereins für Psychiatrie zu München am 21. und 22. September 1916," *Allgemeine Zeitschrift für Psychiatrie* 73 (1917): 162–233.
99 Letter from Generalarzt Georg Friedrich Wilhelm Schultzen, Sanitätsdepartement des Kriegsministeriums, to Gaupp, Archiv der Eberhard-Karls-Universität, Tübingen, Akte Nr. 308/89, "Kriegsneurose"; "Zusammenkunft der Kriegsneurotiker-Ärzte," *Münchener Medizinische Wochenschrift* 65 (1918): 1226-7.
100 Letter from Friedrich K. E. von Ammon, Kriegsministerium to Sanitätsamt, 8. August 1918, BayHStA, Stellv. Gen. Kom. des II. Armee Korps, Bd. 14, Akte 1.

The Ministry of War also suggested that neurosis stations be opened for visits by members of the press. Articles appeared praising the work of Germany's doctors and seeking to dispel rumors of brutal and abusive treatment. An article in the Würzburger *Generalanzeiger* concluded with the following accolade, "We are convinced that anyone who, as we, can have a look at this neurosis station, will say: this is neither a prison nor a torture chamber, rather a modern, exemplary institution, which deserves endless praise and further expansion."[101]

THE CONTINUITY QUESTION

The experience of millions of soldiers in World War I was characterized by the high visibility of doctors; frequent hospital visits, examinations, transfers, and reassignments typified the widespread medicalization of life that occurred during the war, and the nearly five million men who reported wounded and the fifteen million ill testify to the tremendous role that German medicine played in the war.[102] War neurotics were particularly affected by this process, as they were subjected to an enclosed system that guided them from central observation stations through treatment and into the workforce.

Long after the war, medicine continued to play a decisive role in the lives of veterans and their families. Pension questions formed the terrain upon which issues of medical control were contested through the 1920s and one area in which the memory of the war was worked out. For former war neurotics, pension claims were seldom successful; they often meant humiliation by unsympathetic doctors and countless reexaminations. Particularly after a 1926 ruling overturned the legal status of traumatic neurosis, doctors were even less likely to award pensions for the psychological consequences of military duty.[103] Patients responded to these experiences with public demonstrations against doctors known for brutality or stingy pension-practices, and in the November Revolution, rebellions in the neurosis stations led to acts of patient revenge against terrified medical officers.[104]

Treating war neurosis meant the assertion of psychiatric control over issues that lay in a gray area between legal, military, and medical spheres. The

101 "Im Lazarett für Kriegs-Nervenkranke: Eine Besprechung durch Pressevertreter," *Würzburger Generalanzeiger*, Oct. 31, 1918, BayHStA, Stellv. Gen. Kom. des II. Armee Korps, Bd. 14, Akte 1.
102 See Bessel, *Germany After the First World War*, 6.
103 See Eghigian, "Bürokratie"; and Robert W. Whalen, *Bitter Wounds: German Victims of the Great War, 1914-1939* (Ithaca, N.Y., 1984), chap. 4.
104 See the description of the Revolution in Ernst Kretschmer, *Gestalten und Gedanken* (Stuttgart, 1963), 94; also "Beschwerde über Begutachtung und Gutachter," Bundesarchiv, Abteilung Potsdam, Reichsarbeitsministerium, film no. 36027.

medical discourse that elided patriotism, work, and mental health sharpened the political dimensions that had always been a part of medical practice. In such a way, doctors gained control over the fates of thousands of individuals and could use treatment sessions to reinforce their hierarchical superiority and to preach their moral and political values to their patients. At the same time, in the context of increasing manpower needs both in industry and in the field, the goal of individual health was eclipsed by the needs of the "national community," and psychiatrists and neurologists developed a system whose administration of patients paralleled industrial management of matériel. But, as this essay has tried to show, inseparable from this discourse of control was also a discourse of healing. To be sure, the methods involved were often brutal and inhumane, but as we have seen, neurotic soldiers were removed from the field, and in most cases medical treatment brought an end to debilitating symptoms and enabled patients to return to work.

The methods of active treatment developed in World War I were incorporated in the psychiatric reform movement of the 1920s. The implementation of work therapy created a more pleasant and normalized environment for asylum inmates, but it was also part of a rationalized system that responded to Weimar's economic crises by prioritizing the treatment of the mentally ill based on their perceived value to society.[105] Similar ambiguities characterized other Weimar era reform movements such as sex reform and social hygiene, whose genuinely emancipatory strands coexisted uneasily with the controlling supervision of experts and medical professionals.[106] These movements, just as the treatment of neurosis in World War I, should not be seen as precedents for the ethical abominations committed by doctors under fascism, but rather as heralding the often ambiguous role of medical professionals in the modern welfare state.

---

105 See Hans-Ludwig Siemen, "Reform und Radikalisierung der Psychiatrie in der Weltwirtschaftskrise," in Norbert Frei, ed., *Medizin und Gesundheitspolitik in der NS-Zeit* (Munich, 1991): 191–200; Karl-Heinz Roth, "Psychosomatische Medizin und 'Euthanasia': Der Fall Viktor von Weizsäcker," *1999: Zeitschrift für Sozialgeschichte des 20. und 21. Jahrhunderts* 1 (Jan. 1986): 65–99.
106 See Grossmann, "New Woman"; Weindling, "Social Hygiene."

7

Sterilization and "Medical" Massacres in National Socialist Germany

Ethics, Politics, and the Law

GISELA BOCK

The place in the history of medicine in Germany of Nazi sterilization policy and the massacres in which medicine and medical doctors were involved, especially the politics of "euthanasia," is by no means self-evident. Sterilization is a form of birth control that may be contested but is today usually considered legitimate; the concept of euthanasia has oscillated, from the late nineteenth century, between voluntary and nonvoluntary death, between one's own and someone else's control over one's death. The question therefore is that of birth control and death control, of the agents, circumstances, and purposes of such control. Birth and death are multifaceted issues, and many of their aspects are dealt with by medical theory, practice, and the medical profession, particularly in the nineteenth and twentieth centuries. It was (and is) the task of medical theory and practice to help new creatures come into the world and help them and the other human beings to live and survive by curing and healing. But it is not this task that defines the place of sterilization and euthanasia in the history of medicine from 1933 to 1945 but the fact that medical theory and practice largely took an opposite turn. Medicine and many doctors came to be involved in the National Socialist crimes. Furthermore, they were among the most important agents of these crimes, precisely because procreation and death came to be objects of National Socialist policy, of race hygiene, eugenics, or, to use the specifically Nazi term, *Erb- und Rassenpflege* (genetic and racial hygiene). Healing, killing, and the relationship between the two were redefined, and this new relationship finally led to what has been aptly called "medicalized killing."[1] From its

---

1 Robert Jay Lifton, *The Nazi Doctors: Medical Killing and the Psychology of Genocide* (New York, 1986). The relationship of healing and killing is a focus of recent research: *Volk und Gesundheit: Heilen und Vernichten im Nationalsozialismus* (Tübingen, 1982); *Heilen und Vernichten im Nationalsozialismus: Köln und das Rheinland* (Cologne, 1985); Angelika Ebbinghaus et al., eds., *Heilen und Vernichten im Mustergau Hamburg* (Hamburg, 1984). For the concept of and debate on "euthanasia" from the late nineteenth century, see Hans-Walter Schmuhl, *Rassenhygiene, Nationalsozialismus, Euthanasie: Von*

149

beginnings in 1933, the National Socialist regime claimed "the supremacy of the state in the field of life, marriage, and the family." It was first and foremost a claim for state-run birth control, formulated with respect and in the official commentary to the law to "prevent hereditarily diseased offspring" of July 14, 1933, which provided for compulsory and mass sterilizations on eugenic grounds.[2] This kind of supremacy of the state expressed the fact that race hygiene was now elevated to the status of an official doctrine of the regime, which proclaimed the need for a "prevention of worthless life" (*Verhütung unwerten Lebens*) and for its eradication (*Ausmerze*) by means of sterilization. Until 1945 about 400,000 people were sterilized on the basis of this law and its subsequent modifications (including about 40,000 persons in the territories that were annexed beginning in 1938).[3] By 1939 the supremacy over life had come to include the power over death: the policy of "annihilation of life unworthy of living" (*Vernichtung lebensunwerten Lebens*), or euthanasia. Its victims were largely inmates of psychiatric clinics, but also ill people in other institutions, including concentration camps, and between 1939 and 1945 their overall number has been estimated to be about 200,000.[4] The massacre of the ill in particular, but also eugenics at large, were intertwined in important ways with anti-Jewish policies and the genocide of the Jewish people. Medicine and many doctors played a crucial role in all of these National Socialist policies, and they did so to differing degrees in the various phases and strands of these policies.

In the immediate postwar years, studies by Alice Platen-Hallermund, Alexander Mitscherlich, Fred Mielke, and others of the massacre of the ill remained few and far between and were known only to specialists; but in general publications on the policy of eugenic sterilization were usually

---

der *Verhütung* zur *Vernichtung "lebensunwerten Lebens,"* (Göttingen, 1987). Because of the ambiguities of the term I use quotation marks. The translations from German in this chapter are mine.

2 Arthur Gütt, Ernst Rüdin, and Falk Ruttke, *Gesetz zur Verhütung erbkranken Nachwuchses vom 14. Juli 1933 etc.* (Munich, 1934), 5.

3 Gisela Bock, *Zwangssterilisation im Nationalsozialismus* (Opladen, 1986), 232–8. There were almost 400,000 informal denunciations for sterilization in 1934 and 1935 (no overall figures are available for later years), about 430,000 formal applications in 1933–39, 200,000 court decisions in favor of sterilization in 1934–36, almost 200,000 actual sterilizations from 1934 to mid-1937. In the following eight years, probably 160,000 sterilizations were performed in the Germany of the 1937 borders, and 40,000 in the annexed territories (no figures are available for the occupied territories where harsher laws were introduced or for the sterilizations outside the 1933 law). These figures are close to the estimates of the federal ministries of Finance (320,000 within the borders of 1937) and Justice (350,000) in the 1950s and 1960s. Kurt Nowak extrapolates a higher, but improbable, figure of 460,000 in his "Sterilisation und 'Euthanasie' im Dritten Reich," *Geschichte in Wissenschaft und Unterricht* 39 (1988): 331.

4 Ernst Klee; *"Euthanasie" im NS-Staat* (Frankfurt/Main, 1983), 5 (several hundreds of thousands); Götz Aly, ed., *Aktion T 4: 1939–1945: Die "Euthanasie"-Zentrale in der Tiergartenstrasse 4* (Berlin, 1989), 4 ("almost 200,000") and 11 ("over 200,000"). The exact number of the victims until 1941 is known to be 70,273. See Schmuhl, *Rassenhygiene*, 189, 213, 219, 236, 239, 247.

apologetic in tone.[5] But even though serious historical research – by medical scholars, historians, and others – started late,[6] many of the basic facts of the two phenomena with which this chapter mainly deals, sterilization and euthanasia, are by now quite definitely established. Nonetheless, their precise historical and political meaning continues to be contested. The debate focuses on the what, why, how, and when of the various policies and is supported by a growing number of local and regional studies. The respective answers given also imply different views of the positions taken and the roles played by medicine, psychiatry, and doctors in the regime's ideology and institutional and political practice.

Since the early 1980s, when National Socialist eugenics and medicine came to be explored more closely, several authors adopted one of the major Nazi concepts for the genocide of the Jews – the "final solution of the Jewish question" – by identifying race hygiene, sterilization, and especially euthanasia as "the final solution of the social question" (*Endlösung der sozialen Frage*). They believed these policies to be motivated by economic considerations prevailing in a capitalist and imperialist regime, namely, those of utility, efficiency, and profit; in addition, they maintained that the massacre of the Jews was rooted in such economic and utilitarian considerations as well. National Socialist race hygiene has thus been viewed as an integral part of the long-term processes of "modernization" and "rationalization."[7] Other scholars, in particular historians, argue that it was not so much an outgrowth of modernity or modernization but of a crisis of modernity, that it expresses

5   Alice Platen-Hallermund, *Die Tötung Geisteskranker in Deutschland* (Frankfurt/Main, 1948; reprinted: Bonn, 1993), originally in *Hippokrates* 18 (1947) and 19 (1948); Alexander Mitscherlich and Fred Mielke, *Das Diktat der Menschenverachtung* (Heidelberg, 1947), reprinted as *Wissenschaft ohne Menschlichkeit* (1949) and *Medizin ohne Menschlichkeit* (1960ff); Dolf Sternberger and Karl Jaspers et al., "Dokumente zu den Geisteskranken-Morden," *Die Wandlung* 2 (1947): 160–8. For the postwar views on Nazi crimes, see Falk Pingel, "Die NS-Psychiatrie im Spiegel des historischen Bewusstseins und sozialpolitischen Denkens in der Bundesrepublik," in Franz-Werner Kersting et al., eds., *Nach Hadamar: Zum Verhältnis von Psychiatrie und Gesellschaft im 20. Jahrhundert* (Paderborn, 1993), 174–201.

6   See note 1 and *Medizin im Nationalsozialismus: Kolloquien des Instituts für Zeitgeschichte* (Munich, 1988); Michael H. Kater, *Doctors Under Hitler* (Chapel Hill, N.C., 1989); Norbert Frei, ed., *Medizin und Gesundheitspolitik in der NS-Zeit* (Munich, 1991); *Mediziner im "Dritten Reich*," special issue of *Geschichte und Gesellschaft* 14, no. 4 (1990).

7   Karl Heinz Roth and Götz Aly, "Das Gesetz über die Sterbehilfe bei unheilbar Kranken," in Karl Heinz Roth, ed., *Erfassung zur Vernichtung: Von der Sozialhygiene zum "Gesetz über Sterbehilfe"* (Berlin, 1984), 101–79; Karl Heinz Roth, "Ein Mustergau gegen die Armen, Leistungsschwachen und 'Gemeinschaftsunfähigen,'" in Ebbinghaus et al., eds., *Heilen und Vernichten*, 7–17; Götz Aly, "Der saubere und der schmutzige Fortschritt," in Götz Aly et al., *Reform und Gewissen: "Euthanasie" im Dienst des Fortschritts* (Berlin, 1985), 9–78; Götz Aly et al., *Aussonderung und Tod: Die klinische Hinrichtung der Unbrauchbaren* (Berlin, 1985); Klaus Dörner, *Tödliches Mitleid: Zur Frage der Unerträglichkeit des Lebens, oder: die Soziale Frage: Entstehung, Medizinierung, Endlösung – heute, morgen* (Gütersloh, 1988). For a summary and criticism of the "modernization" approach, see Norbert Frei, "Wie modern war der Nationalsozialismus?" *Geschichte und Gesellschaft* 19 (1993): 367–87.

the dark side of modern historical progress, which contains an ambivalent potential not only for humane improvement but also for human destruction, and they point to a "pathology" or an "ambivalence of modernity." Moreover, the late Detlev Peukert has placed the eugenic policies of National Socialism in the context of an overall, eugenic as well as ethnic *Endlösung*, which he, even though rejecting a merely one-dimensional explanation, believed to originate largely in the contemporary "spirit of science," including medical science.[8] Many years ago Karl Dietrich Bracher and, more recently, Dirk Blasius, Peukert, and others have identified Nazi race hygiene as part and parcel of Nazi racism and the complex race policy and have sought to explain the relationship between eugenic racism, in particular sterilization and "euthanasia," and ethnic racism, which focused on the persecution of "alien" ethnic or religious groups, most of all the Jews. Eugenic racism came to be identified as a kind of racism that used scientific means and methods, that is, as scientific racism.[9] Blasius also strongly advocated an approach that places the concept of humane ethics (*Humanität, Menschlichkeit*) at the center of the analysis – the problem of the crisis, undermining, loss, and the end of humane standards – and he does so with reference to Thomas Mann's concept of a "defection from humanity" (*Abfall vom Humanen*).[10] In a similar vein, here I focus on the process of dehumanization and do so by placing medicine and

8   Detlev J. K. Peukert, "Die Genesis der 'Endlösung' aus dem Geiste der Wissenschaft," in *Zerstörung des moralischen Selbstbewusstseins*, ed. Forum für Philosophie Bad Homburg (Frankfurt/Main, 1988), 24–48; Dirk Blasius, "Ambivalenzen des Fortschritts: Psychiatrie und psychisch Kranke in der Geschichte der Moderne," in Frank Bajohr et al., eds., *Zivilisation und Barbarei: Die widersprüchlichen Potentiale der Moderne: Detlev Peukert zum Gedenken* (Hamburg, 1991), 253–68.

9   Karl Dietrich Bracher, "Stufen der Machtergreifung," in Karl Dietrich Bracher et al., *Die national-sozialistische Machtergreifung* (Cologne, 1962), 274–86; Willi Dressen, "Euthanasie," in Eugen Kogon et al., eds., *Nationalsozialistische Massentötungen durch Giftgas* (Frankfurt/Main, 1983), 28 ("Die rassistische Absicht"); Dirk Blasius, "Die 'Maskerade des Bösen': Psychiatrische Forschung in der NS-Zeit," in Frei, ed., *Medizin und Gesundheitspolitik*, 265–85; Peukert, "Genesis der 'Endlösung'"; Peukert, "Alltag und Barbarei: Zur Normalität des Dritten Reiches," in Dan Diner, ed., *Ist der Nationalsozialismus Geschichte? Zu Historisierung und Historikerstreit* (Frankfurt/Main, 1987), 51–61; Peukert, "Rassismus und 'Endlösungs'-Utopie," in Christoph Klessmann, ed., *Nicht nur Hitlers Krieg: Der Zweite Weltkrieg und die Deutschen* (Düsseldorf, 1989), 71–82; Bock, *Zwangssterilisation*, 59–76, 100–115, chap. 6; Bock, "Krankenmord, Judenmord und nationalsozialistische Rassenpolitik: Überlegungen zu einigen neueren Forschungshypothesen," in Bajohr et al., eds., *Zivilisation und Barbarei*, 285–306; Paul Weindling, *Health, Race and German Politics Between National Unification and Nazism, 1870–1945* (Cambridge, 1989); Robert N. Proctor, *Racial Hygiene: Medicine under the Nazis* (Cambridge, Mass., 1988); Stefan Kühl, *The Nazi Connection: Eugenics, American Racism, and German National Socialism* (New York, 1994), 70–2.

10   Thomas Mann to Albert Oppenheimer, Feb. 12, 1949, in Thomas Mann, *Dichter über ihre Dichtungen*, vol. 3: *1944–1955*, ed. Hans Wysling (Passau, 1981), 223. Dirk Blasius, "Die Ordnung der Gesellschaft: Zum historischen Stellenwert der NS-Psychiatrie," in Klaus Dörner, ed., *Fortschritte der Psychiatrie im Umgang mit Menschen* (Rehburg-Loccum, 1984), 13–21; Dirk Blasius, "Das Ende der Humanität: Psychiatrie und Krankenmord in der NS-Zeit," in Walter H. Pehle, ed., *Der historische Ort des Nationalsozialismus* (Frankfurt/Main, 1990), 47–71. See also the title concepts of Mitscherlich's and Mielke's publication.

doctors in their political context. In this context, referring to humane ethics and values – understood as equality of all human beings as well as special care for the ill and the weak – does not mean applying simply an ahistorical moralistic yardstick. Rather the concept is being used as an analytic instrument. Moreover, as will be seen, the concept *Humanität* was by no means alien to the Nazi discourse itself, precisely because this discourse rejected it.

Various explanations have been put forward – some of them contradicting, some complementing, each other – with regard to how Nazi eugenic policies emerged, were put into practice, and were radicalized. Historians have highlighted the transition from "ideas into politics" and thus have underlined the power of ideas or ideology as the origin, cause, and driving force behind radicalization.[11] Others who doubt the power of mere ideas or destructive impulses have adapted the debate on "intentional" versus "structural" explanations of the Holocaust to the analysis of sterilization and euthanasia. They tend to downplay pre-1933 expressions of such ideas as unrealistic metaphors, to find little originality in Nazi race hygienic ideas, to consider them as no more than a "peripheral element of Nazi ideology" and the euthanasia program as "not genuinely National Socialist." In this view, what was specifically National Socialist – and therefore the cause of the events in question – was not ideology, but rather the particular functioning and structure of Nazi political decision making: a cumulative dynamic caused by charismatic legitimation and the chaos of polycratic centers that competed for power.[12] Others have justly pointed out that any explanation should take into account not only ideas but also – and more importantly – institutions and bureaucracies, particularly as factors that lowered the normal moral checks against interference in body and life and raised the destructive potential; the institutions involved in eugenic policies did not so much compete with as reinforce each other.[13] In very recent years, major scholars in the field seem to share – against some rather dogmatic formulas and unilinear explanations – a new emphasis on the multicausality of origins, complexity of transitions, and plurality of meanings.[14] This emphasis also invites an exploration of some

11 See Jeremy Noakes' important article, "Nazism and Eugenics: The Background to the Nazi Sterilization Law of 14 July 1933," published in Roger J. Bullen, Hartmut Pogge von Strandmann, and Antony B. Polonsky, eds., *Ideas into Politics* (London, 1984), 75–94.

12 Schmuhl, *Rassenhygiene*, 132, 360, 370 (quotes). No weight is therefore attributed, e.g., to Hitler's public advocacy of sterilization and extermination of the "weak" in 1929 (152–3).

13 Alfons Labisch and Florian Tennstedt, "Gesundheitsamt oder Amt für Volksgesundheit? Zur Entwicklung des öffentlichen Gesundheitsdienstes seit 1933," in Frei, ed., *Medizin und Gesundheitspolitik*, 51; Alfons Labisch and Florian Tennstedt, *Der Weg zum Gesetz über die Vereinheitlichung des Gesundheitswesens vom 3. Juli 1934*, 2 vols. (Düsseldorf, 1985).

14 Dan Diner, "Rationalisierung und Methode: Zu einem neuen Erklärungsversuch der 'Endlösung,'" in *Vierteljahrshefte für Zeitgeschichte* 40 (1992): 359–82; Dirk Blasius, *"Einfache Seelenstörung": Geschichte der deutschen Psychiatrie, 1800-1945* (Frankfurt/Main, 1994).

perplexing complexities, such as the unexpected discovery that psychiatrist Gerhard Schmidt's famous analysis, written in 1947 and one of the first studies of euthanasia, was not published on the advice of Karl Jaspers and Kurt Schneider. Critics and onetime opponents of euthanasia, they advised Schmidt not to publish his work because they gave a higher priority to supporting the psychiatric profession's search for a new respectability. Schmidt's study was published only in 1965, now with a preface by Jaspers.[15]

Finally, as to the "when," the debate over the specifically historical dimension, that of time and transitions, continuity and discontinuity, continues. Did it all begin in the early nineteenth century or even earlier,[16] with Charles Darwin,[17] or in the late nineteenth century, with Sir Francis Galton, Ploetz, and Schallmayer?[18] Or is the historical divide rather to be identified in World War I and the ensuing cultural and political crises (earlier voices being isolated or a minority, not trends)? Or does the year 1933 mark the substantial divide, signifying the political event that encouraged and enabled destructive features of eugenics and medicine to come to the fore? Is the massacre of the ill begun in 1939 – with the massacres in conquered Poland[19] – essentially an outgrowth of the previous eugenic sterilization policy or should we rather emphasize the profound and obvious differences between state-run birth control and outright murder and, especially, the radicalizing impact of World War II? This chapter therefore focuses on continuities and discontinuities with respect to the year 1933 and the periods before as well as after Nazism's rise to power.

When the Hitler cabinet enacted the law for compulsory sterilization in 1933, the underlying race hygienic or eugenic discourse had already been elaborated in its entirety. It included several elements that highlight the important role of medicine in German eugenics – a role that points to a

15 Gerhard Schmidt, *Selektion in der Heilanstalt, 1939–1945* (Stuttgart, 1965). Kurt Schneider was a prominent member of the medical profession during the Nazi years. See Blasius, "Ende der Humanität"; Blasius, "Psychiatrie und Krankenmord in der NS-Zeit: Probleme historischer Urteilsbildung," in Ralf Seidel and Wolfang Franz Werner, eds., *Psychiatrie im Abgrund* (Puhlheim-Brauweiler, 1991), 126–38. For other scholars who argued against publication of Schmidt's study, see Hendrik van den Bussche, "'Zusammenbruch' und Nachkriegszeit," in Bussche, ed., *Medizinische Wissenschaft im "Dritten Reich"* (Berlin, 1989), 440–1. An excellent update of Schmidt's work on Eglfing-Haar is Bernhard Richarz, *Heilen, Pflegen, Töten: Zur Alltagsgeschichte einer Heil- und Pflegeanstalt bis zum Ende des Nationalsozialismus* (Göttingen, 1987).
16 Dörner, *Tödliches Mitleid*; Karl Heinz Roth, "Mustergau," 15–16, 26.
17 Klee sees the beginning in Charles Darwin's book of 1859, *"Euthanasie,"* 457.
18 Schmuhl, *Rassenhygiene*; Schmuhl, "Sterilisation, 'Euthanasie,' 'Endlösung': Erbgesundheitspolitik unter den Bedingungen charismatischer Herrschaft," in Frei, ed., *Medizin und Gesundheitspolitik*, 295.
19 Klee, *"Euthanasie,"* 95–8; Schmuhl, *Rassenhygiene*, 240–7.

specific strand of "defection from humane values." The cultural and political crisis after World War I, reinforced by the economic crisis of the early 1930s and the perception of a widespread physical, emotional, and mental "degeneration" (*Entartung*), was attributed to the phenomenon called "counterselection" (*Gegenauslese*). Behind the idea of counterselection lay the notion that the progress of modern medicine violates the ancient process of "natural selection" precisely because of its progressive and humane features (although including the premodern ethical imperative of the Hippocratic oath). These humane features were seen as promoting the survival and procreation of the weak, helpless, poor, the "unfit," and "inferior." Medical progress came therefore to be considered as "a series of Pyrrhic victories."[20] Because modern medicine (along with modern welfare reforms, religious charity, and Marxism) was considered to benefit the wrong kind of people, that is, the "inferior" kind, and, moreover, to do so at the cost of the general community, it came to be classified negatively as "humanitarian sentimentalism" (*Humanitätsduselei*).

The notion that modern medicine was interfering with natural selection rose to prominence during the early twentieth century and was elaborated more broadly and deeply after World War I. It took various forms, nuances, and degrees of boldness or mildness, depending on time, place, the individuals who proposed it (among them many doctors), and the larger social context. In addition, it was complemented by five other important notions. First, the features of eugenic "inferiority" – most of all emotional and mental defects – were increasingly defined and classified by psychiatrists and psychiatry as a subdiscipline of medicine. Hence, medicine was to be transformed from an alleged cause of "degeneration" into a tool to be employed against it, from an alleged vehicle of counterselection into an agent of contra-counterselection. Second, those features were increasingly considered to be congenitally transmitted, and psychiatry became a privileged field of human genetics. The heredity discourse turned into heredity fanaticism, a heredity panic, and often enough it served as a global model for explaining all of society's problems. Third, the apocalyptic panic was supplemented by its apparent opposite: a utopia of perfect health, the vision of a world without illness, weakness, suffering, and misery that was proclaimed with revolutionary pathos. Fourth, the individual human being as subject of suffering and object of healing was supplanted by a collectivity to be redeemed, the *Volkskörper*, or ethnic community conceived as an organism; this is where

---

20 Hans-Günter Zmarzlik, "Der Sozialdarwinismus in Deutschland als geschichtliches Problem," in *Vierteljahrshefte für Zeitgeschichte* 11 (1963): 254.

dehumanization was increasingly manifest. Finally and most importantly, these notions included a powerful call to social and political action and expressed a particular kind of human hubris, a belief in human power to realize that utopia. It was the admonition to "return" to the allegedly "natural" selection, to "weed out" (ausmerzen) the unfit and inferior through man-made social and political tools where "nature's" tools were no longer in force. One privileged tool was the prevention of inferior offspring.

Surgical sterilization – known and studied since the turn of the century – as well as euthanasia were heatedly and publicly debated in Weimar Germany. By that time both of them were no longer a theoretical matter but had also become a practical one: Sterilizations on eugenic grounds were performed to some extent but rather secretly, mostly on poor women. Recent research has explored the little-known fact that already during World War I about 70,000 inmates of psychiatric institutions were starved to death or killed by medical means.[21] At the time this was considered a war emergency measure, but it also laid the ground for, and influenced, the public debate that started in 1920 on an "annihilation of life unworthy of living" – the "mercy" killing of ill, insane, or unfit persons.[22] Despite this debate, or rather because of it, sterilization was clearly considered to be the privileged method for reducing the number of inferior people or altogether doing away with them. In the course of the Weimar Republic and particularly its final years, which were marked by economic depression, virtually all strands of eugenic thought agreed on sterilization as the major method of eugenic intervention, and "negative eugenics" took precedence over "positive eugenics," that is, policies concerning child and family welfare. The Prussian Health Council drafted a sterilization bill, which was never enacted, and organized a meeting of seventy-eight experts from many professions, particularly doctors. Held in July 1932, the conference witnessed several National Socialists (among them Leonardo Conti) pleading for outright compulsion and declaring that to be the Nazi position on the matter. Even though the draft of this bill provided for a clause of consent – in contrast to the Nazi sterilization law that followed a year later – the terms of the draft and even more those of the debate left no doubt that what was at stake was not the well-being of individuals but that of the Volkskörper.[23]

21 Hans Ludwig Siemen, Menschen blieben auf der Strecke: Psychiatrie zwischen Reform und Nationalsozialismus (Gütersloh, 1987), 29–33. Siemen's figure is the difference between prewar mortality and the mortality during the war.

22 Karl Binding and Alfred Hoche, Die Freigabe der Vernichtung lebensunwerten Lebens (Leipzig, 1920); Schmuhl, Rassenhygiene, 115–25.

23 Labisch and Tennstedt, Weg zum Gesetz, 252–7; Bock, Zwangssterilisation, 55–8, 80–94; Weindling, Health, 444, 450–7, 522–5. The 1932 draft provided for much wider grounds for sterilization than the 1933 law, even including the healthy carriers of a latent disease.

The activities of the Prussian Health Council, which were widely publicized, contributed to the fact that the aforementioned notions became commonplace, by no means only among members of the Nazi Party, and that the Nazi stand on compulsion was well known. These radical eugenic ideas were widely shared, particularly by doctors, for example, by the Hartmann League. Their underlying premises were shared by virtually all public figures and professional experts, and only a very few actively opposed them, for example, representatives of the physically handicapped.[24] The Reich minister of the interior, Wilhelm Frick, summarized eugenic consensus in his notorious speech of June 28, 1933, to the Expert Advisory Committee on Population and Race Policy, thereby announcing the imminent sterilization law:

Until now we have had an exaggerated type of personal hygiene and welfare for the single individual without any regard for the insights of genetics, selection of life and race hygiene. This kind of modern "humane values" and social welfare for the ill, weak and worthless individual will have enormously cruel effects on the people as a whole and will finally lead to its ruin.... In order to raise the number of genetically healthy progeny we have, first of all, the duty to diminish the expenses for the asocial, inferior and hopelessly genetically ill and to prevent the procreation of hereditarily tainted persons.[25]

With respect to the relationship between the history and the prehistory of our twofold subject, sterilization and euthanasia, two major events seem to mark decisive turning points: World War I opened up its serious prehistory, the transition from single voices and mere forerunners to a powerful trend; and National Socialism's rise to power in 1933 opened up its actual history. With respect to historical causation and agency, we certainly need to emphasize the power of preexisting ideas and mentalities – those prevailing in medicine and human genetics as well as economic ideas about public expenses at a time of depression. But no less significant was the role of political, legal, and institutional power. Even though the eugenic discourse underlying mass sterilization had been elaborated before 1933, largely by doctors and other scientists, its "rise to power" should be located not just in the history of science, in the *Geist der Wissenschaft* (Peukert), but far more importantly in the history of politics, in the *Ungeist der Politik* (Blasius).[26] The first and major

24 E.g., some of the blind, deaf, and crippled; see Bock, *Zwangssterilisation*, 80–1, 279–80; Weindling, *Health*, 480–4.
25 Wilhelm Frick, *Bevölkerungs- und Rassenpolitik im neuen Deutschland* (Langensalza, 1933).
26 Blasius, "Maskerade," 268 (cf. Peukert, "Genesis der 'Endlösung'"); see Blasius's criticism of the notion "tödliche Wissenschaft" set forth by Benno Müller-Hill in his *Murderous Science: Elimination by Scientific Selection of Jews, Gypsies and Others: Germany 1933–1945* (Oxford, 1988). The same may be argued with respect to Dörner's "murderous compassion." See note 7 to this chapter and Blasius, *"Einfache Seelenstörung"*, 182.

single political factor was the rise to power of Adolf Hitler and his party. Whatever would have become of the Prussian Health Council's draft had they not come to power – and we should be aware of the pitfalls of counterfactual history that has often been construed for this case – for it was National Socialism that, in the words of one eugenicist in 1934, "raised race hygiene to the level of an explicit principle of government." It did so by means of the sterilization law, which has aptly been called "the first comprehensive race law of National Socialism."[27] Historically and politically, there is no contradiction in the view that this law was, in the words of one Nazi writer, "the most decisive and revolutionary" among the laws for the "preservation and purification of the race"[28] and the fact that the underlying discourse had been elaborated earlier, by Nazis as well as by non-Nazis and not-yet-Nazis. This was felt most clearly by those medical doctors and scientists who had committed themselves so strongly and early to eugenic sterilization and who were to be its most efficient practitioners, such as Ernst Rüdin who, in 1934, wrote: "It was only through the political work of Hitler that the meaning of race hygiene has become publicly manifest in Germany and it is only due to him that our thirty-year-old dream to put race hygiene into practice, has become a reality."[29] In 1943 he could still conjure up "Hitler's and his followers' everlasting historical merit of having risked undertaking, far beyond purely scientific knowledge, the decisive and pioneering step toward brilliant race-hygienic action in and for the German people."[30] Rüdin represents many doctors and most psychiatrists to whom the year 1933 opened up the opportunity of crossing political as well as ethical boundaries. The psychiatric profession, in particular, accepted this opportunity enthusiastically and expressed "a yearning for the omnipotence of the new rulers."[31]

Among the groups advocating eugenic mass sterilization, medical doctors and psychiatrists formed a powerful lobby. For the doctors who believed in the mission of race hygiene, it usually implied their own mission to help redeem society, to put the interests of the self-defined "community" before the interest of the individual. This meant, in the first place, that their own interest – ideological and professional – happily coincided with the interests of the regime. Yet it should not be forgotten that many other groups recom-

27 Blasius, "Ambivalenzen," 265. The previous quote is from Hermann Werner Siemens, *Vererbungslehre, Rassenhygiene und Bevölkerungspolitik*, 6th ed. (Berlin, 1934), 3.
28 Otto Schwarz and Erwin Noack, *Die Gesetzgebung des Dritten Reiches: Ein Grundriss* (Berlin, 1934), 30 (one of many examples for this assertion among National Socialists).
29 Ernst Rüdin, "Aufgaben und Ziele der Deutschen Gesellschaft für Rassenhygiene," *Archiv für Rassen- und Gesellschaftsbiologie* 28 (1934): 228. For Rüdin, see Blasius, "Maskerade," 271–7.
30 Ernst Rüdin, "Zehn Jahre nationalsozialistischer Staat," *Archiv für Rassen- und Gesellschaftsbiologie* 36 (1943): 321.
31 Blasius, "Maskerade," 272.

mended and lobbied for eugenic mass sterilization, such as welfare organizations, the Associated German Communes, the Evangelical church, and especially the Inner Mission, and the depression of the early 1930s boosted their number. The reason why the sterilization law came about so easily and against so little public criticism was because it promised so many things to so many people: No children from inferior people seemed to mean gains to the communal and other public funds, reduced costs for institutional care, fewer illegitimate children, no more schools for backward children, more funds for the "deserving" unemployed, better health for the population at large. Nevertheless, medicine, psychiatry, and doctors were at the center of the campaign, and they were also at the center of the new institutions and administrations that made the practice of compulsory and mass sterilization possible. The coincidence of doctor's interests and the interests of the regime took on the political form of five major institutional innovations.

The first innovation, and perhaps the most revolutionary, was the establishment of special sterilization courts by January 1934 (there were 223 such courts in 1936). These courts were one of the elements where the Nazi sterilization practice differed from that in other countries that had laws providing for eugenic sterilization. The courts included three judges – only one of them a lawyer, the other two being doctors, usually psychiatrists, human geneticists, population scientists, or anthropologists – and the sentence was passed by majority vote. Doctors had become judges, "medical judges" (*ärztliche Richter*) with the full power of the law behind them – an unheard of development. Doctors exerted legal power over procreation, passing verdicts on life and nonlife. Virtually all better-known eugenicists and psychiatrists sat on such courts at one time or another; others were busy handing in expert advice. It was the fulfillment of an old dream of race hygienists and many doctors who had complained about the lack of power over their patients. In the words of the doctor Arthur Gütt, one of the authors of the sterilization law and its chief executor in the Reich Ministry of the Interior:

The advanced level of surgery enables us to employ the weapon of sterilization in our battle against hereditary diseases! In the same way in which we have succeeded in healing diseases and preventing epidemics, we have now before our eyes the goal to ban the menace of hereditary disease. ... Therefore, the judges and doctors must be aware of their responsibility for the people and the race, because it is in the hands of these two professions that the law has laid the means to re-empower the natural process of eradication and to diminish the hereditary taints in our people![32]

32 Arthur Gütt, "Ausmerze und Lebensauslese in ihrer Bedeutung für Erbgesundheits- und Rassenpflege," in Ernst Rüdin, ed., *Erblehre und Rassenhygiene im völkischen Staat* (Munich, 1934),

Equally important was the law for the unification of the public health system of July 3, 1934, which Gütt also devised. Its purpose was the standardization of public health throughout the Reich, public health now being defined as *Erb- und Rassenpflege* and placed in the hands of newly created "state doctors" (*staatliche Amtsärzte*) who ran the newly created "state health offices" (*staatliche Gesundheitsämter*). By 1943 over 1,000 state health offices had been created, and most of the state doctors were members of the Nazi Party or one of its suborganizations. Their task was to implement what has been called "the three core laws of National Socialist race hygiene": the sterilization law, the "blood protection law" of September 15, 1935, and the "marital health law" of October 18, 1935. The latter two laws were originally intended to be included in one single law: The first of them prohibited marriage and sexual intercourse between Jews (or Gypsies or other "alien races") and non-Jewish Germans, and the second prohibited marriage between eugenically undesirable persons and "hereditarily healthy Germans." Both the sterilization courts and the public health system were entirely new; they would not have come into being if the Weimar Republic had lasted.[33] The state doctors were empowered to search for sterilization candidates and to invite them in for a eugenic examination, which might include, for instance, an intelligence test for "feeblemindedness." These doctors could and did call for police assistance if those who were scheduled to be sterilized did not comply voluntarily.[34] They officially suggested clients to the courts, wrote eugenic affidavits, and often sat on the courts as medical judges, thus combining the functions of prosecutor and judge. Moreover, they collected information for a comprehensive census on the eugenic condition of the German people (*erbbiologische Bestandsaufnahme*). Thus, this reform of the health sector differed, once again, from the sterilization practice in other countries; it rendered the search for sterilization candidates possible and hence the fact that two thirds or three quarters of the sterilized had been living privately, outside institutions.

Third, many medical doctors who were known to be convinced eugenicists were appointed to high government and administrative positions, where they promoted sterilization and later euthanasia. Alongside the eugenicists in the Reich Ministry of the Interior, above all Gütt, were many others in the various state (*Länder*) interior ministries, for example, Ludwig Sprauer in Baden, Eugen Stähle in Württemberg, and Walther Schultze in Bavaria.[35]

182. For the role of the doctors in the courts (and of the courts and the jurists), see Bock, *Zwangssterilisation*, 178–230.

33 Labisch and Tennstedt, *Weg zum Gesetz*, 325, 315–16, 369. Cf. Bock, *Zwangssterilisation*, 187–92.

34 For the use of police force, see Bock, *Zwangssterilisation*, 213, 256–9.

35 Kater, *Doctors under Hitler*, 61, 126–8; Heinz Faulstich, *Von der Irrenfürsorge zur "Euthanasie": Geschichte der badischen Psychiatrie bis 1945* (Freiburg/Breisgau, 1993); Weindling, *Health*, chap. 8.

Furthermore, gynecologists and surgeons – the "masculine heroes of the scalpel"[36] – performed sterilizations in specially selected hospitals. In 1936 there were 108 such hospitals and 144 specially nominated surgeons; their places and names were included in the greatly expanded, second edition of the official commentary on the sterilization law. These institutions and persons encroached, almost daily, on the bodily integrity of women and men, usually against their will. Because the operation was more dramatic on women than on men, some men and many women suffered not only from being defined as inferior, but also from the ensuing complications. About 5,000 persons, mostly women, died in the course or aftermath of the operation, often as a result of the victim's resistance or suicide. In order to diminish such inconveniences, some doctors studied new methods of "bloodless" sterilization; one of these doctors, Carl Clauberg, continued his research in Auschwitz, where he performed sterilization experiments on Jewish, Gypsy, and Polish women.[37] Finally, all doctors and other medical personnel, inside as well as outside medical institutions, were obliged to denounce hereditarily ill and inferior patients, either to the sterilization courts or, from 1934, to state doctors. For this purpose the rights of patients to medical secrecy and the duty of doctors to maintain this secrecy were abolished. Most doctors were instructed at courses for race hygiene throughout the Reich, but in many cases instruction was unnecessary because they not only followed the call but followed it eagerly.

Clearly not every single doctor conformed to the new policy; there were also other views of mental patients and their treatment.[38] There is evidence of numerous cases of hesitance or even resistance.[39] But on the whole, the medical profession and its new institutions represented a major area where dehumanization flourished and where the normal human, moral, and social checks against violent interference with body and life were diminished and even dissolved. It was precisely the institutionalization of race hygiene,

36 Michael H. Kater, "Medizin und Mediziner im Dritten Reich," *Historische Zeitschrift* 244 (1987): 309.
37 See Bock, *Zwangssterilisation*, 372–82, 453–6, and Gisela Bock, "Gleichheit und Differenz in der nationalsozialistischen Rassenpolitik," *Geschichte und Gesellschaft* 19 (1993): 287–8; Monika Daum and Hans-Ulrich Deppe, *Zwangssterilisation in Frankfurt am Main, 1933–1945* (Frankfurt/Main, 1991), 127–30, 156–62.
38 In particular a complementary effort on the part of arriviste, ambitious, and well-connected psychotherapists to compete with psychiatrists by offering the hope of therapeutic repair by means of psychological treatment. See Geoffrey Cocks, *Psychotherapy in the Third Reich: The Göring Institute* (New York, 1985); Geoffrey Cocks, "The Professionalization of Psychotherapy in Germany, 1928–1949," in Geoffrey Cocks and Konrad H. Jarausch, eds., *German Professions, 1800–1950* (New York, 1990), 308–28.
39 Labisch and Tennstedt, *Weg zum Gesetz*, 324; Bock, *Zwangssterilisation*, 288–89. Practical resistance seems to have been more widespread than theoretical resistance on the part of publishing scholars: Weindling, *Health*, 480–4.

mainly in the judiciary and the medical bureaucracy, that precipitated its radicalization and dehumanization. The kind and degree of dehumanization can best be grasped from the outcries and protests, and the lives and deaths of the victims – half of them women, half of them men, and including Jews, Gypsies, Poles, and blacks. It seems that a higher proportion of the ethnic minorities were sterilized than of the ethnic majority.[40] Compulsory mass sterilization had many gender-based features besides the gendered death rate, such as the gender-specific tests of eugenic inferiority. Women were tested as to their capability and willingness to perform domestic as well as occupational work, men as to their occupational performance; women, but not men, as to their capability of raising children; women's irregular sexual behavior was investigated, but men's was not. Particularly young women deplored the loss of their future as mothers. One of them wrote, in somewhat old-fashioned terms: "It is depressing that the innocent people are butchered. ... But God knows it is the most wicked sin in the world if a human being is deprived of its nature, just as if the root is cut from a tree which then dies."[41]

What had been attacked, by doctors and nondoctors, as the sentimental humanitarianism of modern medicine disappeared in the context of steril-ization policy; it was considered obsolete and was replaced by another type of modernity that claimed to substitute the harshness of a "nature" lost for-ever. Traditional ethical values were replaced by a "new ethics" of "value" and lack thereof with respect to a racially defined community. Sometimes this new ethics was not even claimed to be based on nature but rather on man-made values to which life, birth, and death had to be accommodated. Fritz Lenz wrote in 1943 that

[t]hese values are not taken over from nature, they do not follow from natural selec-tion. If they did, we might indeed believe it to be quite acceptable when low-talented Germans have more children than talented ones. Yet if we, as race hygien-ists, consider such a situation as highly undesirable and call it counterselection, we presuppose a value measure which does not follow from the natural processes themselves. Rather we interpret the natural processes according to our own values.[42]

Lenz wrote this at the time when the partial defection from humane values had turned into their definite rejection. In the process that led from the pol-icy of sterilizing the unfit to the policy of massacre, medicine and doctors played a decisive role. What were the historical causes of this process, its logic,

40 Bock, *Zwangssterilisation*, 351–68; Daum and Deppe, *Zwangssterilisation in Frankfurt am Main*, 164–70; Hansjörg Riechert, "Im Schatten von Auschwitz: Die nationalsozialistische Sterilisationspolitik gegenüber Sinti und Roma," Ph.D diss., University of Bochum, 1993.
41 Sterilization trial record in Staatsarchiv Freiburg, Gesundheitsamt Lörrach no. 544.
42 Fritz Lenz, "Gedanken zur Rassenhygiene (Eugenik)," *Archiv für Rassen- und Gesellschaftsbiologie* 37 (1943): 85. Cf. Renate Rissom, *Fritz Lenz und die Rassenhygiene* (Husum, 1983).

and dynamics? Was the massacre of the ill a mere extension of a sterilization policy in which killing, or at least the potential for killing, was contained from the beginning; or was there a process of genuine and continuous radicalization between 1933 and 1939; or was the policy of massacre rather based on, and inspired by, new and more immediate factors, issues, and attitudes that arose in the late 1930s and early 1940s?

In 1935 the medical officer at the Württemberg Ministry of the Interior, Stähle, felt the need for justifying publicly the deaths resulting from compulsory sterilization, which had caused widespread unrest and public criticism. He weighed them against the fate of people who would fall victim to the alleged crimes of the insane (he obviously forgot that sterilization did not prevent crimes but births), and he compared the sterilization deaths to soldiers' sacrifice of their lives for the community in World War I.[43] In October 1939 Stähle repeated his old line in a conversation with Herbert Linden, a high officer in the Reich Ministry of the Interior and responsible for sterilization. Linden justified the impending massacres by pointing to the insane asylum inmates in World War I who had died of tuberculosis, as a result of hunger, and had thereby infected "curable" patients; Stähle agreed and added: "If at times of war thousands of young and healthy people have to sacrifice their lives for the community, this sacrifice can also be expected on the part of the incurably ill."[44]

This kind of argument suggests a direct continuity between the sterilization discourse of the 1930s and the euthanasia discourse and practice dating from 1939: the assumption that compulsory eugenic sterilization necessarily led to euthanasia and that the former also implied the latter. This assumption is confirmed by the brevity of time, barely six years, that was required for the "prevention of worthless life" to turn into its "annihilation" and that has been called the incubation period of euthanasia. There are various indications that the transition period was even shorter.[45] The psychologist and historian Robert Jay Lifton underscores the fact that "sterilization was a forerunner of mass murder," although adding significantly, in view of other countries that introduced eugenic sterilization, that this happened "only in Germany."[46] Euthanasia has been identified as the "logically next step" to

43 Egon Stähle, "Unfruchtbarmachung und Weltanschauung," *Ärzteblatt für Württemberg und Baden* 2, no. 7 (1935): 1.
44 Egon Stähle (in a trial of 1947), quoted in Klee, *"Euthanasie,"* 90.
45 See esp. Hitler's conversation with Wagner in 1935 (Mitscherlich and Mielke, *Medizin ohne Menschlichkeit* [1978], 183–4) and Nitsche's hint at early killing in asylums (Klee, *"Euthanasie"*, 47). See also Schmuhl, *Rassenhygiene*, 178–81 ("Der Zeitraum von 1933 bis 1938 als Inkubationsphase der 'Euthanasieaktion'").
46 Lifton, *Nazi Doctors*, 22.

follow sterilization policy.[47] Many authors consider the introduction of eugenic abortion in 1935 as a step in radicalization, even though the consent of the pregnant woman was required – at least officially, although not always in practice – and abortion on eugenic grounds is widely accepted today without constituting a link to (mass) murder.[48] The continuity and relative smoothness of transition from state-run birth control to state-run death control, an almost uninhibited radicalization is evident in many instances: Most importantly, in the concept of "inferiority" itself, the deadly metaphors of eugenic language, in the institutions and institutional dynamics emanating from bureaucratic efficiency, the personnel (all supporters and practitioners of euthanasia had also supported race hygiene and sterilization), the deaths through sterilization, the gradual decline of ethical arguments against killing that resulted from the previous interference in bodily integrity and the acceptance of death through sterilization, and the transition from sterilization to the killing of babies and children in the first phase of euthanasia that many understood as postnatal anti-natalism. For those condemned to sterilization, the one officially accepted alternative was voluntary confinement in a closed psychiatric asylum, which often led to their death in the course of euthanasia.[49] Yet at the same time, stress should also be laid on the independence of sterilization policy as a specific form of population policy, that is, anti-natalism, and the profound difference between birth prevention and massacre (or, in the terminology of the period, between *Fortpflanzungsauslese* and *Vernichtungsauslese*). The continuity of discourse and practice, as well as their fundamental discontinuity, has been aptly expressed in the formula of sterilization as "extermination without massacre."[50] Yet logical continuity of discourse and historical continuity do not always coincide: Not everywhere did a radical eugenic sterilization discourse lead to massacre,[51] and not necessarily the same kind of people became victims of sterilization and euthanasia (sterilization was

---

47 Michael H. Kater, "Die Medizin im nationalsozialistischen Deutschland und Erwin Liek," *Geschichte und Gesellschaft* 16 (1990): 460.

48 Except for important strands within the Catholic Church. See Klaus Dörner, "Nationalsozialismus und Lebensvernichtung" (1967), reprinted in Klaus Dörner, *Diagnosen der Psychiatrie* (Frankfurt/Main, 1975), 67; Klaus Dörner, "NS-Euthanasie: Zur Normalisierung des therapeutischen Tötens," in Klaus Dörner, ed., *Fortschritte der Psychiatrie im Umgang mit Menschen* (Rehburg-Loccum, 1984), 108; Lothar Gruchmann, "Euthanasie und Justiz im Dritten Reich," *Vierteljahrshefte für Zeitgeschichte* 20 (1972): 239–40; Bock, *Zwangssterilisation*, 96–100, 382–9, 436–8; Schmuhl, *Rassenhygiene*, 161–4. Writing before World War II, David Victor Glass saw abortion on eugenic grounds in Germany as a "liberalization" of the current abortion law. See his *Population Policies and Movements in Europe* (1940; reprinted: London, 1967), 183.

49 See Bock, *Zwangssterilisation*, 262–4, 347–51, 372–89; Bock, "Gleichheit und Differenz," 299–300.

50 Schmuhl, *Rassenhygiene*, 40 ("Ausrottung ohne Massenmord").

51 On the United States, see Kühl, *Nazi Connection*.

programmatically and actually performed on people with relatively minor troubles, so-called *leichte Fälle*).

In addition, historical continuity of discourse is not necessarily identical with historical causation or agency, and logical continuity may coexist with historical discontinuity. This appears to result from recent studies that point to new aspects of the history of medicine and psychiatry along their own internal dynamics, often on a local or regional level, and to factors in the radicalization that hint at a more complex and differentiated picture than the assumptions that imply a unilinear, long-term development. By the mid-1930s, it became obvious that eugenic sterilization disappointed the high-strung hopes on which medical enthusiasm had been built, especially the vision that a decrease in inferior procreation would diminish the need for (costly) asylums. For a variety of reasons, some of which apparently linked to National Socialism's insistence on a certain kind of "normality," from 1933 to 1939 the number of inmates in psychiatric institutions increased by 30 percent, reaching 340,000. Contrary to what eugenic enthusiasm had assumed and announced, a high percentage of those inmates who were sterilized could not, or were not allowed to, be discharged because they were, or were considered to be, long-term patients. At the same time, the cost and care per patient decreased enormously, leaving the inmates in evermore abject misery and with an increasing death rate. Equally importantly, the prestige of psychiatry and psychiatrists decreased at a similar rate, and it did so precisely because of the widespread eugenic propaganda against the unfit and worthless. Now the effect of this propaganda began to backfire on the psychiatric profession itself and to undermine its sacrosanct legitimacy; in the words of Valentin Falthauser, later one of the major euthanizers, an increasing "hatred against the asylums" had emerged by the mid-1930s.[52] In 1939 Rüdin complained about the "devaluation" of his profession and the loss of its attraction for young doctors (although he continued without remorse to insist on eugenic sterilization as the "great deed of the German state and people").[53] Outside the asylums the open relief for the emotionally and mentally handicapped, a major acquisition of the Weimar reforms,[54] practically collapsed (since its main function after 1933 had become the search for sterilization candidates), and inside the institutions the overcrowding and deprivation both shifted and reinforced the division between the curable – who were offered, or subjected to, an "active therapy" – and the incurable, or long-term

52 Quoted in Siemen, *Menschen*, 141; see also 144 and chap. 3.
53 Quoted in ibid., 133.
54 See Hans-Ludwig Siemen, "Die Reformpsychiatrie der Weimarer Republik," in Kersting et al., eds., *Nach Hadamar*, 98–108.

patients. A new stage in the old and much-debated psychiatric problem and procedure of selecting between curable and incurable people had been set in motion. It developed its own dynamics and led to a search for drastic solutions.[55]

Against this background the explanation of the rise of euthanasia gains a new dimension: The motives and goals of its agents were not only, or perhaps not so much, the result of long-standing eugenic ideas on racial and genetic improvement but of immediate, short-term needs closely linked to the "needs" of the profession. Furthermore, the military requirements of World War II, especially for military hospitals, were gaining new prominence among the various strands that led to euthanasia and to its historical explanation. Recently the fact that the first T-4 killing centers were located in southwestern Germany has been plausibly attributed to its geomilitary situation, and the additional fact that apparently more hospitalized people in southwestern Germany fell victim to the massacres than in the north has been attributed to the earlier beginning, linked to the blitzkrieg against France. At this time the directors of psychiatric institutions did not yet know the aim of the deportation and therefore did not hesitate much letting their inmates depart.[56] In particular the decentralized phase of euthanasia from 1942 to 1945 may therefore be viewed not just as a continuation, under a better cover-up, of the highly centralized "Action T-4" (which had officially been stopped in 1941) but as a war measure and a renewal of the mass starvation of inmates during World War I.

Since the 1980s the historical conceptualization of National Socialist psychiatry and the euthanasia doctors has been shaped by the discovery that its major agents were not "reactionary" but "progressive" and "modern." This insight had largely been forgotten after its articulation by Alice Platen-Hallermund in 1948: "We must confront the strange fact that precisely some psychiatrists who were interested in therapy and men of practical commitment, such as Kurt Schneider, Heyde, and Hermann Paul Nitsche, came to fight for the euthanasia of the mentally ill."[57] The key elements that support this notion are three. First, the medical agents of death, among whom also Falthauser should be mentioned, had been well known as reformers in the

---

55 Siemen, *Menschen*, 161. See also Hans-Walter Schmuhl, "Kontinuität oder Diskontinuität? Zum epochalen Charakter der Psychiatrie im Nationalsozialismus," in Kersting et al., eds., *Nach Hadamar*, 112–36. "Active therapy" included Insulin-, Cardiazol-, *Elektroschock* and work. Cf. Siemen, *Menschen*, 183; Angelika Ebbinghaus, "Kostensenkung, 'aktive Therapie' und Vernichtung," in Ebbinghaus et al., eds., *Heilen und Vernichten*, 136–46; Schmuhl, *Rassenhygiene*, 261ff.
56 Faulstich, *Von der Irrenfürsorge*, 270ff.
57 Platen-Hallermund, *Tötung Geisteskranker in Deutschland*, 14. She also wrote about the continuation of killing after 1941, which many believe to be a recent discovery.

1920s and were not wavering in their therapeutic optimism, even in the 1940s. They continued to stress modern "active therapy" for those patients who were believed to be curable, but these methods were often extremely aggressive and far from being benign. Second, several documents were discovered, the most important of them dating from 1941 and 1943 and in which the psychiatrists and euthanizers – de Crinis, Schneider, Hans Heinze, Rüdin, Nitsche – planned the future of psychiatry after the anticipated victory.[58] They established a startling and frighteningly close link between healing and killing: euthanasia being understood as a way for emptying institutional space of incurable patients, as a precondition for curing the curable and productive patients; their vision was opposed, in part at least, to the goal of those who wished the space to be emptied for military hospitals and the victims of bombing raids. Third, such strategies were conceived as a method for upgrading the psychiatric profession, for rescuing it, in Nitsche's words, from being considered "inferior" (just like its patients).[59] For instance Rüdin, Nitsche, and others worried, on the one hand, about the future of psychiatry if it was to be confined to eliminating the unfit[60]; on the other hand, the apparent need for disposing of them by death – in order to create space as well as to leave only patients who were worth the therapeutic efforts of professionals – turned them into "professional killers."[61]

These elements seem to require a view of the killing experts not as uncontrolled and irrational murderers but as cool planners of "progress" through rational and scientific methods, devoid of ethical, or simply humane, considerations. But there are some significant differences between the larger historical interpretations drawn from these phenomena. Peukert and Blasius explain them as resulting from a profound crisis of modernity, modernization, and the bourgeois belief in progressive civic reform, a crisis that was more pronounced in Germany than elsewhere, as the barbarism that appears to be a possibility – though by no means a necessity – contained within civilization.[62] Other authors identify this kind of mass murder as intimately

58 Especially "Gedanken und Anregungen betr. die künftige Entwicklung der Psychiatrie" (1943), sent by Nitsche to Brandt on June 26, 1943. An extract was first published in Hans-Ludwig Siemen, *Das Grauen ist vorprogrammiert: Psychiatrie zwischen Faschismus und Atomkrieg* (Giessen, 1982), 154–6; partly published also in Dörner, ed., *Fortschritte der Psychiatrie*, 212–17, and in Aly et al., *Reform und Gewissen*, 42–8. See also Schmuhl, *Rassenhygiene*, 378n.37, 452 n.4.
59 Nitsche's complaints to Brack (1941, 1942) quoted in Schmuhl, *Rassenhygiene*, 274, 276.
60 Plans for the future of psychiatry seem to have been also driven by competition from psychotherapists at the Göring Institute (see Cocks, *Psychotherapy in the Third Reich*, and "Professionalization of Psychotherapy") and by psychologists: Ulfried Geuter, *Die Professionalisierung der deutschen Psychologie im Nationalsozialismus* (Frankfurt/Main, 1984).
61 Lifton, *Nazi Doctors*, 491.
62 Peukert, "Genesis der 'Endlösung'"; Blasius, "Ambivalenz." Bajohr et al., eds., *Zivilisation und Barbarei* is dedicated to Peukert's memory.

coupled with, or even a form of, modernization and reform; take for rational and "economically useful" what the euthanizers presented as such; and see reform as an integral part of National Socialist massacres and the massacres as "the other side of the coin" of reform. Thus, they tend to blur important boundaries between mass killing and other forms of maltreatment or even humane reforms.[63] But the depressing fact that healing and killing went hand in hand in those dark times and in the minds of the euthanizers should not, from the point of view of ethical commitment, lead historians to assume that the relationship between healing and killing is, or was, a "dialectical" one.[64] Instead, the radical contradiction between the two, the "perversion" of the first in the second[65] must be explained, the "healing-killing paradox" should be highlighted precisely as a paradox and conflict[66] and likewise the specific kind of professionalization that produced professional killers. From this point of view, we are dealing with a "peculiar simultaneity of healing and killing,"[67] a complex web of simultaneous professionalization and "deprofessionalization,"[68] medicalization of killing and "demedicalization" of the profession.[69] Yet for the purpose of overall historical explanation, concepts such as dehumanization and the decline and loss of humane ethics may be more plausible, precisely because they do not circumvent, but highlight, the ethical and anti-ethical values in question and because they underscore why and how mental patients came to be considered as less than human beings. The agents of death – such as Falthauser – knew well why, when they felt the need to justify themselves, they conjured up a new ethics that upheld that "acting in terms of euthanasia cannot be a crime against humanity, but precisely the opposite," namely, acting "as a true and conscientious doctor" who "liberates" from their suffering those who "have sunk to the level of animals."[70] From the point of view of ethical standards, one striking element in the thought of the euth-

---

63 See note 7 to this chapter. Schmuhl has juxtaposed the "structuralist" model underlying his *Rassenhygiene* with the conceptual framework of "modernization": Schmuhl, "Reformpsychiatrie und Massenmord," in Michael Prinz and Rainer Zitelmann, eds., *Nationalsozialismus und Modernisierung* (Darmstadt, 1991), 239–66; Schmuhl, "Sterilisation, 'Euthanasie,' 'Endlösung'"; for criticism of the "modernization" hypothesis, see Blasius, *"Einfache Seelenstörung"*, 185–91; Christof Dipper, "Modernisierung des Nationalsozialismus," *Neue Politische Literatur* 36 (1991): 450–6.

64 Schmuhl, *Rassenhygiene*, 261. In fact, the publications and exhibitions catalogues with the title *Heilen und Vernichten* usually do not deal with healing, but with discrimination and annihilation.

65 Kater, "Medizin und Mediziner," 303, 344.

66 See, e.g., Lifton, *Nazi Doctors*, 430.

67 Siemen, "Reformpsychiatrie der Weimarer Republik," 107.

68 Kater, "Medizin und Mediziner," 352; and Kater, "Doctor Leonardo Conti and His Nemesis: The Failure of Centralized Medicine in the Third Reich," *Central European History* 18 (1985): 321.

69 Wolfgang Petter, "Zur nationalsozialistischen 'Euthanasie,'" in Wolfgang Michalka, ed., *Der Zweite Weltkrieg* (Munich, 1989), 821.

70 Falthauser in 1948, quoted in Siemen, *Menschen*, 192. See also Pfannmüller's statement, "Ich bin kein Mörder," quoted in Richarz, *Heilen, Pflegen, Töten*, 198.

anizers was one that was at the roots of the larger race-hygienic discourse: their hubris as well as hypocrisy; their belief in the "totalitarian fiction" of a hygienic utopia, of a world without misery and disease; and their belief in their own vocation to produce it. Like the agents of the genocide against the Jewish people, they claimed, for the sake of the "total realization" of this fiction, the "right to determine who should and who should not inhabit the world."[71]

The discourse of eugenicists and euthanizers, as well as the parallels and overlapping of eugenics with the persecution of Jews and the Holocaust, confirms what Platen-Hallermund stated in the late 1940s:"Regardless of all arguments of the adherents and advocates of euthanasia, euthanasia was never a medical but exclusively a political problem."[72] Lifton has coined the concept of "doubling" in order to explore the psychological functioning of the medical killers in Auschwitz. This concept has been criticized by historians as too psychological and individualistic and therefore risking evasion of the political, social, and institutional dimensions, or as inappropriate for the euthanasia killers, because they practiced "mass murder without conscience of guilt" and had no "division of consciousness" or self, having themselves so intimately linked reform and destruction.[73] Yet on the one hand, individual dispositions of the victimizers are far from being irrelevant – for instance, in view of the fact that some psychiatrists, such as Hans Roemer, director of the famous asylum at Illenau, were enthusiastic supporters of sterilization but stopped short of supporting euthanasia[74] – and social history no longer focuses just on overall processes and structures but also on individual perceptions and mentalities. On the other hand, the concept of doubling may well be understood as pointing to the one overall as well as specific, social as well as political feature of National Socialism that, irrespective of the admitted and obvious multiplicity of origins, causes, and motivations that coincided to produce large-scale and systematic mass murder, produced and shaped race hygienic policies as well as the much larger massacres following euthanasia – the politics of racism.

If taken in a more metaphorical sense, beyond its potential for insight into the victimizer's self and as an indication of the functioning of Nazi politics, doubling may be understood as the mental, social, and political mechanism that was at the roots of Nazi racism, particularly in its institutionalized form

71   Hannah Arendt, *The Origins of Totalitarianism* (New York, 1966), 391–2, 474–9; Hannah Arendt, *Eichmann in Jerusalem* (London, 1984), 279.
72   Platen-Hallermund, *Tötung Geisteskranker in Deutschland*, 9.
73   Blasius,"Maskerade"; Hans-Walter Schmuhl, "Die Selbstverständlichkeit des Tötens: Psychiater im Nationalsozialismus," *Geschichte und Gesellschaft* 16 (1990): 417–20, 432–3, 436.
74   Faulstich, *Von der Irrenfürsorge*, 237ff; Klee, *"Euthanasie,"* 274.

as race policy and race bureaucracy. On this level it implies a "doubled" treatment of human beings according to their apparently or allegedly different value, along the division between "inferiority" and "superiority" on ethnic and eugenic grounds. Taken to its extreme, it means that some human beings are perceived and treated as human beings, whereas other human beings are perceived and treated as less than that or even as the opposite. Obviously, race policy is not a simple but a complex phenomenon. Under National Socialism it was directed against ethnic "aliens" (Jews, Gypsies, Slavs, blacks), as well as against the "worthless" within the national or ethnic community. It is useful and necessary to distinguish, historically as well as analytically, between eugenic racism and ethnic, especially anti-Jewish, racism, and therefore it has been appropriate to treat eugenics – from sterilization to euthanasia – separately from the most spectacular form of National Socialist race policy, the persecution and destruction of the European Jews.[75] But it is equally useful and necessary to explore and analyze their common grounds, their commonalties, and their interactions.[76] The reason why in National Socialist Germany – different from other countries where eugenic sterilization was legalized, sometimes even with compulsion clauses, and where anti-Semitism and racism existed – eugenic sterilization became a mass phenomenon, a "population" policy in the strict sense, and why mass sterilization led to massacre, may be identified in the fact that National Socialism conceived it ideologically and practiced it institutionally as an integral part of its overall race policy.

The persecution and destruction of European Jewry has been largely explained – although with significant differences over the profound causes and agency – in terms of a radicalization that led from economic, political, and cultural discrimination and segregation to systematic massacre. But equally impressive has been the suggestion of, and the research on, the fact that the most systematic, scientific, bureaucratic, industrialized, anonymous, and therefore the most dehumanizing, antihuman form of killing – the gas vans and gas chambers – has been derived from the massacre of eugenically defined groups and was transferred from Hadamar to Auschwitz, where doctors figured prominently among the killers.[77] The mental and political vision of systematic mass killing has been developed not only in the mass-shooting of Jews in the conquered territories but also in the step from systematic

75 An example is Schmuhl, *Rassenhygiene*, 29–30, 383 n.16.
76 See, e.g., Bock, *Zwangssterilisation*, 59–75, 100–3, 354–68, 452–5.
77 For this transition, see esp. Lifton, *Nazi Doctors*; Peukert, "Genesis der 'Endlösung'"; Christopher R. Browning, "Genozid und Gesundheitswesen," in Christian Pross and Götz Aly, eds., *Der Wert des Menschen: Medizin in Deutschland, 1918–1945* (Berlin, 1989), 316–27; Klee, *"Euthanasie,"* 367–79; Schmuhl, *Rassenhygiene*, 240–60.

"prevention" to systematic "annihilation" of "worthless" life, that is, in the context of eugenic racism, to be then employed for the purpose of ethnic racism. The two were not separate and did not, in the strict sense, follow each other but overlapped and interacted in various ways.[78] The "Jewish Question" was translated into medical imagery: Eugenic sterilization did not exclude Jews but included many of them, and euthanasia included the first systematic massacre of Jews, without even a selection between the curable and incurable.[79] Eugenic racism has been a major and driving force behind the radicalization of ethnic racism, even though originally the assumption of a "twisted road to Auschwitz" has not taken it into account[80] and regardless of the fact that some euthanizers may have disagreed with the extension of their own deadly visions to the Jews.

Sterilization and "euthanasia" in the history of National Socialist medicine may be placed in their larger social and political context in the following ways. First, the extremely short road from compulsory and mass sterilization to the massacre of the ill can, in part, be explained by the internal dynamics of the medical profession, but even more important is the political, institutional, and mental power of the National Socialist policy of racism. Doctors were seen – and many of them saw themselves – as the agents of racial, ethnic, as well as eugenic, purity and finally of genocide. Second, the twisted but short road from the persecution of Jews and Gypsies to their systematic physical destruction passed largely through the eugenic massacre of the ill. Third, both massacres were forms of National Socialist race policy, distinctive but interacting and sharing a similar imagery. It seems therefore plausible to identify the massacre of the ill, as does Lifton, as "a prior, smaller genocidal

---

78 Kater, *Nazi Doctors*, 177-83 ("The Medicalization of the 'Jewish Question'").
79 Henry Friedlander, "Jüdische Anstaltspatienten im NS-Deutschland," in Aly, ed., *Aktion T4*, 34–44; Lutz Raphael, "Euthanasie und Judenvernichtung," in Christina Vanja and Martin Vogt, eds., *Euthanasie in Hadamar: Die nationalsozialistische Vernichtungspolitik in hessischen Anstalten* (Kassel, 1991), 79–90; Christine-Ruth Müller and Hans-Ludwig Siemen, *Warum sie sterben mussten: Leidensweg und Vernichtung von Behinderten aus den Neuendettelsauer Pflegeanstalten im "Dritten Reich"* (Neustadt/Aisch, 1992), 68–70, 128–9; Friedemann Pfäfflin et al., "Die jüdischen Patienten der Psychiatrischen und Nervenklinik des Universitätskrankenhauses Hamburg (1927–1945)," in Friedemann Pfäfflin et al., eds., *Der Mensch in der Psychiatrie* (Berlin, 1988), 101–28; Christiane Hoss, "Die jüdischen Patienten in den rheinischen Anstalten zur Zeit des Nationalsozialismus," in Matthias Leipert et al., *Verlegt nach unbekannt: Sterilisation und Euthanasie in Galkhausen, 1933–1945* (Cologne, 1987), 60–76; Manfred Klüppel, *"Euthanasie" und Lebensvernichtung am Beispiel der Landesheilanstalten Haina und Merxhausen* (Kassel, 1985), 28–31; Bettina Winter, "Die Heil- und Pflegeanstalt Heppenheim von 1914 bis 1945," in *Psychiatrie in Heppenheim ... 1866–1992* (Kassel, 1993), 83–6.
80 Karl A. Schleunes, *The Twisted Road to Auschwitz: Nazi Policy Toward German Jews, 1933–1939* (Urbana, Ill., 1970); Hans Mommsen, "Die Realisierung des Utopischen: Die 'Endlösung der Judenfrage' im 'Dritten Reich,'" *Geschichte und Gesellschaft* 9 (1983): 381–420.

event."[81] Yet I would hesitate to classify the eugenic strand of racism, including euthanasia, simply as genocide.[82] For historical as well as analytical reasons, we need to determine not only common grounds, commonalties, and interactions but also differences – among victims, among perpetrators, and among policies. Complexities should not be all too lightly collapsed into identities. Moreover, because the German people clearly did not perceive sterilization and euthanasia as an attack on themselves as a people – despite some remarkable criticism and opposition – the adoption of the concept of genocide for euthanasia appears to be mistaken.[83] Fourth, at the roots of National Socialist race policy is a doubled vision of humanity and human beings – a more or less modern, more or less normal twentieth-century welfare state for the "valuable" kind, and discrimination, persecution, and finally massacre of the "unworthy" kind. In the minds of their propagators, these were two sides of the same coin, intimately linked, for instance, in the notion that costly welfare for the valuable could be had, and paid for, only by suppressing the eugenically and ethnically "alien." But in other people's minds, including historians', this link is not compelling. The democratic European welfare states demonstrate clearly that welfare measures need not be accompanied by inhumane and anti-human policies.[84] National Socialism, including its medical dimensions, should not be conceived as a modern welfare state,[85] but rather as its perversion – a regime where the hubris of medical utopianism and racial purity put an end to humane ethics.

81 Lifton, *Nazi Doctors*, 479. The German translation has "kleiner Genozid" (*Ärzte im Dritten Reich* [1988], 581).
82 As does Schmuhl, "Sterilisation, 'Euthanasie,' 'Endlösung,'" 296, 300-1, 308.
83 This has justly been pointed out by Norbert Frei in his introduction to *Medizin und Gesundheitspolitik*, 15.
84 For some comparisons, see Gisela Bock and Pat Thane, eds., *Maternity and Gender Policies: Women and the Rise of the European Welfare States, 1880s–1950s* (London, 1991).
85 Christoph Sachsse and Florian Tennstedt, *Der Wohlfahrtsstaat im Nationalsozialismus* (Stuttgart, 1993). Based on the interpretation of Nazi racism as an "Endlösung der sozialen Frage," the authors argue that National Socialism was a welfare state and that it differed only in degree, not in kind, from other and democratic welfare states (273–8).

8

The Old as New

The Nuremberg Doctors' Trial and Medicine in Modern Germany

GEOFFREY COCKS

On October 25, 1946, Brigadier General Telford Taylor, Chief of Counsel for War Crimes, filed an indictment before Nuremberg Military Tribunal I charging twenty-three German defendants with "murders, brutalities, cruelties, tortures, atrocities, and other inhuman acts."[1] Known officially as "The Medical Case," the subsequent proceedings also became known as "The Doctors' Trial" because twenty of the defendants were physicians. On August 20, 1947, fifteen of the defendants were declared guilty. The next day seven were sentenced to death and five to life imprisonment. The charges encompassed four crimes: the Jewish skeleton collection, the project to kill tubercular Polish nationals, the "euthanasia" program, and medical experiments on civilian and military prisoners. The experiments included the following: high altitude; freezing; malaria; mustard gas; sulfanilamide treatment of gas gangrene; bone, muscle, and nerve regeneration and bone transplantation; potability of sea water; epidemic jaundice, typhus, and other vaccines; poisoned food and bullets; phosphorus incendiary bombs; biochemical treatment of sepsis with phlegmon; blood coagulation with polygal; toxicity of phenol; chemical, surgical, and X-ray sterilization. The victims included Germans, Russians, Czechs, Ukrainians, Poles, Yugoslavs, Jews, Roma, Jehovah's Witnesses, communists, theologians, resistance fighters, mental patients, so-called asocials, men, women, and children. The exact numbers are impossible to determine, but according to trial documents, approximately 3,500 people were used as test subjects. At least 800 died, as many as 400 of the 1,100 test subjects in the Dachau malaria tests alone.[2]

The human experiments constituted the bulk of the charges, and this chapter will attempt to show that their origins and aims stemmed from the social

---

1 Trials of War Criminals Before the Nuernberg Military Tribunals Under Control Council Law No. 10 (Washington, D.C., 1950), I:8 (hereafter cited as TWC I, TWC II). I am grateful to Michael Geyer, Richard Evans, Margaret Anderson, and Charles McClelland for their helpful comments on this essay.
2 TWC I:289.

173

and professional trajectories of medicine in the history of modern Germany. These dynamics in turn demonstrate some problematic structural and attitudinal features of modern Western history in general and thus can alter our understanding of the place of German history in the history of the West. The Nuremberg Doctors' Trial, therefore, has significance even beyond the history of Nazi atrocities, the extent and limit of international justice, and the fragility of medical ethics.

It might seem at first that there is little to say about these acts from the perspective of law, ethics, or history. The cases at Nuremberg were simple and straightforward. They involved the murder of the involuntary subjects of medical experimentation.[3] Even the Nuremberg Code, which declared that "certain basic principles must be observed in order to satisfy moral, ethical, and legal concepts"[4] in medical experimentation on human beings, was originally ghettoized as "a good code for barbarians but an unnecessary code for ordinary physician-scientists."[5] In other words, the actions of the Nazi doctors were an aberration from well-established and well-observed principles of medical practice and research. They were clearly and unambiguously contrary to medical as well as general ethics. And when it comes to history, what do these atrocities tell us about the Third Reich – and Germany – that we do not already know?

In the realm of law, the Medical Case at Nuremberg is significant in two fundamental ways. First of all, it was the first in a series of trials. In 1947 doctors charged with experimenting on human beings at Sachsenhausen and Auschwitz were tried in Berlin and Cracow, respectively. In East Germany trials were held in 1966 in Berlin and Magdeburg for like crimes committed at Neuengamme and Auschwitz. West Germany had held its own Sachsenhausen trial in Cologne in 1962.[6] But the reach of trials has been distinctly limited. Only a few of the many individuals involved in medical crimes have been brought to justice, not to mention the even more wide-

---

3   Michael A. Grodin, "Historical Origins of the Nuremberg Code," in George J. Annas and Michael A. Grodin, eds., *The Nazi Doctors and the Nuremberg Code: Human Rights in Human Experimentation* (New York, 1992), 139; Rainer Osnowski, ed., *Menschenversuche: Wahnsinn und Wirklichkeit* (Cologne, 1988).
4   *TWC* II:181.
5   Jay Katz, "The Consent Principle of the Nuremberg Code: Its Significance Then and Now," in Annas and Grodin, eds., *Nazi Doctors and the Nuremberg Code*, 228.
6   Gerhard Baader, "Menschenexperimente," in Fridolf Kudlien, ed., *Ärzte im Nationalsozialismus*, (Cologne, 1985), 177; Brigitte Leyendecker and Burghard F. Klapp, "Deutsche Hepatitisforschung im Zweiten Weltkrieg," in Christian Pross and Götz Aly, eds., *Der Wert des Menschen: Medizin in Deutschland, 1918–1945* (Berlin, 1989), 270; Günther Schwarberg, *The Murders at the Bullenhuser Damm*, trans. Erna Rosenfeld and Alvin Rosenfeld (Bloomington, Ind., 1984), 112–19; Donald M. McKale, "Purging Nazis: The Postwar Trials of Female German Doctors and Nurses," *Proceedings of the South Carolina Historical Association* (1981): 156–70.

spread unpunished complicity in the sterilization and murder of mental patients by the Nazis.[7] Moreover, legal actions cannot address the issue of those in medical authority who said or did nothing on the basis of suspicion or knowledge of what was going on in the camps and asylums. Much of the controversy over Alexander Mitscherlich's documentation of the Doctors' Trial arose from Mitscherlich's contention that knowledge and tolerance of medical atrocities extended deep and high into the ranks of the medical profession.[8] Many members of the medical leadership in West Germany in particular had continued or built careers in the Third Reich.

Second, the Nuremberg Code became the cornerstone for national and international legislation concerning human experimentation in research and treatment. The World Medical Association, founded in 1947, codified standards for human experimentation in the successive Declarations of Helsinki in 1964, 1975, 1983, and 1989. But whereas the original Nuremberg Code has as its first principle the "voluntary consent of the human subject,"[9] the Helsinki guidelines have made what many see as ethically dubious concessions at the expense of this first principle to the political and military requirements of states as well as to the medical and scientific interests of doctors and researchers.[10] Even these strictures are often not honored in the breach. The U.S. military employed four of the acquitted Doctors' Trial defendants both before and after their acquittal.[11] Debates have raged over the value and use of data from the Dachau experiments.[12] More recently,

7 Hans-Walter Schmuhl, *Rassenhygiene, Nationalsozialismus, Euthanasie: Von der Verhütung zur Vernichtung "lebensunwerten Lebens," 1890–1945* (Göttingen, 1987); Michael Burleigh, *Death and Deliverance: "Euthanasia" in Germany c. 1900–1945* (Cambridge, 1994); Dirk Blasius, "Psychiatrischer Alltag im Nationalsozialismus," in Detlev J. K. Peukert and Jürgen Reulecke, eds., *Die Reihen fast geschlossen: Beiträge zur Geschichte des Alltags unterm Nationalsozialismus* (Wuppertal, 1981), 367–80.

8 Alexander Mitscherlich and Fred Mielke, *Wissenschaft ohne Menschlichkeit: Medizinische und Eugenische Irrwege unter Diktatur, Bürokratie und Krieg* (Heidelberg, 1949), v, 6, 279–98. This theme dominates the biomedical division of the recently opened Holocaust Museum in Washington, D.C.; see *Journal of the American Medical Association* 268 (1992): 575–6.

9 *TWC* II:181.

10 Katz, "Consent Principle," 231–4; on legitimate challenges to Western individualism from Eastern and Southern cultures incorporating communal values, see Robert J. Levine, "Validity of Consent Procedures in Technologically Developing Countries," in Zenon Bankowski and N. Howard Jones, eds., *Human Experimentation and Medical Ethics* (Geneva, 1982), 16–30.

11 Linda Hunt, "U.S. Coverup of Nazi Scientists," *Bulletin of the Atomic Scientists* 41 (1985): 21–3; see also Stefan Kühl, *The Nazi Connection: Eugenics, American Racism, and German National Socialism* (New York, 1994); and Christian Pross, "Nazi Doctors: Criminals, Charlatans, or Pioneers? The Commentaries of the Allied Experts in the Nuremberg Doctors Trial," in Charles G. Roland et al., eds., *Medicine Without Compassion, Past and Present: Fall Meeting, Cologne, September 28–30, 1988* (Hamburg, 1992), 253–84.

12 Robert L. Berger, "Nazi Science – The Dachau Hypothermia Experiments," *New England Journal of Medicine* 322 (1990): 1435–40; see also the exchange in *Lancet* 151 (1946): 798, 830, 961; ibid., 152 (1947): 143; and the prophetic novel by Josephine Bell, *Murder in Hospital* (London, 1941). Not surprisingly, West German medical journals of the period (e.g., *Münchener medizinische Wochenschrift,*

evidence has surfaced of experimentation on athletes and mental patients in the former German Democratic Republic.[13] And in December 1990 the U.S. Food and Drug Administration "granted the Department of Defense a waiver from the informed consent requirements of the Nuremberg Code and existing federal law and regulations to use unapproved drugs and vaccines on the soldiers involved in Desert Shield."[14] Most recent are the revelations concerning American plutonium experiments conducted between 1946 and 1956 on less than fully informed human subjects.

When it comes to ethics, the Nazi doctors were guilty of violating two fundamental principles: "the prohibition against inflicting suffering on human beings and the Kantian categorical imperative prohibiting the use of persons as mere means to the ends of others."[15] Such moral imperatives provide the basis for arguments in favor of the universal application of a code of ethics for doctors and researchers. We are right to reserve special condemnation for doctors who cause and observe suffering and death. The invocation of an ethical imperative is also a necessary and effective response to the arguments from ethical and cultural relativism, from precedent, and from legal positivism, all of which were advanced by the defense at Nuremberg. Such principles are also especially vital in a modern age of professional functionalism and individual and corporate careerism. The Nuremberg defendants argued that as medical experts they could not be held responsible for judging matters of politics or law. This was more than an attempt to obscure the fact that it was mostly they as members of an influential scientific, medical, and military community who had initiated the experiments. It was also an obversion of an especially arrogant, destructive, and militarized Nazi medical "generalization of expertise" to which doctors among professionals everywhere have been particularly prone.[16]

The Doctors' Trial also tells us a great deal about history, about the history of professionalized medicine in Germany, about the history of Germany in general, and about one of the trajectories in the modern history of the West

Deutsche medizinische Wochenschrift, Medizinische Klinik) do not discuss "The Doctors' Trial"; cf. Viktor von Weizsäcker, "'Euthanasie' und Menschenversuche," *Psyche* 1 (1947–48): 68–102. Only recently have the Japanese begun to confront similar human experiments carried out by the infamous Unit 731; see Ian Buruma, *The Wages of Guilt: Memories of War in Germany and Japan* (New York, 1994), 162–3, 189, 194.

13 Steven Dickman, "East Germany: Science in the Disservice of the State," *Science* 245 (1991): 26–7; see also Annette Tuffs, "Germany: Horror Hospital," *Lancet* 338 (1991): 624.

14 George J. Annas, "The Nuremberg Code in U.S. Courts: Ethics versus Expediency," in Annas and Grodin, eds., *Nazi Doctors and the Nuremberg Code*, 216.

15 Ruth Macklin, "Universality of the Nuremberg Code," in Annas and Grodin, eds., *Nazi Doctors and the Nuremberg Code*, 255.

16 See Geoffrey Cocks, "Partners and Pariahs: Jews and Medicine in Modern German Society," *Leo Baeck Institute Yearbook* 36 (1991): 195–6.

as a whole. In Germany doctors played an inordinate role in the development and application of racial biology both before and after the advent of the Nazis.[17] The defendants at Nuremberg were at some pains to avoid mentioning any professional or individual allegiance to Nazi racial aims. In this they were not alone. In Mario Puzo's 1955 novel about occupied Germany, *The Dark Arena*, a U.S. Army civilian personnel officer in Frankfurt laments, "Never in the Party, never in the SA, never in the Hitler Youth. Christ, I'm dying to meet a Nazi."[18] At the Doctors' Trial, this type of behavior reached one of its many low points when Karl Gebhardt denied knowledge of the purpose of the camps, blamed atrocities there on "the negative selection of... scum, conscripts, [and] foreigners," and defended the honor of "the decent Waffen SS."[19] Such disingenuous denial also, however, alerts us to motivating factors other than Nazi beliefs among these men (and one woman). The same is true of their rationalizations. Aside from attempting whenever possible to distance themselves from the experiments which had caused injury and death, the defendants vainly attempted to justify their actions. Several of these arguments had to do with the status of the human subjects: The prisoners in the experiments had been condemned to death; they were volunteers; they offered themselves in expiation for their crimes; those subjected to life-threatening experiments had been promised commutation if they survived. The defense also offered four arguments having to do with obedience to authority: It was wartime; the government had power and authority over the defendants; they had a right and a responsibility to help defend their country; there was no law in Germany or anywhere else against human experimentation. This last argument from authority was linked to an argument from precedent: Human experimentation had a long history. Finally, there was the argument from utility: The few must be sacrificed to save the many during a total war in which the lives of thousands of German soldiers and civilians were threatened by enemy action and by disease. This utilitarian argument was also in accord with the Nazi ideal of *Gemeinnutz geht vor Eigennutz* (public good has priority over individual good), which was applied to military triage of German wounded during World War II.[20]

The prosecution at Nuremberg was forced to concede that there had been precedents for human experimentation. Cross-examination by the defense of

---

17 Paul Weindling, *Health, Race and German Politics Between National Unification and Nazism, 1870–1945* (Cambridge, 1989).
18 Mario Puzo, *The Dark Arena* (New York, 1955), 45.
19 *TWC* II:146.
20 Johanna Bleker, "Zum Problem der Krankensichtung in der deutschen Wehrmachtsmedizin im Zweiten Weltkrieg," in Samuel Mitja Rapoport and Achim Thom, eds., *Das Schicksal der Medizin im Faschismus* (Berlin, 1989), 184–7.

prosecution expert witness Dr. Andrew Ivy also elicited the fact that the American Medical Association guidelines for human experimentation presented as evidence for the prosecution dated from 1946.[21] But the prosecution was hardly defenseless on this score. Aside from powerful arguments ranging from Western moral philosophy and the Hippocratic oath to the ethical bankruptcy of the Nazi racism that informed the experiments, the prosecution was able to cite a preexisting ordinance regulating experiments on human beings. There was only the one, but it had been promulgated in 1931 – in Germany.

On February 28, 1931, the Reich Interior Ministry published a circular concerning "Richtlinien für neuartige Heilbehandlung und für die Vornahme wissenschaftlicher Versuche am Menschen" (guidelines for novel treatment and for the undertaking of experiments on humans).[22] These guidelines, expanding on a similar Prussian directive from 1900, required, among other restrictions, consent of the patient for any nonemergency innovative therapy and of the subject of any nontherapeutic research.[23] There was debate at Nuremberg about whether these guidelines had the force of law. The Nazi regime apparently never specifically revoked these guidelines, but no such specific revocation would have been required. The Nazis abolished the Reichsgesundheitsrat, the five-man council that had issued the guidelines. More importantly, the Nazis destroyed the ethical autonomy of physicians upon which the guidelines were based. The *Reichsärzteordnung* (Reich Physicians' Ordinance) of 1935, which declared that medicine was no longer a trade but rather a profession, subordinated the doctor to the dictates of the state, the will of the *Volk*, and what was termed the individual physician's own "gesundes Volksempfinden" (healthy national instincts).[24]

However, the 1931 guidelines have a history of their own that allows us to place the Doctors' Trial in a more extensive and fruitful context. Like the Prussian directive of 1900, the Reich circular of 1931 was largely the result of public outcry over well-publicized instances of medical malfeasance by doctors and hospitals. In the 1890s the cause célèbre was that of the dermatologist Albert Neisser of Breslau, who had inoculated four children and three adolescent female prostitutes with syphilis serum. In 1930 a Social Democratic member of the Reichstag, Dr. Julius Moses, decried the deaths

21 *TWC* II:85.
22 *Reichsgesundheitsblatt* 6 (1931): 174–5; *TWC* II:83.
23 Hans-Martin Sass, "Reichsrundschreiben 1931: Pre-Nuremberg German Regulations Concerning New Therapy and Human Experimentation," *Journal of Medicine and Philosophy* 8 (1983): 99–111; Pross and Aly, eds., *Der Wert des Menschen*, 92; on the Prussian directive, see Grodin, "Historical Origins of the Nuremberg Code," 127–8.
24 *Reichsärzteordnung* (Berlin, 1943), 7, 11.

of seventy-five children in Lübeck whose pediatricians were experimenting with tuberculosis vaccines.[25] By this time the medical establishment had already become extremely worried about the rising tide of public criticism. There was the danger that restrictions might be placed on their ability to try new treatments and to perform necessary medical research. In addition, German law as a whole was only gradually coming to reflect the need of doctors and medical researchers to experiment on patients and subjects.[26] The 1931 circular, therefore, was designed not to hinder experimental therapy and research but rather to allow it. This is clear from the first guideline:

> In order that medical science may continue to advance, the initiation in appropriate cases of therapy involving new and as yet insufficiently tested means and procedures cannot be avoided. Similarly, scientific experimentation involving human subjects cannot be completely excluded as such, as this would hinder or even prevent progress in the diagnosis, treatment, and prevention of diseases.[27]

These guidelines thus represented the success of doctors in establishing legally the principle of medical expertise and control within the bounds of law and traditional morality. The guidelines left enforcement to the individual doctor. They also expressed what must have been widespread agreement among doctors concerning the rights of patients and research subjects. Although the guidelines did contribute to the growing asymmetry of power and authority between doctor and patient, it seems fair to say that most doctors in Germany – even in wartime – would have been averse to the gross violations of human rights that were involved in the concentration camp experiments. There is even evidence in published proceedings of the Doctors' Trial that there were degrees of culpability among the defendants that reflected not only function and fear but also reservation. Of course, many doctors acquiesced in, or at least did not protest, these same illegal and unethical acts. In any case, the doctors on trial at Nuremberg could hardly have been unaware of this debate or unaffected by the conditions occasioning it. These physicians were representative of

---

25 Grodin, "Historical Origins of the Nuremberg Code," 127, 129.
26 Alfons Stauder, "Die Zulässigkeit ärztlicher Versuche an gesunden und kranken Menschen," *Münchener medizinische Wochenschrift* 78 (1931): 108. The same complaint was made by socialist physicians about the Nazi law banning vivisection. See, e.g., "Die Vivisektion des Proletariats" [1934], *Internationales Ärztliches Bulletin: Zentralorgan der Internationalen Vereinigung Sozialistischer Ärzte, Jahrgang I-VI (1934–1939)*, Beiträge zur Nationalsozialistischen Gesundheits- und Sozialpolitik, no. 7 (Berlin, 1989), 47–50. On Stauder's leading role in the *Gleichschaltung* of the medical profession, see Michael H. Kater, *Doctors Under Hitler* (Chapel Hill, N.C., 1989), 182–4.
27 Grodin, "Historical Origins of the Nuremberg Code," 130; see also Friedrich Müller, "Die Zulässigkeit ärztlicher Versuche an gesunden und kranken Menschen," *Münchener medizinische Wochenschrift* 78 (1931): 104–7. The complete German text of the circular is in Sass, "Reichsrundschreiben 1931," 107–9.

the mainstream of German medicine, not aberrant demons imposed by the Nazi regime upon the medical profession. They may not have been the cream of the German medical profession, but they came from the same bottle. Gerhard Rose, for one, was director for tropical medicine at the Robert Koch Institute. Karl Gebhardt, for another, had been an assistant at the University of Munich to Germany's leading surgeon, Ferdinand Sauerbruch, and since 1925 had specialized in reconstructive surgery and rehabilitation at Hohenaschau and Hohenlychen.[28] Their varying allegiances to Nazi racial ideals, along with their ambition and the prevailing political, social, and military conditions, simply led these doctors to reject humane standards.

But two broader historical conditions also worked significant influences on these doctors. The first was the rapid and pervasive medicalization of modern German society during the twentieth century. Doctors and medicine simply became more important and powerful during the period. This was common throughout the Western world; everywhere doctors and medicine began to play significant roles in the lives of individuals and in society. The second major historical influence on the Nazi doctors was the Nazis' own marked hypersensitivity to health and illness.

Whereas in earlier times illness and disease were closely linked in time with death and thus were matters of individual fate, modern medicine (and public sanitation and health policy) began to render illness and disease a matter of organized prophylaxis and treatment. As a result, for the first time the sick person became a social entity with an actual and perceived identity.[29] The ramifications of this development included significant social conflict. During the Weimar Republic, many doctors believed that their status and well-being were threatened by certain political and economic forces and trends. Historian Michael Kater has documented the large percentage of doctors who were led as a result into varying degrees of allegiance to National Socialism. Doctors on the political right warned of a "crisis in medicine" that was "variously construed as the bureaucratization, specialization, or scientization of medicine."[30] Often mixed into this were complaints about materialism, urbanism, and the pernicious influence of Jewish physicians.

28 U.S. Nuernberg War Crimes Trial, Record Group 238, Microcopy M-887, roll 29, frames 538–9; National Archives, Washington, D.C.; "Vermerk über die Besichtigung der klinischen Abteilung für Sport- und Arbeitsschäden der Heilanstalten Hohenlychen," R 89 13499, 129–33, Bundesarchiv Koblenz; Karl Gebhardt, "Allgemeines zur Wiederherstellungschirurgie," *Zentralblatt für Chirurgie* 63 (1936): 1570–6.
29 Claudine Herzlich and Janine Pierret, *Illness and Self in Society*, trans. Elborg Forster (Baltimore, Md., 1987).
30 Robert N. Proctor, *Racial Hygiene: Medicine Under the Nazis* (Cambridge, Mass., 1988), 69.

The political left criticized what they saw as capitalist inegalitarianism and the greedy hostility of the doctors' lobby toward the state health insurance system. This discontent was aggravated at the end of the decade by the ongoing increase in health premiums and decline in payments, even though businesses and government continued to pour increasing amounts of money into the system until at least 1930.[31] This situation – one not unfamiliar in the West today – was commented on regularly and angrily in a survey psychoanalyst Erich Fromm conducted among German blue- and white-collar workers in 1929.[32] Controversies among proponents and opponents of natural health, homeopathy, and *Schulmedizin* (academic medicine) also raged, though more across and within political, social, and occupational boundaries than along them.

Relationships between patients and doctors were also problematic. By and large, doctors gained state-sanctioned expert authority – "practitioner control" – over their patients. The perverse extremity of this trend would be reached by Nazi human experimentation. People in general tended to like their own doctors, but to be suspicious of, or even hostile to, doctors as a group. (This is not unlike the present situation in the United States.) We have already referred to long-standing public unease over medical experiments on patients and the doctors' success in protecting themselves by issuing guidelines for therapeutic and nontherapeutic experimentation in 1931. Historian Edward Shorter has argued that during the twentieth century doctors in the West gradually built a reputation for caring and competence in the minds of patients. For the first time, doctors were able to diagnose, treat, and even cure illness. According to Shorter, it was after World War II that the impersonality of modern technical medicine began seriously to erode this generally happy relationship. Shorter's model holds generally true for Germany, but as we have seen, patients' and the public's attitudes toward doctors – and doctors' attitudes toward patients and the public – were deeply ambivalent. The mutual distrust Shorter demonstrates for the period after 1945 is clearly evident in Germany during the interwar period.

The Third Reich only made things worse. Doctors were brought under the control of the state, educational standards in medicine deteriorated, and the many Jewish general practitioners and specialists in Germany and Austria were barred from practice altogether in 1938. The introduction in the 1930s

---

31   David Abraham, *The Collapse of the Weimar Republic: Political Economy and Crisis*, 2d ed. (New York, 1986), 241.
32   Erich Fromm, *The Working Class in Weimar Germany: A Psychological and Sociological Study*, ed. Wolfgang Bonss and trans. Barbara Weinberger (Cambridge, Mass., 1984). The analysis of responses to questions about health and illness was not published.

of medically effective mass market drugs enhanced the popularity of doctors, but at the same time it tended to make them the passive dispensers of comfort or cure instead of their active agents. During the war doctors were in even greater demand because the Nazis required *Atteste* (certification) from physicians in order for people to miss work or obtain extra rations. But the growing vigilance of the authorities for slackers and malingerers (and doctors' cultivation of them) as well as chronic shortages of drugs diminished public appreciation of, and reliance upon, increasingly overworked and inexperienced doctors. Doctors, largely products of an authoritarian past now aggravated by an authoritarian present, often regarded patients as irresponsible in any number of ways.[33]

Nazi hypersensitivity to matters of health and illness was inherent in Nazi racism, with its obsession with a hierarchy of races based on specific physical and mental characteristics. The Nazis' social Darwinism added the component of struggle against inferior races. Even war itself, as the emotional and practical solution to the problem of inferior races, was inherently problematic for the Nazis. In 1944 Reichsgesundheitsführer Leonardo Conti, echoing the concern of early race hygienist Alfred Ploetz and the antiwar stance of the Monist League before World War I, worried about the "dysgenic" effects of war whereby the fittest die at the front while the less fit burden already strained medical services at home.[34] The Nazis' obsession with strength expressed a preoccupation with weakness and threats to the physical integrity of the body. During the nineteenth century, disease had become a pervasive metaphor for the "unnatural," whereas the rising anti-Semitism of the time drew upon a long-standing association in the minds of many Europeans between Jews and illness.[35] The disease imagery of Hitler's *Mein Kampf* and the bloody misogynist fantasies of members of the Freikorps are two major cases in point.[36] On the basis of comparatively few responses to the questions "Are you afraid of illness?" and "Why (not)?" as well as a few other related questions in his survey of 1929, Fromm concluded that Nazi voters (and the most active members of the Communist Party, or KPD) betrayed a greater

---

33 Meldungen aus dem Reich, May 9, 1940, Microcopy T-175, roll 259, frame 1485, and Oct. 2, 1941, roll 261, frames 4928–31, National Archives; Jahresgesundheitsbericht, Gesundheitsamt Grevenbroich-Neuss, Jan. 31, 1940, Reg. Düsseldorf 54341, Nordrhein-Westfälisches Hauptstaatsarchiv, Düsseldorf; Edward Shorter, *Bedside Manners: The Troubled History of Doctors and Patients* (New York, 1985).

34 Leonardo Conti, "Stand der Volksgesundheit im 5. Kriegsjahr," 15, Reg. Aachen 16486, Nordrhein-Westfälisches Hauptstaatsarchiv, Düsseldorf.

35 Sander L. Gilman, "Jews and Mental Illness: Medical Metaphors, Anti-Semitism, and the Jewish Response," *Journal of the History of the Behavioral Sciences* 20 (1984): 150; Susan Sontag, *Illness as Metaphor* (New York, 1978), 74.

36 Klaus Theweleit, *Male Fantasies*, 2 vols., trans. Erica Carter, Stephen Conway, and Chris Turner (Minneapolis, Minn., 1987 and 1989).

sense of hopelessness and internal conflict.[37] For example, Questionnaire 204 is that of a Nazi voter from Frankfurt am Main who saw Germany controlled by "the Jew" and who answered the questions about fear of illness with "Ja" and "Da sie für uns nichts gutes Einbringen" (nothing good comes of it).[38]

The Nazis' problems were aggravated from the start by the fact that the overall health of the German population had been adversely affected by the effects of malnutrition and the associated health and developmental problems stemming from World War I, the inflation of 1923, the Depression, and the Nazis' own martial activities in the 1930s.[39] These problems had in turn aggravated the already widespread significant health problems among Germans in the economically deprived classes. We must also remember that the Germans by and large constituted a society long concerned with matters of individual and collective *Sauberkeit* (cleanliness). Mobilization for war created a shortage of doctors, particularly among specialists, so much so that the misogynist Nazis were forced to admit unprecedented numbers of women into the medical schools and even to toy with the idea of allowing Jewish physicians to treat non-Jewish patients.[40] The war also led directly to the experiments on human beings in the concentration camps. The shortage of doctors, medical students, and military cadets as sources of traditional volunteers was advanced by the defense at Nuremberg as an additional compelling reason to use camp inmates.[41] In Russia, German soldiers were exposed to bitter cold, which, together with the Luftwaffe's concern for airmen downed at sea, led to the hypothermia experiments.[42] Heavy casualties from gas gangrene on the Eastern front led to the sulfanilamide experiments.[43] The increasingly high operational ceilings attained by enemy aircraft led to the high-altitude experiments.[44] The exposure of German troops in Poland and Russia to typhus, malaria, jaundice, and cholera led to the vaccine experiments.[45]

---

37 Erich Fromm papers, 1929–49, series 3: International Institute for Social Research, B. The German Worker Under the Weimar Republic, box 12, F.5, Unsorted Fragments of Drafts in German, Cont'd, "Bearbeitung zu Frage 415/16 auf Seite 5a," New York Public Library.

38 Ibid., box 13, Tabulations of Questionnaires, F. 5, no. 201–10.

39 Wehrwirtschafts-Inspektion VII (Munich), 1937, Microcopy T-77, roll 248, frames 824–8, National Archives; Friedrich Kortenhaus, "Verschlechterung der Volksgesundheit?" *Münchener medizinische Wochenschrift* 79 (1932): 1964–5.

40 Reichsminister des Innern to Regierungspräsident Frankfurt/Oder, Aug. 23, 1941, p. 3, Pr. Br. Rep. 3 B Nr. 178, Staatsarchiv Potsdam (now Landeshauptarchiv Brandenburg); Cocks, "Partners and Pariahs," 197–200.

41 *TWC* I:323, 326, 330, 492–3.

42 Ibid., *TWC* I:266.

43 Ibid., *TWC* I:356.

44 Ibid., *TWC* I:142.

45 Ibid., *TWC* I:494, 508. On the cholera experiments carried out on prisoners of war in Russia, see Fridolf Kudlien, "Begingen Wehrmachtsärzte im Russlandkrieg Verbrechen gegen die Menschlichkeit?" in Pross and Aly, eds., *Der Wert des Menschen*, 343.

There was" also an important domestic aspect to Nazi concern over the
vulnerability of German soldiers to dangerous infectious diseases. The Nazis
worried that not just slave laborers but returning soldiers from the East would
be sources for new epidemics in Germany.[46] This concern was based on the
outbreak of epidemics in Germany during World War I, largely as a result of
widespread malnutrition. It also rested on the assumption that Germans were
more vulnerable because German public hygiene had rendered such diseases
relatively rare. It was also thought that peoples in the East had built up toler-
ances against such scourges. This view reflected Nazi emphasis on biology,
their typical unconcern with the suffering of others, a studied ignorance of
the role played by the disruptive effects of war, occupation, and exploitation,
and a desire to use this suffering for propaganda about the "unhygienic"
lifestyles of "inferior" races. It was in fact Nazi concern over threats to the
health of resident Germans as a result of the poor conditions under which
Jews were forced to live that played an important role in the creation of the
ghettos in Poland.[47] The German home front in fact never suffered from
epidemics during World War II. This was due to the ruthless segregation of
Eastern prisoners, an efficient mobilization of military and civilian health
agencies, and the fact that the Germans were able to feed themselves at the
expense of the many countries they occupied. Vaccinations, supported by
the German drug industry, played only a small role. The German people
suffered from the multiplication of common ailments, occasioned and aggravated by wartime conditions, especially in the large cities under attack from
the air.[48] Illness also spread because it became one means of what Martin
Broszat more broadly called *Resistenz*[49]: in this case the largely unpolitical
mitigation and avoidance of unpleasant and inconvenient obligations.

The principal ethical lesson contained in the history of the Doctors' Trial
at Nuremberg concerns the dangers of social corporatism. Modern Germany
consistently displayed such a corporatist ethic in its political and social organization. This solidarity can produce benefits for the whole and protect the

---

46 Deutscher Gemeindetag Berlin to Deutscher Gemeindetag Düsseldorf, Sept. 1, 1942, RW 53/466,
    Nordrhein-Westfälisches Hauptstaatsarchiv, Düsseldorf.
47 Christopher Browning, "Genocide and Public Health: German Doctors and Polish Jews,
    1939–1941," *Holocaust and Genocide Studies* 3 (1988): 21–36.
48 Jahresgesundheitsbericht, Stadtkreis Krefeld, Feb. 23, 1944, Reg. Düsseldorf 54291I, Nordrhein-
    Westfälisches Hauptstaatsarchiv, Düsseldorf; see also United States Strategic Bombing Survey,
    Morale Division, Medical Branch Report, *The Effect of Bombing on Health and Medical Care in
    Germany* (Washington, D.C., Oct. 30, 1945).
49 Martin Broszat, "Resistenz und Widerstand: Eine Zwischenbilanz des Forschungsprojekts," in
    Martin Broszat et al., eds., *Bayern in der NS-Zeit* (Munich, 1981), 4:691–709; for an instance of such
    "resistance" – and also reliance upon the popular amphetamine Pervitin – see Heinrich Böll's mem-
    oir, *What's to Become of the Boy? Or: Something to Do with Books*, trans. Leila Vennewitz (New York,
    1984).

members of the group against the depredations of individuals, as was the case with the German health-care system. But it can also lead to organized violation of the rights of individuals and of groups inside and outside the larger group in the name of solidarity. Corporatism cultivates a sense of duty, degrees of conformity, and even fanaticism. In Germany corporatism was part of a similarly generalized historical tradition of illiberalism that significantly affected the professions. These dynamics played a role in the Holocaust and among the doctors who performed experiments on human beings. This is not to say that the careerism and venality even more common as abuses within the liberal ethos were absent among these doctors.[50] And it is not to say that other large economic and political forces were not also responsible for these crimes.[51] But corporatism was the most pervasive phenomenon affecting the groups and individuals involved in these atrocities.

There is also a historical lesson in this story, one that allows us to see the old *Sonderweg* controversy in a new way. The lesson lies in the fact that the corporate tradition in Germany anticipated certain corporatist features of Western postliberal industrial statism. In the twentieth century, corporatism became a major feature of, among other things, the professionalization of society. The organization of the interests of experts and their employers was accelerated by the growth of the state as a source of money to be granted and regulation to be influenced. These trends were magnified by the two world wars and the resultant "military-industrial complex." The world wars, which came about chiefly as a result of German difficulties, miscalculations, and ambitions, accelerated the "economic militarization" of modern societies throughout the West. The growth in scale and influence of what historian Michael Geyer has called the "organization of violence" by the modern state[52] helped further the trend toward corporate professional and technical service to the state. The growing influence of corporate bodies attempting to monopolize knowledge and technology marginalized the power of political parties and the public. Professionals became an important element of a postliberal state of large interlocking public and private institutions and organized interests.

---

50 See the example of Sigmund Rascher discussed in Kater, *Doctors Under Hitler*, 125–6.
51 Achim Thom, "Verbrecherische Experimente in den Konzentrationslagern – Ausdruck des anti-humanen Charakters einer der faschistischen Machtpolitik untergeordneten medizinischen Forschung," in Achim Thom and Genadij Ivanovic Caregorodcev, eds., *Medizin unterm Hakenkreuz* (Berlin, 1989), 397–9.
52 Michael Geyer, "The Past as Future: The German Officer Corps as Profession," in Geoffrey Cocks and Konrad H. Jarausch, eds., *German Professions, 1800–1950* (New York, 1990); see also Michael S. Sherry, *In the Shadow of War: The United States since the 1930s* (New Haven, Conn., 1995).

Germany, therefore, did not follow a *Sonderweg* in the sense of a departure from a political standard achieved in the West. The false dichotomy between the "peculiar" and the "modern" that liberal historians have imposed upon German history was a function of the American and Western European struggle with their own political and social ambiguities. These were projected onto "the other" in the form, first, of Germany, particularly as a result of the two world wars, and then of Russia, particularly during the Cold War.[53] There was no "special path" in German history because there was no path that had led to an ideal liberal democracy in the West. Instead, in the West and in Germany there were elements of various political and social realities, including liberal democracy. But Germany, like any nation, has its own history and culture. And it was precisely some of that which was peculiar in kind and degree – here the military and professional corporatism preserved chiefly by Bismarck's *kleindeutsch* answer to the German question – that evolved under other conditions in Western nations in the twentieth century. Geyer has argued that the traditional portrayal of two Germanies, one rational and industrial, and the other militaristic and backward, was a function of "a corporate *pax Americana* and of 'America' as the imaginary fulfillment of the Western course of (liberal capitalist) development."[54] To the extent that the concept "nation" is a meaningful one for historians, there was of course only one Germany. The question is how to evaluate the specific conditions of German history without reducing that history to a function of Western ideological concerns. Germany was not the antipode of political developments in the West. Germany also was not simply a somewhat more illiberal version of the Western bourgeois state.[55] Part of the problem is that the primary subject matter of each of these approaches to German history – "premodern" elites and modern bourgeoisie, respectively – determines the nature and scope of the findings. If one studies the feudal one finds the feudal. If one studies the bourgeois one finds the bourgeois. Understanding Germany on its own unitary terms, however, permits us to avoid a static dichotomy posed around the standard of a liberal model and scale of modern historical development.

53 The "domino effect" used by the United States to describe the spread of Communism was in part a carryover from World War II descriptions of the inexorable spread of German and Japanese military expansionism.

54 Michael Geyer, "Looking Back at the International Style: Some Reflections on the Current State of German History," *German Studies Review* 13 (1990): 113.

55 David Blackbourn and Geoff Eley, *The Peculiarities of German History: Bourgeois Society and Politics in Nineteenth-Century Germany* (New York, 1984). On the distinctiveness of German liberalism, see Dieter Langewiesche, *Liberalismus im 19. Jahrhundert: Deutschland im europäischen Vergleich* (Göttingen, 1988).

In Germany strong traditions of corporatism in society and state had been preserved and strengthened by the unique manner of German state building through the unification of Germany by Prussia.[56] As in the West, powerful new commercial and industrial interests in the Reich, too, displayed inherent corporate instincts. Bismarck, like Napoleon III in France and Benjamin Disraeli in England only with more success, harnessed the new political forces of liberalism and democracy in service to old standards and structures of paternalistic governance. Less successful was his attempt to woo the working class to the paternalistic state by means of a state health insurance system. Even Wilhelm II, that bumbling avatar of Prussianism, maintained some degree of royal authority through a striking and effective mix of old and new methods of rule.[57] This paternalism of thought and deed in Germany contrasts with the liberalism of England during the same period, where greater economic and political individualism helped create the greater effectiveness of political parties and Parliament and also greater disparities between rich and poor.[58]

The process of professionalization itself was also problematic along these same lines. The growing power of the professions in Germany was advanced by a traditional German respect for learning, the rapid industrialization of Germany, growing technical sophistication in disciplines like medicine, and in the end, the Nazi demand for such organized technical expertise for purposes of racial selection, social control, and military expansion. Professions in the West, however, have traditionally been associated with liberal ideals such as individual liberty, a free market, meritocracy, and representative government. Had, therefore, German professionals represented a challenge to corporate traditions in Germany? This was most certainly not the case with the medical profession since 1869, when liberal Berlin physicians had completed a successful effort to establish medicine legally as a free trade rather than as a profession. From the founding of the Reich in 1871 onward, doctors (and, to one degree or another, most other professions) confronted and courted a powerful state bureaucracy. In the case of medicine, Bismarck's construction of a state health insurance system and the subsequent growth of socialist influence within it prompted aggressive collective action among doctors in defense of their interests. Such action included the threat of strikes to improve the position of doctors in the *Krankenkassen* (sickness funds) system, a campaign to gain recognition from the state as a profession (achieved

56 John Breuilly, "State-Building, Modernization and Liberalism from the Late Eighteenth Century to Unification: German Peculiarities, Liberalism, and Modernization in Wilhelmine Germany," *European History Quarterly* 22 (1992): 257–84, 431–8.
57 Thomas A. Kohut, *Wilhelm II and the Germans: A Study in Leadership* (New York, 1991).
58 Kenneth Barkin, "Germany and England: Economic Inequality," *Tel Aviver Jahrbuch für deutsche Geschichte* 16 (1987): 200–11.

with ambiguous political and professional effects in 1935), and ongoing attempts to regulate the market for physicians' services. Moreover, during the twentieth century–and especially with the national and economic disasters following World War I–many doctors were radicalized toward the political right. More generally, the German experience of professionalization has alerted historians not only to what the "liberal" professions in Germany confronted, but also to what liberal professions are, or at least have become. Thus the recent study of the German experience of professionalization has contributed to an established critique of the Western ideal type of the liberal professional.

Historian Charles McClelland has argued that "the German experience of professionalization, with its complicated tangle of private sphere and bureaucratically controlled dimensions, may prove more typical of professionalization throughout the twentieth-century world than the Anglo-American 'model.' "[59] International legislation on human experimentation enhancing professional, state, and military claims at some expense of patients and subjects is a relevant example in the field of medicine. The trend toward "professional neocorporatism" began in late Imperial Germany, according to historian Konrad Jarausch, when "professionals participated in the bourgeois shift from liberal to national attitudes," assuming a "postliberal" position based on a "rising tide of 'academic illiberalism.' "[60] This shift away from liberalism aggravated the tendency among professionals everywhere in the twentieth century toward using "the state to secure income and social position" and "rejecting its control over practice and organization."[61] In Germany this process drew upon an especially strong tradition of institutionalized corporatist thought, practice, and feeling at all levels of polity and society. Such a tradition encouraged both the obedience to state authority in pursuit of professional recognition and the defense of the profession's own corporate interests against the state and against competitors and clients. Particularly in medicine, even the enlightened liberal scientific ethic of individual and social improvement through technical and therapeutic

---

59   Charles E. McClelland, *The German Experience of Professionalization: Modern Learned Professions and Their Organizations from the Early Nineteenth Century to the Hitler Era* (Cambridge, 1991), 10.

60   Konrad H. Jarausch, *The Unfree Professions: German Lawyers, Teachers, and Engineers* (New York, 1990), 24. This characterization employs a historical Central European meaning of "corporatism" as calling for a sociopolitical order based on *Berufsstände*. The prefix "neo" indicates the postliberal thrust of the attempt to reintroduce premodern elements into high industrial society (269n. 97). It can also be argued that no such turn from "liberal" to "national" was necessary to produce the type of corporate behavior Jarausch describes. Such an argument views liberalism as inherently corporate rather than as a more or less Western "ideal type" corrupted by special German conditions.

61   Ibid., 24.

intervention and prevention itself could help advance even inhumane state imperatives.[62]

Nazi Germany occasioned a fatal confluence of these trends and traditions. Genocide and *Krankenmord* were the direct result of Nazi racism. For genocide no other rationale or rationalization was advanced. The murder of the mentally and physically ill could be and was rationalized on the grounds of mercy or, especially during the war, utility. The experiments on human beings were racist in that they at least implicitly accepted the racist categorization of prisoners they used, in particular the Jews, Poles, and Russians upon whom the most dangerous experiments were usually conducted. But even though they were occasioned, informed, and exacerbated in effect by racism, these experiments, unlike those perpetrated by Josef Mengele and others at Auschwitz, were primarily military in origin and nature, thus providing ready rationalizations that have been defended and echoed at other times and places. The great majority of the doctors on trial at Nuremberg were in the military: Seventeen of twenty-three were members of either the Luftwaffe, the army, or the Waffen SS. Most were not career military, but they worked on behalf of the military and had also subscribed to the militaristic ethos of the Nazi Party and its affiliated organizations. During the war, as members of a military band of brothers, the Nuremberg doctors' professionalized corporatist instincts were intensified by a militaristic regime engaged in a campaign of racial expansion and extermination. They were thus relatively insulated from the atomization and individual competitiveness caused by Nazi dissolution of traditional social groupings.[63]

Moreover, the individuals who conducted the experiments were in great measure acting on principles and practices long embedded in their culture, their society, and their military identity. These principles and practices were then reinforced by much that was happening around them in the Third Reich. These doctors had been born, raised, educated, and in some cases had established themselves professionally before the Nazis came to power. Each one of them, had, as a child, youth, and young adult, internalized values, habits, and attitudes of an Imperial Germany at the height of its powers and in the depths of its final crisis. World War I had an especially significant effect on

62 Michael Hubenstorf, "'Aber es kommt mir doch so vor, als ob Sie dabei nichts verloren hätten': Zum Exodus von Wissenschaftlern aus den staatlichen Forschungsinstituten Berlins im Bereich des öffentlichen Gesundheitswesens," in Wolfram Fischer et al., eds., *Exodus von Wissenschaften aus Berlin: Fragestellungen–Ergebnisse–Desiderate: Entwicklungen vor und nach 1933*, Akademie der Wissenschaften zu Berlin Forschungsbericht, no. 7 (Berlin, 1993), 444–55; Alfons Labisch, *Homo Hygienicus: Gesundheit und Medizin in der Neuzeit* (Frankfurt/Main, 1992), 133.

63 Detlev J. K. Peukert, *Inside Nazi Germany: Conformity, Opposition, and Racism in Everyday Life*, trans. Richard Deveson (New Haven, Conn., 1987), 236–42.

doctors and psychiatrists, who were drafted in unprecedented numbers to deal with the staggering physical and mental casualties of industrial warfare. Military service itself only aggravated the authoritarianism common among doctors as increasingly effective and sought-after experts in matters of life and death. The same was even truer in World War II, especially on the embattled home front. By that time doctors had become even more therapeutically effective, largely through the medical and surgical advances of World War I, as well as the introduction of a wide range of drugs in the 1930s. The increasing initiative of patients only heightened doctors' defense of their prerogatives and authority, now backed up by ruthless Nazi wartime sanctions.

To be sure, the Nuremberg doctors tended to be younger members of the medical profession who had been radicalized by the cultural and professional disruptions of World War I and its outcome, the inflation of 1923, and the *Weltwirtschaftskrise* (world economic crisis) of 1929. All of them were either in their twenties or thirties i.n 1933: Pediatrician Herta Oberheuser, who assisted Karl Gebhardt with the sulfanilamide experiments at Ravensbrück, was twenty-two in that year; Sigmund Rascher, who conducted the high-altitude experiments at Dachau, was twenty-four then. Such doctors were especially susceptible to Nazi propaganda promising national renewal and opportunities – professional and otherwise – for disillusioned yet ambitious youth. The drastic political change of 1933 itself provided opportunities for many people on the way up within, or on the margins of, any establishment to establish themselves, often at the expense of departed Jewish colleagues, in positions of influence.[64]

The effects of all these experiences were intensified by the Nazi environment after 1933. In power were men violently acting out a "personal agony of armour-plated self-discipline."[65] In a very real sense, the Nazis were already at war from 1933 onward. Although the Nazis may have atomized German society by dissolving traditional social groupings, the competitive "hierarchical continuum of achievement"[66] also allowed groups such as doctors to advance their corporate interests in both service and sacrifice to the state. It was a system that "foster[ed] the egotism of both individuals and groups."[67] The war cut both ways, creating an environment of individual "survivalism" and of shared purpose and misery.[68] The professional, military, political, and

---

64 See, e.g., Geoffrey Cocks, *Psychotherapy in the Third Reich: The Göring Institute* (New York, 1985).
65 Peukert, *Inside Nazi Germany*, 169; Theweleit, *Male Fantasies*; Michael Burleigh and Wolfgang Wippermann, *The Racial State: Germany, 1933-1945* (Cambridge, 1991).
66 Peukert, *Inside Nazi Germany*, 95.
67 Michael Geyer, "The Nazi State Reconsidered," in Richard Bessel, ed., *Life in the Third Reich* (Oxford, 1987), 59.
68 Cf. Tilla Siegel, "Wage Policy in Nazi Germany," *Politics and Society* 14 (1985): 37; Christa Wolf, *Patterns of Childhood*, trans. Ursule Molinaro and Hedwig Rappolt (New York, 1984), 200.

national identities of the doctors experimenting on human beings fused under the pressures of war into a hard alloy of interest, duty, desire, allegiance, and rationalization. The very extremities of the camps and the condition of the people in them magnified the effects of Nazi racial propaganda.[69]

But the professional culture of the Nuremberg doctors had shaped them along the lines of a corporatist and statist professional ethos that antedated World War I and anticipated general Western developments. These various corporate contexts reinforced each other during World War II. Their authority as medical experts over their test subjects reproduced in extreme measure their increasingly hard-won authority over their patients. The doctors operated under the aegis of that most brutally powerful of state institutions, the military, whereas the war itself mobilized their loyalty to the nation. All of these corporate identities and loyalties tore at their capacity to make individual judgments about the individuals at their mercy. These doctors were not creatures simply of National Socialism and World War II, but of the history of modern Germany and the West. Germany, as a result of its own "peculiarities" and the forces of modernization, was an early postliberal state and society beset by a series of exceptional crises after 1914.[70] In 1930 conservative politicians, military men, and bureaucrats assumed control of the Weimar Republic and three years later handed Hitler the keys to power.[71] The combination of these traditions and crises brought out the worst in German institutions and attitudes and permitted the worst to wield power. Among these worst were the doctors tried at Nuremberg. Their stations at the brutal intersection of the military, the medical profession, and the concentration camp system produced extreme actions, which are nonetheless telling of multiple aspects of German and Western history in the modern era.

69 For an argument for a similar phenomenon among German soldiers in Russia, see Omer Bartov, *Hitler's Army: Soldiers, Nazis, and War in the Third Reich* (New York, 1991).

70 For an analysis restricted to economic corporatism, see Werner Abelshauser, "The First Post-Liberal Nation: Stages in the Development of Modern Corporatism in Germany," *European History Quarterly* 14 (1985): 285–318. By concentrating on "corporatist interest mediation" (287), Abelshauser posits a dichotomy between authoritarian "state" corporatism and "democratic welfare" corporatism that understates the historical confluence in modern German society and culture of "preliberal" and "postliberal" corporatist institutions and attitudes.

71 Detlev J. K. Peukert, *The Weimar Republic: The Crisis of Classical Modernity*, trans. Richard Deveson (New York, 1992), 280.

9

The Debate that Will Not End

The Politics of Abortion in Germany from Weimar to National Socialism and the Postwar Period

ATINA GROSSMANN

The current ongoing debates and dilemmas about abortion in united Germany, in both the "new" and the "old" states of the Federal Republic, are shadowed and shaped by a long history of conflict. It is a history marked – at least since the inclusion of Paragraphs 218–20 (which criminalized most abortions) in the penal code of the new German Reich in 1871 – by continuous controversy and attempts at regulation, albeit with many different permutations.[1] The story is punctuated by sharp breaks in policy under different political regimes, but also – and perhaps above all – by a continually selective conditional approach, in which attitudes to abortion were mainly determined not in terms of rights but by assessments of social and economic conditions as well as of individual "fitness" and "health." This chapter sets a context for discussion of the present unclear situation by following briefly some continuities and shifts from the Weimar campaigns for the abolition of Paragraph 218 through the Third Reich and then into the multiple changes of the postwar period. It also argues a point that should be self-evident but that seemingly needs to be continually revisited, especially in light of the wealth of newly open archival material now accumulating: The lines of continuity – of social control and social anxiety – that so preoccupy historians of modern Germany, especially those concerned with medicine and hygiene, look different if one follows the history of German abortion and birth control politics into the post-World War II period and beyond a narrative concluded by the descent into National Socialism and the Holocaust.

* Portions of this chapter have appeared in my *Reforming Sex: The German Movement for Birth Control and Abortion Reform* (New York, 1995).

1 For a discussion of criminalization starting with the Bamberger Halsgerichtsordnung of 1507, see Michael Gante, *Par. 218 in der Diskussion: Meinungs- und Willensbildung, 1845–1976* (Düsseldorf, 1991), 10–22; see also Günter Jerouschek, "Zur Geschichte des Abtreibungsverbots," in Gisela Staupe and Lis Vieth, eds., *Unter anderen Umständen: Zur Geschichte der Abtreibung* (Berlin, 1993), 11–26.

WEIMAR

The most dramatic moment in the history of German abortion politics, and one that in many ways continued to define the parameters of debate at least throughout the period of reform in the 1970s, came with the (well-known and much documented) 1931 Communist-led "Wolf-Kienle" campaign. This highly visible militant mass mobilization demanded women's right to abortion and the repeal of Paragraph 218, as well as the immediate release of the two physicians arrested for performing or providing medical certificates for numerous abortions. The militance and momentum of the campaign and its broad appeal to women of all classes provided a space for highly public and pointedly feminist interventions unique in the history of German sex reform. The politics of "Your Body Belongs to You" (*Dein Körper Gehört Dir*), never a standard part of political, medical, or eugenic arguments for abortion, slipped into the conflict in late Weimar and managed temporarily to disrupt, if not displace, the dominance of class-struggle politics and a consensus about the importance of healthy motherhood and eugenically fit offspring in sex reform discourse. Yet, despite slippage into rights rhetoric, for most reformers the right to choice in sexual and reproductive matters was never inalienable. In their generally needs-based (rather than rights of either woman or fetus) discourse of collective welfare – whether of class, *Volk*, or nation – if and when a state were adequately to fulfill its social welfare promises, it would then have the right to regulate childbearing. This proposition would quickly be borne out by the Soviet recriminalization of abortion in 1936, by the social health claims of the National Socialists in Germany, and eventually by the shifting abortion policies followed by the postwar East and West German states.

Despite the intense activity, both within a medical profession that increasingly demanded that its professional prerogatives to make decisions about terminating pregnancy be protected and as part of the popular movement, the campaign to change the law failed. The embattled Weimar Republic insisted on maintaining on the books a law that was highly unpopular and persistently flouted. Hardly anyone believed that the law could substantially prevent abortions, and most policymakers doubted that, at least at a time of economic crisis, government intervention could really influence reproductive decisions. Still, except for the Communist Party or KPD, all political parties supported some form of criminalization as a sign of the government's commitment to raise the birth rate and police sexual morality at a time when conventions in those areas seemed to be collapsing. Thus, it is important to understand the abortion controversy not only in terms of eugenic and population politics but also as the most visible part of the larger debate about values, ethics, and a "new morality" associated with the emergence of a "new woman."[2]

NATIONAL SOCIALISM

After January 1933, the long-term sex reform goal of legalizing sterilization and guaranteeing physicians' right to perform medically and eugenically necessary abortions was realized by the Nazis, *but* under conditions that specifically denied any possibility of compatibility between social fitness and individual control – the sex reform dream – and gave coercive power to doctors and the state. Restrictions on abortion and birth control that had been loosely and irregularly enforced during the Weimar years were tightened and enforced according to more specifically racial and eugenic criteria. On May 26, 1933, seven years after the reform of Paragraph 218 had eliminated Paragraphs 219 and 220 prohibiting any kind of publicity or education regarding abortion or abortifacients, they were reintroduced into the penal code. For the Nazis, the destruction of the sex reform movement – which had demanded legal abortion, sex- and birth-control-counseling, and mass access to contraceptives – the purges of Jewish and leftist doctors, and the enforcement of laws criminalizing abortion were all interdependent and necessary to the rebirth of the *Volk*.

Until recently our knowledge about abortion policies and practices in the Third Reich has been remarkably limited. Based on her pathbreaking research on forced sterilization, Gisela Bock has argued that during this period, "*Gebärzwang* [compulsory childbearing] did not go beyond what was usual before 1933, after 1945, or in other countries," and insisted that the true "novelty" of Nazi policy was its extreme anti-natalism.[3] But the excellent new (and ongoing) research of the Berlin historian Gabriele Czarnowski is now documenting a far more differentiated and complex situation. The Nazis launched a massive campaign to eliminate voluntary abortions, whether performed by doctors, midwives, or pregnant women themselves, at the same time as abortions deemed medically and, particularly, eugenically or racially necessary were legalized, tolerated, and in some cases brutally coerced. Anti-natalist policies were indeed strengthened when the 1933 sterilization

2 See Atina Grossmann, "Abortion and Economic Crisis: The 1931 Campaign Against Par. 218," in Renate Bridenthal, Atina Grossmann, and Marion Kaplan, eds., *When Biology became Destiny: Women in Weimar and Nazi Germany* (New York, 1984), 66–86; and chap. 4 of my book, *Reforming Sex: The German Movement for Birth Control and Abortion Reform 1920 to 1950* (New York, 1995).

3 Gisela Bock, "Antinatalism, Maternity, and Paternity in National Socialist Racism," in Gisela Bock and Pat Thane, eds., *Maternity and the Rise of the European Welfare States, 1880s–1950s* (London and New York, 1991), 242.

law was amended in June 1935 to institutionalize the link between eugenic sterilization and abortion: Abortions, even of advanced pregnancies, certified as necessary on medical and mostly eugenic grounds by medical commissions of the Reichsärztekammer were declared legal; if ordered on eugenic grounds, they had to be followed by sterilization. But unlike sterilization, these abortions were technically dependent on women's consent. Provocatively, Bock argues therefore that, after the new regulations sanctioning medically and eugenically indicated abortions, "abortion was now no longer prohibited" in Germany.[4]

Coercive pro-natalism was, however, by no means absent from – and indeed was absolutely central to – the Nazi agenda, which had after all been characterized from the outset by thundering against abortion as a crime against the *Volk*. As Czarnowski aptly puts it, "The prohibition on abortion and directly or indirectly compulsory abortion co-existed."[5] At the same time in 1935 that certain abortions were legalized, midwives and doctors were also required, as they had not been in Weimar, to report all miscarriages, premature births, and medically indicated terminations. Abortions were strictly regulated by state-appointed medical commissions; state control and the power of certain segments of the medical profession were greatly increased. But women's freedom to maneuver, as well as that of physicians who during Weimar had been willing to provide women with affidavits of medical necessity, was drastically reduced. Furthermore, the "Guidelines for interruption of pregnancy and sterilization on health grounds," issued by the Reichsärztekammer in 1936, greatly narrowed the medical criteria allowing therapeutic abortions. Whereas in Weimar, medical necessity – sanctioned by a 1927 Reichsgericht ruling – had provided sympathetic doctors with a rather large loophole, especially in cases of heart, lung, and psychiatric disorders, the Nazis clearly intended their indications to be primarily eugenic, and medical only in very severe cases.

The notion that abortion was now for the first time legal would have come as quite a surprise to the numerous physicians who were attacked as abortionists, often for referrals or procedures allegedly conducted years earlier, or the many women who found their abortion networks – whether through doctors, midwives or lay abortionists – under relentless attack. Especially women physicians with their large female clientele, as well as Jewish and politically outspoken doctors who had worked in birth control and sex

---

4 Gisela Bock, *Zwangssterilisation im Nationalsozialismus: Studien zur Rassenpolitik und Frauenpolitik* (Opladen, 1986), 99.
5 Gabriele Czarnowski, "Frauen als Mütter der 'Rasse': Abtreibungsverfolgung und Zwangs-sterilisation im Nationalsozialismus," in Staupe and Vieth, eds., *Unter anderen Umständen*, 59.

counseling centers, were particular targets of the regime's tougher enforcement of antiabortion laws, subjected to intimidating interrogations and repeated entrapment attempts, both before and after 1935.[6]

For Weimar sex reformers, the shock of denunciation, imprisonment, and exile was exacerbated by the simultaneous dramatic shifts in the abortion policies of the Soviet Union. Indeed, the Soviet recriminalization of abortion in 1936 brought to leftist Paragraph 218 opponents a similar kind of shock and confusion that the Nazi-Soviet Pact did for others three years later (although given the contingent nature of their own arguments for legal abortion, they perhaps should not have been so surprised). The June 27, 1936, decree "In Defense of Mother and Child" abrogated the revolutionary reform of November 1920, when the young Soviet Union had become the first nation to legalize abortions performed in hospitals by physicians, and now prohibited abortion except on medical or eugenic grounds. Recriminalization came, as it would again in the Soviet-dominated German Democratic Republic, or GDR, in 1950, after a period of legality justified by a state of (postwar and postrevolution) emergency and wrapped into what Wendy Goldman has called a "larger campaign to promote 'family responsibility,'" equality of the sexes, and protection of motherhood.[7]

In Germany in January 1941, coercive pro-natalism was sharpened by the so-called Himmler police ordinance that banned the importation, production, or sale of any material or instrument likely to prevent or interrupt pregnancy; an attack not only on abortion but also on contraception. Only condoms were exempted upon army request because of their role in combatting venereal disease. By 1943 the skyrocketing incidence of illegal abortion under wartime conditions led to the incorporation into Paragraphs 218 and 219 of a paragraph that allowed for the death penalty to be imposed, "[i]f the perpetrator through such deeds continuously impairs the vitality of the German *Volk*." Further restrictions were also imposed on contraception and unauthorized sterilization.[8] Czarnowski has now discovered that these

---

6   This is a common theme in memoirs by émigré women physicians. See, e.g., Wolfgang Benz, ed., *Das Tagebuch der Hertha Nathorff: Berlin-New York, Aufzeichnungen, 1933–1945* (Frankfurt/Main, 1988), 82–3; Henriette D. Magnus Necheles, "Reminiscences of a German-Jewish Woman Physician," (Chicago, 1940), original deposited in Houghton Library, Harvard University; reworked and translated by Ruth F. Necheles (New York, 1980), 49; Edith Kramer and Lydia Ehrenfried (both unpublished memoirs, Leo Baeck Institute, New York); and Rahel Strauss, *Wir lebten in Deutschland: Erinnerungen einer deutschen Jüdin, 1880-1933* (Stuttgart, 1961), 139.

7   Wendy Goldman, "Women, Abortion and the State, 1917-1936" in Barbara Evans Clements et al., eds., *Russia's Women: Accommodation, Resistance, Transformation* (Berkeley and Los Angeles, 1991), 244; see also Janet Evans, "The Communist Party of the Soviet Union and the Women's Question: The Case of the 1936 Decree 'In Defence of Mother and Child,'" *Journal of Contemporary History* 16, no. 4 (Oct. 1981): 757–75.

8   Henry P. David, Jochen Fleischhacker, and Charlotte Höhn, "Abortion and Eugenics in Nazi

penalties were indeed carried out on abortionists during the war, especially – but not only – on Polish women in occupied Poland who performed
abortions on "German" women. For example, Ludwika W. was executed in
German-occupied Warthegau for having performed voluntary abortions on
four *Volksdeutsche*, or ethnic German women. The court was not interested
however in the six cases in which she had aborted Polish women.[9]

The most salient feature of all Nazi abortion policy was its clear selectivi-
ty – both in terms of "race" and decisionmaking. Voluntary abortions, desired
by women themselves and not state-sanctioned for reasons of the health of
the *Volk*, were severely repressed – up to and including the death penalty for
those performing the abortions (including doctors, but usually midwives).
Abortions on racially, physically, and mentally valuable women were to be
stamped out. Abortions on the racially undesirable and unfit were coercively
performed according to decisions of the same medical commissions that
determined sterilizations and were generally not severely punished if performed illegally.

The other side of the harsh wartime regulations limiting abortion and
access to contraceptives was the secret directives permitting abortions on
foreign forced laborers as well as on the growing number of German women
who became pregnant, via consensual sex or rape, by foreign workers or prisoners of war. Already in 1940 the minister of the interior issued a confidential
memo instructing local health offices to consider "voluntary" abortions
beyond those legalized by the 1935 amended Law for the Prevention of
Hereditary Disease, for example, where there was suspicion of hereditary
defect not covered by that law, or in "urgent, proven" cases of rape or undesirable racial combinations (with someone *artfremd*). Again, sterilization was
recommended as a follow-up.[10]

As the war dragged on and more and more foreign, especially female, workers from the conquered territories in the East were forced to work in the
Reich, coercive abortion policies became more horrific. Until the end of
1942, female forced laborers (approximately 2 million of the 7.7 million
POWs and foreign laborers working in the Reich in 1944) who became pregnant were sent home. But in the spring of 1943, the Reichs Medical Führer
together with the Ministry of Health and the Reichs Commissar for the
Consolidation of the German *Volk* (*Reichskommissar für die Festigung des*

Germany," *Population and Development Review* 14, no. 1 (March 1988): 96–7; see also Hans
   Harmsen, "Notes on Abortion and Birth Control in Germany," *Population Studies* 3 (1950): 402.
9 Capital punishment was also imposed on "commercial abortionists" in the *Altreich*; see Czarnowski,
   "Frauen als Mütter," 67–8; see also David, "Abortion," 98.
10 Bundesarchiv Koblenz (hereafter cited as BArch[K]), Schumacher collection 399.
   Reichsministerium des Innern, Sept. 19, 1940, secret memo to health offices and local governments.

deutschen Volkstums, or RKF) began organizing abortions of "unworthy" fetuses on a massive scale. If the father was allegedly of German blood, the decision about whether to perform an abortion on a foreign worker (*Ostarbeiterin*) was made by a commission of the Reich medical chamber, together with the SS and RKF. If pregnancies were deemed worth continuing, the newborns were then forcibly taken from their mothers and handed over to *Lebensborn* homes for "Germanicization"; some were placed into special camps where they invariably died of starvation and maltreatment.[11]

By the beginning of 1945, the issue of abortions on "German" women took on new urgency. The encroaching Red Army had advanced to such a point that the possibility of mass "violations" of German women by Soviet troops was acknowledged and indeed widely propagandized as part of a campaign to keep both the military and home fronts intact. The Ministry of Interior not only sanctioned extralegal abortions in cases of rape but even suggested the establishment "in large cities [of] special wards for the care of such women."[12] This suspension of Paragraph 218 in cases of alleged rape by the "racially alien" Soviet soldiers, coupled with continued insistence on the fundamental criminality of abortion (albeit minus the draconian 1943 regulations), was to survive the fall of the Third Reich and last into the postwar years.

ABORTION IN POSTWAR DIVIDED GERMANY

No sooner had the guns been stilled than abortion instantly reemerged as a pressing public and personal issue. The chaotic social conditions in defeated Germany and the immediate problem of pregnancies resulting from mass rapes committed by Red Army soldiers as they fought their way West into Berlin forced a harsh confrontation with Paragraph 218. The Nazi regime had, as we have seen, prepared for the possibility of extralegal abortions of "Slav" or "mongol" fetuses. The regime's collapse now led to a virtual suspension of Paragraph 218 as doctors worked feverishly in the spring and summer of 1945 to abort pregnancies caused by rape.

It has been suggested that perhaps one out of every three of the about one and a half million women in Berlin at the end of the war were raped; many, but certainly not all, during the notorious week of "mass rapes" from April

11 See Michael Burleigh and Wolfgang Wippermann, *The Racial State: Germany, 1933–1945* (Cambridge, Mass., 1991), 73; see also Czarnowski, "Frauen als Mütter," 68–71; Michaela Garn, "Zwangsabtreibung und Abtreibungsverbot: Zur Gutachterstelle der Hamburger Ärztekammer," in Angelika Ebbinghaus, Heidrun Kaupen-Haas, and Karl Heinz Roth, eds., *Heilen und Vernichten im Mustergau Hamburg: Bevölkerungs- und Gesundheitspolitik im Dritten Reich* (Hamburg, 1984), 39.

12 Reichsministerium des Innern to Reichsministerium der Justiz, express letter, Berlin, Feb. 26, 1945 in BArch(K) R22/5008, pp. 107–8.

24 to May 5 as the Soviets finally secured Berlin. One recent estimate claims that up to two million German women were raped by Red Army soldiers.[13] Serious research on this extraordinarily complex and overdetermined topic is just beginning, but for our purposes the significant problem is less the actual scope of the rapes than their immediate public coding as social health and population political problems that required medical intervention.[14]

Driven by a complicated set of racist, eugenic, health, and humanitarian motives, and with the support of the Protestant bishop, doctors in Berlin quickly decided to suspend Paragraph 218 and perform abortions on raped women who wanted them. And as one woman doctor later reported, "they all wanted them."[15] The ad hoc decision was quickly institutionalized by a highly organized medical and social hygiene system that never completely broke down, at least in the cities. Throughout most of the first year after May 1945, medical commissions composed of three or four physicians attached to district health offices approved medical abortions – almost up until the very last month of pregnancy – on any woman who certified that she had been raped by a foreigner, usually but not always a member of the Red Army. With dubious legality but with virtually full knowledge and tolerance by all relevant – both German and occupation – authorities, with the consent of the Protestant – although not the Catholic – church, abortions in the period directly after the end of the war were performed it would appear on a fast assembly line.[16] Indeed, the Berlin *Sonderregelung* on abortions after rape was

---

13 Helke Sander and Barbara Jöhr, eds., *Befreier und Befreite: Krieg, Vergewaltigungen, Kinder* (Munich, 1992), 48, 54–5; see also Erich Kuby, *Die Russen in Berlin 1945* (Bern, 1965), 312–13.

14 See Atina Grossmann, "A Question of Silence: The Rape of German Women by Occupation Soldiers," *October* 72 (Spring 1995): 43–63; see also Ingrid Schmidt-Harzbach, "Eine Woche im April: Berlin 1945: Vergewaltigung als Massenschicksal," *Feministische Studien* 2 (1984): 51–65; Erika M. Hoerning, "Frauen als Kriegsbeute: Der Zwei-Fronten Krieg: Beispiele aus Berlin," in Lutz Niethammer and Alexander von Plato, eds., *"Wir kriegen jetzt andere Zeiten": Auf der Suche nach der Erfahrung des Volkes in nachfaschistischen Ländern: Lebensgeschichte und Sozialkultur im Ruhrgebiet 1930 bis 1960* (Bonn, 1985), 327–46; Annemarie Tröger, "Between Rape and Prostitution: Survival Strategies and Chances of Emancipation for Berlin Women after World War II," in Judith Friedlander et al., eds., *Women in Culture and Politics: A Century of Change* (Bloomington, Ind., 1986), 97–117; Albrecht Lehmann, *Im Fremden ungewollt zuhaus: Flüchtlinge und Vertriebene in Westdeutschland, 1945–1990* (Munich, 1991), 151–69

15 Anne-Marie Durand-Wever, M.D., "Mit den Augen einer Ärztin: Zur Kontroverse zwischen Professor Nachtsheim und Dr. Volbracht," *Berliner Ärzteblatt* 83, no. 14 (1970): Sonderdruck (n.p.n).

16 See the remarkable files on "Interruption of Pregnancy" in Landesarchiv Berlin (hereafter cited as LAB), Rep. 214/2814/220–1 and 2740/156 (Bezirksamt Neukölln), discussed in Grossmann, "A Question of Silence." E.g., of 141 pregnancies (35 in unmarried women) approved for termination by the Neukölln health office July 6–24, 1945, two to three months after the height of sexual violence, 16 were in the second month, 27 in the second to third, 71 in the third, 14 in the fourth, 6 in the fourth to fifth, 6 in the sixth, 1 in the sixth to seventh. From Nov. 8, 1945, through Feb. 1, 1946, seven to nine months later, of the 256 pregnancies approved for termination, 4 were in the first to second month, 34 in the second, 26 in the second to third, 87 in the third, 15 in the third to fourth, 38 in the fourth, 4 in the fourth to fifth, 22 in the fifth, 3 in the fifth to sixth, 15 in the sixth, 1 in the sixth to seventh, 6 in the seventh, 1 in the seventh to eighth (from Rep. 214/2814/220).

quickly extended to many Western zones, according to resolutions passed by leading doctors and jurists meeting in Marburg in Hessen (*Marburg Beschluss*) on May 15, 1945.[17]

Legal abortions were performed in public hospitals at public cost. The doctors in charge of the health offices were newly installed antifascists; in Berlin, several were Jewish. But at least some of the doctors on the commissions approving the abortions and probably many of those performing them in hospitals were former committed Nazi Party members who had been (temporarily) suspended from private practice and forced to serve in public positions as part of their denazification proceedings. It seems likely that the techniques used to abort women at extremely late stages of pregnancy had previously been tested on wartime foreign female forced laborers.[18]

These circumstances and the recent background of Nazi-sanctioned abortions in case of rape have led some historians to characterize these postwar abortions as a continuation of Nazi race policy.[19] But again the picture is more complicated and overdetermined, the discontinuities at least as dramatic as the continuities. In interpreting the rape experience to officials and also to themselves and their friends or family, and in making their case for abortion in the affidavits, women (and the medical authorities approving the abortions) relied on a mixed legacy of Weimar and National Socialist population policy discourses, as well as current occupation policy. They repeatedly referred to both the social and racial/eugenic grounds on which their abortion should be sanctioned – despite the presumably compelling and popularly known fact that neither of those indications, but only rape by an occupation soldier, was recognized as justifying an "interruption." Women and their doctors, both female and male, did draw from the Nazi racial hygiene discourse that banned alien (*artfremd*) offspring (indeed when rapes by other occupation forces were certified, the perpetrator was frequently identified as Negro if American, or North African if French). Rapes by Red Army soldiers had after all not only been prepared for in Nazi public health policy but also massively prefigured in Nazi propaganda. Horrific images – notably in newsreels – of subhuman and animalistic invaders raping

Obviously, as one doctor noted in his diary in the summer of 1945, in addition to the many approved abortions performed on the gynecological ward, there continued to be "many illegal abortions by quacks," at least some of "which are then admitted infected into the hospital" (unpublished diary, Dr. Franz Vollnhals, by kind permission of Mrs. Itta Vollnhals).

17 See the useful summary of the legal situation in East and West Germany in Gante, *Par. 218 in der Diskussion*, 24–55.

18 See Burleigh and Wippermann, *Racial State*, 263.

19 See esp. Schmidt-Harzbach, "Eine Woche im April" (also reprinted in Sander and Jöhr, *Befreier und Befreite*); and Hoerning, "Frauen als Kriegsbeute."

German women had been a vital part of the Nazi war machine's feverish (and successful) efforts to bolster morale on the Eastern and home fronts. Women availed themselves of the richly provided Nazi racial imagery of the barbarian from the East, especially the Mongol from the far East.[20] For example, in an affidavit to the Neukölln health office dated July 24, 1945, a woman wrote:

I hereby certify that at the end of April this year during the Russian march into Berlin I was raped in a loathsome way by two Red Army soldiers of Mongol/Asiatic type.[21]

But women (and their doctors) also hearkened back in narrative terms to the social hygiene, sex reform and maternalist discourses of the Weimar welfare state – which predated Nazi racialist formulations and would outlast them – and framed the abortion issue in terms of medical, social, and eugenic indications. Women matter-of-factly and pragmatically asserted their right to terminate pregnancies that were not socially, economically, or medically viable – in the name of saving the family or preventing the birth of unwanted or unfit children. Invoking this discourse of social (not moral or racial) emergency – the problem of any unwillingly pregnant woman who could not take care of a child or another child – another woman wrote on August 6, 1945:

I have three children aged five to eleven years. My husband as a former soldier is not yet back. I have been bombed out twice, fled here in January from West Prussia and now request most cordially that I be helped in preventing this latest disaster for me and my family.

Moreover, in the affidavits that women submitted to health offices, multiple and overlapping voices all talked at once, often in the same document. In an interesting indication of the dissimultaneity of social welfare understandings in the immediate postwar period, many statements freely mixed the social necessity language characteristic of the Weimar debates on Paragraph 218 (which had however never actually been instituted during Weimar or National Socialism) and the racial stereotypes popularized by the Nazis, with threats of suicide or descriptions of serious physical ailments that might have legitimated a medical indication under any regime. A letter from August 20, 1945:

On the way to work on the second Easter holiday I was raped by a Mongol. The abuse can be seen on my body. Despite strong resistance, my strength failed me and I had to let everything evil come over me. Now I am pregnant by this person, can only think about this with disgust and ask that I be helped. Since I would not even

20 See, e.g., *Deutsche Wochenschau*, nos. 755/9 and 10, 1945, and 739/46/1944, in BArch(K), film archive.
21 All depositions quoted from LAB Rep. 214/2814/220 (Bezirksamt Neukölln).

consider carrying this child to term, both my children would lose their mother. With kind greetings.

Thus, in a matter-of-fact, but also desperate, manner, women mobilized existing discourses, entangled them, and deployed them to tell their own story for their on own purposes. Initially this strategy was remarkably effective (and not only in Berlin where my own research has been centered). But by the end of 1946, with the immediate emergency overcome and civil and occupation authority more tightly in place, criteria for legal abortion tightened, especially in the Western sector, and the already high illegal abortion rate climbed even further.

Parallel and deeply connected – but without explicit reference – to the postwar rape experience of so many German women, the Weimar debate on abortion that had been abruptly silenced by the Nazi takeover quickly resumed. This was especially evident in the Soviet zone, which took a much more aggressive role than the West in structuring social and population policy. The press was again filled with speak-outs and interviews, women's conferences convened, students debated, and provincial parliaments argued about abrogating Paragraph 218 and instituting new regulations.[22] Friedrich Wolf's anti-218 drama *Cyankali*, which had inspired such passionate discussion and demonstrations in the late Weimar period was restaged almost immediately; this time, as one reviewer noted, the entire *Volk* shared the working-class misery portrayed.[23] Wolf himself, returned from Soviet exile, interjected himself into the "urgent" debate and recycled his dramatic call in *Cyankali*: "[A] law that makes criminals of 800,000 women a year is no longer a law." But now with socialism supposedly within reach, Communists – as well as Social Democrats – expected that their long-time vision of happy healthy mothers who no longer required abortions would soon be fulfilled.[24] In contrast to Weimar, even for the most committed reformers, the discussion no longer focused on abolition of Paragraph 218, but on the limited, contingent, and transient conditions under which abortion would be justified.

Undoubtedly influenced by memories of the "loathsome" abortions performed in the aftermath of the *Zusammenbruch*, abortion reform advocates now revised their pre-1933 call for full legalization. The anti-Nazi physician

---

22 E.g., "Diskussionen um den Paragraphen 218," *Neue Zeit*, Dec. 25, 1946; see the extensive collections of press clippings in Stiftung Archiv der Parteien und Massenorganisationen der DDR im Bundesarchiv (hereafter cited as BArch[Sapmo]), Zentral Komitee (hereafter cited as ZK) der Sozialistische Einheitspartei Deutschlands (hereafter cited as SED), IV 2/17/29.

23 Walter Lennig, *Berliner Zeitung*, March 3, 1947 in BArch(Sapmo), ZK der SED, IV 2/17/29, 63.

24 Dr. Friedrich Wolf, "Der Par. 218 und die soziale Indikation," *Neues Deutschland*, Dec. 17, 1946, in BArch(Sapmo), ZK der SED, IV 21/17/29; see also Paul Ronge and Friedrich Wolf, *Problem Par. 218* (Rudolstadt, 1946–7).

Dr. Anne-Marie Durand-Wever, probably the most prominent abortion rights activist to have remained in Germany, now insisted that, although "[t]here are cases in which an interruption must be performed [notably rape],"[25] "no woman's body, no woman's soul can endure such repeated operations."[26] "Woman's health," she asserted, "was her most valuable possession ... also the most valuable capital of the nation."[27]

By the end of the Third Reich and the war, therefore, the abortion question was even more difficult to resolve than before. Communists and socialists were now more explicit about the limits set on a woman's individual right to control her body. In the 1931 campaign, the KPD had touted the benefits of legalization for female health and fertility and carried, albeit reluctantly, the banner "Your body belongs to you." After twelve years of National Socialism, and very importantly, the 1936 Soviet retreat on legalized abortion, that old slogan was dismissed as anarchistic and individualistic; the goal now was to construct a law that could reconcile the state's need for the preservation of the "biological and moral foundations for the continuation of the *Volk*" with its need for realistic (*lebensnah*) laws.[28] Only a few liberal bourgeois feminists like the former Democratic Party (now Liberal Democratic) activist Katharina von Kardorff still insisted, as they had during Weimar, that Paragraph 218 left women with "one leg in the grave and the other in the penitentiary."[29]

Despite some direct and much indirect reference to the immediate past of mass rape and Nazi racial policies, postwar public speech for the most part recirculated, in limited and refigured form, Weimar debates about reform and legalization as well as the easily available model of the Soviet recriminalization. With the exception of some Christian Democratic critics who referred to Auschwitz as justification for their antiabortion stance (one of the rare references to Nazi extermination),[30] the recent past of genocide and forced anti-natalism remained for the most part unarticulated. In familiar language, reformers again asserted that women determined to terminate a pregnancy would do so no matter what the cost and noted the irrationality

---

25 Anne-Marie Durand-Wever in Demokratischer Frauenbund Deutschland (hereafter cited as DFD) Bundesauschuss, Sept. 24, 1948. BArch(Sapmo), DFD archives.
26 Anne-Marie Durand-Wever, *Bewusste Mutterschaft durch Geburtenregelung* (Rudolstadt, n.d. [1946 or 1947]), 30.
27 Durand-Wever in DFD Bundesauschuss, Sept. 24, 1948.
28 SED statement in *Für Dich* 1, no. 18 (Dec. 12, 1946): 3.
29 *Kurier*, Dec. 13, 1946. A few other dissenting voices pleading for women's right to decide, at least within the first trimester, appear in letters to the editor of journals or in the SED files. BArch(Sapmo), ZK der SED, IV 2/17/29.
30 See, e.g., *Frauen Telegraf*, no. 217/1, Dec. 21, 1946, 7, quoting Hermann Frühauf in *Frankfurter Hefte*, collected in BArch(Sapmo), ZK der SED, IV 2/17/29. See also transcripts of debates in the Landtag of Saxony-Anhalt in 1947, in Käthe Kern's collected papers, BArch(Sapmo), Nachlass 145/50, 43.

of unenforceable laws, the social health consequences of botched abortions, and unfit or unwanted offspring, the severity of the (temporary) crisis, and the necessity of contraception as an alternative to abortion. Finally, they assured that under happier circumstances women would certainly revert to their maternal roles.

In the Soviet zone, where the reform of Paragraph 218 was actively pursued (and where numerous exiles initially returned, hoping to resurrect some Weimar sex reform initiatives such as clinic-based medical care (*Ambulatorien*), and marriage- and sex-counseling centers) a revamped motherhood-eugenics consensus emerged within the newly formed (in April 1946) Socialist Unity Party (SED). Rejecting full decriminalization, it favored legalization of the social, in addition to medical, eugenic, and ethical (rape and incest), indication; it also championed extensive pro-natalist measures, such as "adequate protection of mothers" and the establishment of childcare centers."[31] The goal was not "to abolish Paragraph 218 but to make it superfluous."[32] Adding a nationalist twist to maternalist Weimar KPD and Social Democratic rhetoric about women's natural and only temporarily repressed wish for children, and surely influenced by fears about a population shift to the West, SED and social welfare officials affirmed that "Germany needs children, if they can be raised under humane conditions, so that they can become carriers of the new democratic life."[33] They explicitly counterposed this "ethic of healthy and natural motherhood" to the militarist (not the racial) intentions of National Socialist ideology.[34] The conflict between individual rights and collective welfare that had so bedeviled Weimar sex reformers was decided in favor of the latter, but in contrast to the Western zones, defined as including – at least under the present unstable conditions of postwar emergency – broad access to legal abortions.

By the end of 1947, in the Soviet zone, the long-time sex reform and Communist Party goal of abolishing Paragraph 218 was achieved – briefly. New laws legalizing socially, ethically, and medically indicated abortions, approved by a commission of doctors and lay representatives from trade unions and women's groups, were promulgated in the separate state parliaments of the Sowjetische Besatzungszone (SBZ); in Saxony in June, Brandenburg and Mecklenburg in November, and Thuringia in December

---

31 Abt. Frauenausschüsse to the Vorstand of the SED, Oct. 2, 1946, BArch(Sapmo), ZK der SED, IV 2/17/29; see also *Für Dich* 1, no. 19 (Dec. 22, 1946): 8; and ibid., 1, no. 20 (Dec. 29, 1946): 4.

32 Notes in Käthe Kern's collected papers, BArch(Sapmo), Nachlass 145/50.

33 Eva Kolmer, "Frauenschutzgesetz – nicht Par. 218," *Pressedienst*, Jan. 29, 1947, BArch(Sapmo), ZK der SED, IV 2/17/28.

34 E.g., Saxon marriage counseling guidelines, *Richtlinien für Ehe- und Sexualberatungsstellen*, Sept. 17, 1946, Saxon Ministerium für Arbeit und Sozialfürsorge, Nr. 1810, Staatsarchiv Dresden.

(only Saxony-Anhalt did not accept the social necessity indication). Fierce resistance by Christian Democratic (CDU) and some Liberal Democratic (LDP) delegates blocked the SED goal of uniform rules, but still the Soviet zone achieved what Weimar sex reformers had never been able to accomplish before 1933: the abolition of even the reformed 1926 version of Paragraph 218. The SED paper *Neues Deutschland* proudly announced that "the deathknell [hour] of the quack" had sounded.[35]

Yet, the tentative and cautious tone of the debate and the continuing assumption that once conditions had normalized women would willingly bear children for family, state, and *Volk* had set the political and rhetorical parameters within which the social indication could be eliminated only a few years later by the newly established German Democratic Republic. As in the Soviet Union in 1936, the discourse of social emergency and need that had so often been invoked to justify legalizing abortion and other sex reform measures was now deployed to justify recriminalization. As in the Soviet Union, the necessary conditions for the "healthy upbringing" of children – including the protection and equality of women – were now declared assured and indeed promoted by a variety of pro-natalist social welfare measures.[36] As in the Soviet Union in the 1930s, authorities argued that legalization had led to a veritable "abortion addiction." It had failed to fulfill the oft-stated promises of reform: to promote the "will to children" or reduce the dangers of illegal abortions.[37] On September 27, 1950, Paragraph 11 of the Law for the Protection of Woman and Children and for the Rights of Women recriminalized abortion by abolishing the social indication that had so recently been adopted.

---

35 *Neues Deutschland*, Sept. 27, 1947, in BArch(Sapmo), IV 2/17/29, 83. Paragraphs 218, 219, and 220 of the criminal code were abolished, as was the 1935 amendment to the sterilization law sanctioning eugenic abortions, the 1943 law that provided a possible death penalty for abortion, and the 1941 Himmler police ordinance. Crimes justifying ethical indication had to be reported in two weeks, and abortions after the first trimester had to be strictly medically indicated. Additionally (and in contrast to states in the Western zones, which in some cases limited themselves to suspending the genetic health courts), S(oviet) M(ilitary) A(dministration) Order Nr. 6 of Jan. 8, 1946, formally abrogated the Law for the Prevention of Hereditarily Diseased Offspring. See also Kirsten Poutrus, "'Ein Staat, der seine Kinder nicht ernähren kann, hat nicht das Recht, ihre Geburt zu fordern': Abtreibung in der Nachkriegszeit 1945 bis 1950," in Staupe and Vieth, eds., *Unter anderen Umständen*, 73–85.

36 See, e.g., the conditions laid out by Oberstaatsanwalt Hilde Benjamin, *Mitteilungen der juristischen Arbeitskommission im Zentralen Frauenausschuss*, 3 Folge, Juristische Grundlagen für die Diskussion über den par. 218. Abt. Frauenausschüsse bei der Deutschen Verwaltung für Volksbildung in der SBZ, Berlin, Feb. 27, 1947. BArch(Sapmo), DFD archives.

37 K. H. Mehlan, M.D., "Die Abortsituation in der DDR," in *Internationale Abortsituation: Kongress 5-7 Mai 1960* (Leipzig, 1961), 57, 59. In 1950, e.g., the SBZ recorded 311,000 births, 26,360 legal abortions, and ca. 84,000 illegal abortions. In 1951, after passage of the law, the birth rate rose only modestly to 318,000, but the number of legal abortions dropped drastically to 5,037, the estimated number of criminal abortions to 68,000, 59.

Paragraph 11 provoked "very lively" protest from local SED and women's groups at meetings that became so "impassioned and outraged that there was a tumult and a halt had to be called." Women workers attacked the law for expecting them to "bear children only for the state." "Why," they demanded, "do they want so many children – that would be like with Hitler."[38] For their part, Communist officials pointed to the positive measures incorporated in the law and tried to persuade disgruntled women "that we have after all, from the side of the state, done everything possible, to facilitate birth." They contended that, "our *Volk* has to be renewed, not – like Hitler said it – in order to generate soldiers for war, but in order to … assure its continuation in the future."[39] According to a GDR logic, which both appropriated and distanced itself from nationalist and *völkisch* language (and indeed was shared across the border in the Federal Republic), the state's demand for babies was deplorable if made for militarist purposes, but acceptable in the name of strengthening the *Volk*.

But the rank and file were apparently not impressed, and Communists, especially women's activists, were hard pressed to explain the party's turn-around.[40] The conviction that abortions were justified when socially necessary was deeply ingrained among German women, and many in the East remembered the Weimar KPD's singular and resolute position against Paragraph 218. As one disappointed woman doctor noted: "[T]he thought processes of the law … were hard to follow – this must be said in all honesty – especially for those many women and men who had determinedly waged the decades long struggle against Paragraph 218."[41] Or as another women's functionary sighed, "One cannot always do full justice to real life with paragraphs."[42]

FEDERAL REPUBLIC

In West Germany the prohibitions on abortion were more continuous. After the initial informal loosening of Paragraph 218 in the very immediate aftermath of war, the few remaining birth-control (and abortion) supporters explicitly distanced themselves from the radical demands of their (now mostly exiled) Weimar forebears. When the West German family-planning organization Pro Familia was formally established in 1952 – under the leadership of

---

38 SED Landesverband Brandenburg report on factory meeting in Teltow to ZK der SED, Frauenabteilung, Oct. 26, 1950, BArch(Sapmo), ZK der SED, IV 2/17/29.

39 Jenny Matern, Bundesvorstandssitzung, June 11-12, 1951, BArch(Sapmo), DFD archives.

40 See DFD Bundesvorstandssitzung, June 11-12, 1951, Berlin, DFD archives. See also letters and discussion in BArch(Sapmo), ZK der SED, IV 2/17/30.

41 Notes in Elfriede Paul papers, BArch(Sapmo), Nachlass 229/13.

42 Notes for Women's Conference speech, May 28, 1947, in Kern Nachlass 145/50, 125.

Hans Harmsen, the only prominent Weimar sex reformer to have collaborat-
ed actively with the National Socialists and their sterilization programs – the
well-worn specter of the "abortion scourge" was once again invoked as the
justification for contraception and family planning. But the terminology
had shifted away from sex reform and birth control or even from the already
deradicalized term "family planning," to the yet more benign and obscure
(and discreetly Latin as befitted anything to do with sex) name Pro Familia.[43]

1960s TO THE PRESENT

After the upheaval of the immediate postwar years and the renewed commitment to criminalization in both Germanies after 1950, the issue was relatively dormant until the mid-1960s. By then the GDR government was
urging more lenient interpretation of the law by the abortion commissions,
apparently laying the groundwork for relegalization in 1972, which would be
accompanied, as criminalization had been in 1950, by pro-natalist benefits. It
had again become clear that broad access to abortion was essential to East
Germany's program of economic integration of women into the workforce
while simultaneously raising the birth rate.[44] In the West also, strict enforcement lapsed in the late 1960s, and the Grand Coalition under Willy Brandt
brought renewed attention to abortion politics, both in and out of parliament.

But not until the 1970s did a new generation of feminists excavate the
history of the Weimar campaigns, reprinting Käthe Kollwitz's and Alice
Lex-Nerlinger's posters and republishing anti-218 tracts. In many ways,
their mobilization bore a remarkable resemblance to the 1931 campaign,
recycling many of the tactics pioneered forty years earlier, of self-incrimina-
tion campaigns and speak-outs, rallies, petition drives and delegate conferences. In June 1971, 375 prominent women announced in the popular
magazine *Stern* that they had had abortions. Inspired by simultaneous movements in France and United States, but clearly influenced by the Weimar
heritage just being uncovered, the speak-out set off a wave of demonstrations,
not unlike those that swept Germany in the spring of 1931.[45]

---

43 See Sabine Schleiermacher, "Racial Hygiene and Deliberate Parenthood: Two Sides of
    Demographer Hans Harmsen's Population Policy," *Issues in Reproductive and Genetic Engineering* 3,
    no. 3 (1990): 201–10; see also Heidrun Kaupen-Haas, "Eine deutsche Biographie: der
    Bevölkerungswissenschaftler Hans Harmsen," in Ebbinghaus, Kaupen-Haas, and Roth, eds., *Heilen
    und Vernichten,* 41–4; Grossmann, *Reforming Sex*, chap. 8.

44 See confidential memo Re. Par. 11 Gesetze über den Mutter und Kinderschutz und die Rechte der
    Frau vom 27 Sept. 1950, March 1965, Ministerium für Gesundheitswesen, BArch(Sapmo), DFD
    archives.

45 See Joyce M. Mushaben, "Feminism in Four Acts: The Changing Political Identity of Women in
    the Federal Republic of Germany," in Peter H. Merkl, ed., *The Federal Republic at Forty* (New York,
    1989), 76–109.

In 1973 West Germans, prodded by both the GDR's action and the women's movement, settled on the so-called indication model, which legalized abortions after women submitted to a "counseling session" and two physicians had certified the procedure as medically or socially necessary; Pro Familia's counseling centers played a key role in offering women access to those indications. In 1974 the Social Democratic and Free Democratic majority in the Bundestag narrowly passed a bill that aimed to legalize – on the GDR model – abortion on demand in the first trimester. In April 1975 the Supreme Court, at the behest of Christian Democratic state governments, and the CDU/CSU parliamentary faction, overturned the new reform law and vowed to "uph[o]ld the state's obligation to see pregnancy carried to full term ... " – and indeed cited the memory of Nazi crimes to justify that obligation.[46] In East and West Germany, the trimester and indication models continued to confront each other.

When unification came in October 1990, the two parts of Germany could not agree on a single standardized ruling, as the various German states had not been able to agree after 1945. An interim agreement allowed the status quo to continue in both the West and former East for a transitional period of two years. In the summer of 1992, after fourteen hours of debate, the Bundestag by a substantial 356 to 283 margin voted in a compromise bill that allowed first-trimester abortions on demand provided that women underwent compulsory counseling.[47]

In May 1993 the German Supreme Court struck down that compromise as unconstitutional on the grounds that it violated the state's obligation to protect human life. According to the court, women had to be informed that "the unborn child has its own right to life" and that abortion was fundamentally illegal even though they and their doctors would not be prosecuted for terminations performed in the first trimester. Outraged women's advocates charged that, in practice, Germany was returning to a situation not dissimilar to that of Weimar Berlin, where many technically illegal abortions were not prosecuted and where, in the absence of health insurance funding (except in cases of demonstrated rape, medical necessity, or clear expectation that the child would be handicapped), women who paid had access to medical

---

46   Ibid., 92; For an excellent analysis of the 1975 decision, helpful also in understanding the 1993 verdict and the relative weakness of rights rhetoric and the positing of the fetus as a human life requiring protection, see Douglas G. Morris, "Abortion and Liberalism: A Comparison Between the Abortion Decisions of the Supreme Court of the United States and the Constitutional Court of West Germany," *Hastings International and Comparative Law Review* 11 (1988): 159–245.

47   For a brief summary of the abortion debate since the 1970s, see Myra Marx Ferree, "The Rise and Fall of 'Mommy Politics': Feminism and Unification in (East) Germany," *Feminist Studies* 19, no. 1 (Spring 1993): 89–115.

abortions, and all others might be subject to the dubious ministrations of "quacks."[48] This time however, it seems there is no going back, and state governments and private foundations quickly responded by establishing funds to assure that no women could be denied an abortion because of lack of money or insurance. The outrage and anxiety seem to have quickly subsided.[49]

Arguably, the lack of clear or aggressive feminist response to the May decision and the new regulations it forces has something to do – along with multiple contemporary factors – with the emphasis in current historical scholarship on the anti- rather than pro-natalist aspects of Nazi population policy. More attention has recently been focused on forced sterilization and abortion (of the "unfit" and "unGerman") than on the encouragement of "Aryan" motherhood and the elimination of repression of voluntary abortion; furthermore, there has been much new publicity about the often brutally late (albeit desired) abortions performed on pregnant German victims of rape by occupation soldiers after World War II.

Be that as it may, interpretations of the new situation are in any case mixed: In a certain sense, the introduction of a trimester model in the West – with compulsory counseling – is an improvement over the previous indication model; the slow introduction of ambulatory vacuum abortion procedures in the East was an improvement over a situation in which women were entitled to abortion on demand – a benefit they had come to take for granted – but often under uncomfortable and humiliating conditions.

Still, the fact remains that abortion for women in Germany today is a favor for the needy, not a right. The Supreme Court of the land has determined that both doctor and woman must be constantly aware that they are committing an illegal – but not prosecutable (*rechtswidrig aber straffrei*, provided the appropriate time and counseling provisions are met) – act of killing that can be sanctioned only if a woman's "level of tolerable burden" (*Opfergrenze*) has been crossed. The verdict and the guidelines for its enforcement are quite clear in their intent. In the words of the Berlin Senate's Health Administration: "Counseling is in the service of the unborn child. It must be driven by the effort to encourage women to continue their pregnancy and to open their eyes to the possibilities for a life with the child."[50]

---

48   Stephen Kinzer, "German Court Restricts Abortion, Angering Feminists and the East," *New York Times*, May 29, 1993, 1.
49   Mechthild Küpper, "Nach Weimar führt kein Weg zurück," *Wochenpost*, no. 34, (Aug. 19, 1993): 8.
50   Senatsverwaltung für Gesundheit Berlin, "Die Neuregelung der Beratung bei Schwangerschaftskonflikten nach dem Urteil und der Anordnung des Bundesverfassungsgerichts vom 28 Mai 1993," 5. This language is remarkably similar to the cozy tone of the letters of rejection sent to GDR women requesting medically or eugenically indicated abortions after 1950, "We

Furthermore, the power of doctors and medical technology over women's lives is only increased by these regulations; doctors performing abortions (who must not have any connection with the institution that did the counseling) now have a greater responsibility to assure that proper counseling has been carried out (at least three days earlier) and that they can take upon themselves the burden of carrying out an illegal if necessary act. The stress on term rather than on indication requirements places greater pressure on determining the exact stage of pregnancy, which in turn leads to more routine reliance on technology such as ultrasound scans. Finally, the physician is now also called upon to decide whether their patient "can truly personally affirm" (*innerlich bejaht*) the termination of pregnancy.[51]

The story is certainly not over. Paragraph 218 remains on the books, and abortion remains an unresolved, highly contested issue in united Germany. It is not at all clear how long the German electorate, medical profession, courts, and parliament will sustain the current "illegal but not punishable" prescription. The ongoing story of German abortion politics – truly the debate that will not end – must also raise for us new questions for the continually vexed debates about continuity and discontinuity, peculiarity and comparability, in the development of the modern German welfare state, as well as about differences and similarities between East and West after 1945.

are sure that after you have recovered from the initial shock, you will look forward to your little child [*Kindchen*]" (BArch[Potsdam], DQ 1, DDR Ministerium für Gesundheitswesen).

51   Ibid., 14. See also the full text of the verdict, "Das Urteil des Bundesverfassungsgerichts zum Schwangerschaftsabbruch vom 28. Mai 1993," *Juristen Zeitung*, Sonderausgabe, June 7, 1993.

10

The Sewering Scandal of 1993 and the German Medical Establishment

MICHAEL H. KATER

For Hans Mommsen on his sixty-fifth birthday

I

In 1933, fifty-nine years before he was elected president of the World Medical Association for a one-year term, a young German medical student joined Heinrich Himmler's black-shirted SS, and one year later the Nazi Party.[1] His name was Hans Joachim Sewering, and he had come from his home town of Bochum to enroll at the University of Munich. Sewering joined those Nazi organizations of his own accord. Whereas male university students, for the sake of university admittance until the Röhm Putsch in June 1934, had to demonstrate a working affiliation with the SA, the SS, and the Nazi Party did not call for compulsory membership. Sewering was therefore not typical. In the period from 1933 to 1945, only 6 percent of male students of medicine joined the SS, and only 29 percent the party, and like Sewering, they did so for careerist, less than for ideological reasons.[2] Sewering certainly exhibited opportunism when he took up residence at the Munich headquarters of the university-affiliated SA storm troopers (SA-Hochschulamt) on Theresienstrasse.[3]

After graduating with a doctor of medicine degree in April of 1941, Sewering entered the *Wehrmacht* (armed forces), but he was found to be unfit for service and discharged in the summer of 1942. Thereupon he began to work at Schönbrunn sanatorium near the town of Dachau, north of Munich, which specialized in the care of tuberculosis patients. When he arrived there, the institution had been nearly emptied after the evacuation, to a "euthanasia" killing center, of most of its patients. Whereas the euthanasia (T-4) program had officially been stopped in 1941, so-called wild euthanasia, that

---

1 Hans Joachim Sewering, born Jan. 30, 1916, in Bochum. SS-Sturm 2/I/31 entry date: Nov. 1, 1933; SS no.: 143000. NSDAP entry date: Aug. 1, 1934; NSDAP no.: 1858805. MF, SS file Sewering, Berlin Document Center (hereafter cited as BDC).
2 Table 5.5 in Michael H. Kater, *Doctors Under Hitler* (Chapel Hill, N.C., 1989), 257.
3 SS file Sewering, BDC.

is, local and regional killing activities not officially authorized but nevertheless tolerated by Berlin, continued until 1945. The euthanasia center next to Schönbrunn was Eglfing-Haar, where between January 1943 and June 1945 a total of 444 patients were murdered, mostly through controlled starvation.[4]

Documentary evidence[5] shows that Dr. Sewering himself became involved in at least one case of euthanasia selection when on October 26, 1943, he signed an order regarding the fourteen-year-old patient Babette Fröwis, who suffered from mental retardation and epilepsy, but had been cared for without much ado by the nuns of the Schönbrunn Catholic order for the last nine years. In Sewering's referral paper, Babette was said to be "very unruly" and hence unsuitable for Schönbrunn; she was therefore to be transferred to Eglfing-Haar.[6] Two weeks later she died there, officially of pneumonia, but most probably after an overdose of phenobarbitol. Because it was clear to the sisters that any transfers to Eglfing-Haar would lead to a violent death for their charges, a death they deplored but could not prevent,[7] it stands to reason that Sewering, too, must have known about the consequences of his action.

On September 7, 1946, Hans Joachim Sewering, M.D., who by the end of the Third Reich had joined two more Nazi organizations,[8] was denazified by the American authorities in a Dachau court. These authorities, laboring under pressure and suffering both from a lack of knowledge regarding the operation of the Nazi system and all manner of deception daily perpetrated upon them by German suspects, did what today can only be described as an incomplete job, in that they denazified too many people too quickly on the basis of false or porous evidence.[9] In the case of the Sewering hearing, only three of his four Nazi affiliations were known to the judges, and they were not familiar with his professional work in Schönbrunn. Not bothering to check, they accepted his mendacious explanation that without membership in the SS he would not have been allowed to pursue university studies, and

4   Reichsärztekammer, Sewering, BDC; "Die Pressestelle des Ordinariates München meldet," Jan. 22, 1993, author's private archive (hereafter cited as author's PA); *Süddeutsche Zeitung*, Jan. 23–4, 1993; *Der Spiegel*, Jan. 25, 1993, 196.
5   Hans Joachim Sewering, "Ärztliches Zeugnis" for Babette Fröwis, Oct. 26, 1943; "Niederschrift über die Aufnahme der Babette Fröwis," Eglfing, Nov. 1, 1943; death certificate Fröwis, Eglfing, Nov. 18, 1943, all private archive of Dr. Hans Halter, Berlin. *Der Spiegel* editor Halter based his first article on the Sewering-Fröwis case on those documents in *Der Spiegel*, May 22, 1978, 84–8.
6   Quotation from Sewering's statement, printed in *Der Spiegel*, Jan. 25, 1993, 196.
7   "Die Pressestelle des Ordinariates München meldet," Jan. 22, 1993, author's PA.
8   The Nazi welfare organization NSV (*Nationalsozialistische Volkswohlfahrt*) and the university alumni union NS-Altherrenbund (PK Sewering, BDC).
9   See Hajo Holborn, *American Military Government: Its Organization and Politics* (Washington, D.C., 1947); Harold Zink, *American Military Government in Germany* (New York, 1947); Lutz Niethammer, *Entnazifizierung in Bayern: Säuberung und Rehabilitierung unter amerikanischer Besatzung* (Frankfurt/Main, 1972).

they believed his assurances that upon the point of associating himself with the SS and NSDAP he had been politically innocent, soon came to regret his "political error and increasingly distanced himself from the party."[10] However, the assessment by one of Sewering's Nazi area supervisors alone, that "in political and social respects he was without blemish," rendered in August of 1942 and available from the captured Nazi records, could have taught the Americans differently.[11] By naive and ill-advised judges, then, Sewering was classified as a "group II activist," ordered to pay a fine of 1,500 marks, and held responsible for the cost of the trial.[12] This meant that the doctor was now formally exonerated and free to follow a fresh professional and, if he so wished, political career in the new, western-zone democracy.

In the postwar German medical establishment, Sewering rose quickly. Choosing to remain in Dachau, he established there an institution for the treatment of infectious diseases as well as a profitable pulmonological practice. Simultaneously, he entered medical politics from his party of choice, the right-of-center Christian Socialist Union (CSU), later to be led by Franz Josef Strauss. In short order Sewering became a functionary in the union of German public health-care panel physicians (1952), president of the Bavarian Physicians' Chamber, and executive member of the Federal Chamber of Physicians (*Bundesärztekammer*, or BÄK) in Cologne (both in 1955). In 1968 he was appointed honorary professor of social medicine at Munich's Technical University. As of 1959 he was also a delegate to the World Medical Association (WMA), an executive member there since 1966, and its treasurer in 1971. The most important function came his way in October 1973, when the BÄK elected him its president. Already by this time he held so many offices that colleagues were dubbing him the "Emperor of Bavaria." No physician in Germany was more powerful.[13]

Sewering's unquestionable right-wing leanings clinched a decision made by the caucus of the WMA while he was its treasurer and the BÄK representative on its executive board. In 1981 the WMA readmitted to its membership the Medical Association of South Africa, which had left the world organization in 1975 because of a universal condemnation of its racist "apartheid" policies after Steve Biko's violent death. The German WMA delegation under Sewering's leadership played a disproportionately large part

10 "Judgment in the case against Dr. Hans Sewering," Sept. 7, 1946, private archive of Michael J. Franzblau, San Francisco (hereafter cited as PA Franzblau).
11 "Ausführliches Gesamturteil," sign. Kreispersonalamtsleiter, Munich, Aug. 13, 1942, PK Sewering, BDC.
12 "Judgment in the case against Dr. Hans Sewering," Sept. 7, 1946, PA Franzblau.
13 Munzinger-Archiv, Institut für Zeitgeschichte München (hereafter cited as IZM); Hermann Kater, ed., *Politiker und Ärzte: 600 Kurzbiographien und Portraits*, 3d ed. (Hameln, 1968), 325–6.

in the readmittance process because it, together with the Americans and Japanese, was in control of the WMA by dint of a majority of votes.[14] Since 1978, because of alleged improprieties in patient billing procedures, Sewering had already been succeeded as head of the BÄK by Dr. Karsten Vilmar, a surgeon originally from Bremen.[15] Increasingly, younger, more democratic-minded physicians in the Federal Republic who resented Sewering's Nazi past, his right-wing machinations and old-boy network tactics, not to mention his billing practices, were striving to rid themselves of his influence on the BÄK board. Hence in May of 1989, at the annual BÄK convention in Berlin, younger delegates criticized his stand, as evidenced in the South Africa affair, and proposed a motion to prevent Sewering from international travel on behalf of the German medical establishment. But this motion was defeated by the old German medical stalwarts. Sewering's staunch supporter during this interlude was his successor, Vilmar.[16]

Again it was Vilmar who, as chief German representative at the Forty-fourth World Medical Assembly of the WMA in Marbella, Spain, proposed Treasurer Sewering's candidacy as president-elect on September 28, 1992. Sewering's rival candidate was the relatively unknown Dr. J. G. Cardonna of Colombia, and so on October 1 the high-profile German was voted into office by a majority of fifty-three to nine, with nine abstentions.[17] A few weeks later, news about this event had reached concerned physicians outside the WMA in Germany, Israel, and Canada. Hence the German professor of family medicine at Göttingen University, Professor Michael M. Kochen, the son of Polish Holocaust survivors, agreed with his Israeli colleague at the University of Tel Aviv, Professor Michael Weingarten, that Sewering's appointment to the WMA, an organization that had been founded in 1947 in reaction to Nazi medical crimes,[18] was scandalous. In collaboration with a Canadian colleague, Professor William E. Seidelman, then of McMaster University in Hamilton, Ontario, they started searching for a way to annul

14 Winfried Beck, "The World Medical Association Serves Apartheid," *International Journal of Health Services* 20 (1990): 185–91. After an absence from the WMA for several years in the 1970s, the AMA returned to it in 1979.
15 Munzinger-Archiv, IZM. For a biography of Vilmar, born in 1930, see *Wer ist Wer?: Das deutsche Who's Who*, 25th ed. (Lübeck, 1986), 1371.
16 Minutes of proposal of Dr. Fuchs-Hammoser and subsequent discussion, proceedings of 92. Deutscher Ärztetag, Berlin, May 2–6, 1989, private archive of Howard Wolinsky, Chicago (hereafter cited as PA Wolinsky).
17 Summary minutes, 44th World Medical Assembly, Marbella, Spain, Sept.-Oct. 1992, PA Franzblau; Howard Wolinsky, "Ex-Nazi's World Role an Issue for AMA," *Chicago Sun-Times*, June 13, 1993.
18 Sharon Perley et al., eds., "The Nuremberg Code: An International Overview," in George J. Annas and Michael A. Grodin, eds., *The Nazi Doctors and the Nuremberg Code: Human Rights in Human Experimentation* (New York and Oxford, 1992), 154–5.

the appointment.[19] Even though those three physicians were Jewish, the affair was not just a matter of concern to Jews. Non-Jewish colleagues were also contacted, including the historian of medicine at Freiburg University, Professor Eduard Seidler, and myself. I was alerted by William Seidelman, who had been familiar with my ongoing work in the history of Nazi medicine for several years.[20] Although Kochen and Weingarten knew enough about Sewering's past to be concerned, they had been informed by Seidelman that the case was written up in greater detail in two publications of my own, dating from 1987 and 1989. I then sent copies of those publications to Göttingen and Tel Aviv.[21]

By the beginning of 1993, enough explosive material had filtered down from the German–Canadian discussions to the Americans, in particular, the delegates of the American Medical Association (AMA) in Chicago.[22] At a regular executive meeting scheduled for January 7 in Palm Springs by Dr. Raymond Scalettar, the first ever Jewish chairman of its board of trustees, the AMA executive, at Scalettar's insistence, came to demand the withdrawal of Sewering's WMA candidacy. Forthwith, the AMA communicated a formal request to that effect to Dr. André Wynen, the Belgian secretary-general of the WMA. In a subsequent press release, Dr. Scalettar said that the AMA was "deeply disturbed about these grave allegations," because "the personal activities of the WMA officers must in all respects reflect the highest ideals of medicine and adhere to the highest standards of medical ethics." The AMA officers gave notice to the WMA that, if their request were not complied with, the AMA would oppose Sewering's candidacy in future WMA meetings.[23]

In the following two weeks and parallel to the actions of the AMA, concerned professional groups in the United States, Canada, and Germany

19 Kochen to Weingarten, Göttingen, Nov. 23, 1992 (copied to Seidelman, then in Hamilton, Ontario), private archive of William E. Seidelman, Toronto, Ontario (hereafter cited as PA Seidelman).
20 Kochen to author, Göttingen, Dec. 2, 1992; Kochen to Seidler, Göttingen, Dec. 8, 1992, both author's PA.
21 The publications dealing with Sewering's Nazi past are: Michael H. Kater, "The Burden of the Past: Problems of a Modern Historiography of Physicians and Medicine in Modern Germany," *German Studies Review* 10 (1987): 41; Kater, *Doctors Under Hitler*, 3–4.
22 This is the recollection of AMA officer Dr. Raymond Scalettar, in telephone conversation with author, Washington, D.C., Jan. 31, 1994. Reportedly, on Jan. 5, 1993, the Boston University medical ethicist Michael A. Grodin, alerted by William Seidelman, informed Dr. James S. Todd, AMA Executive Vice-President, of Sewering's record (Wolinsky, "Ex-Nazi's World Role an Issue for AMA"; author's telephone conversation with Dr. Seidelman, Hamilton, Ontario, Feb. 3, 1994).
23 Todd to Wynen, Chicago, Jan. 7, 1993; AMA news release, Chicago, Jan. 16, 1993 (quotation), both author's PA; Hutar to Wynen, Chicago, Jan. 8, 1993, PA Seidelman. The circumstances of the Palm Springs meeting were confirmed in author's telephone conversation with Dr. Michael Franzblau, San Francisco, Jan. 30, 1994, and with Dr. Raymond Scalettar, Jan. 31, 1994.

worked hard to have the Marbella decision rescinded, by applying appropriate pressure both to the WMA and the German Federal Chamber of Physicians. Michael Kochen composed English- and German-language texts for international news releases destined for Associated Press, Reuters, and the *NewYork Times*, among others.[24] In Canada, William Seidelman informed the director-general of the Canadian Medical Association that it might be best for all concerned, including the WMA, if the BÄK handled the matter internally and impelled Sewering to withdraw from the presidency.[25] In the United States, the German-American pediatrician Hartmut Hanauske-Abel sent a "physicians' protest," underwritten by reform-minded German colleagues, to the editor of the prestigious British medical journal, *The Lancet*.[26] As well, the Boston-based group "Physicians for Human Rights," supported by many American doctors, issued its own strong protest to the WMA, urging it "to revoke its decision" regarding Sewering's presidency.[27]

Sewering, Vilmar, and their entourage from the BÄK now were on the hot spot. What made matters worse for them after the American initiative of January 7 was that Kochen's news release had indeed reached the major international press channels; questions were now also being asked from within Germany. Therefore, before responding to the AMA's demands, they tried to strengthen their lines of defense. On January 11, 1993, they secured an assurance from Schönbrunn's current director that Sewering could not have been involved in Nazi euthanasia, for if he were guilty, the nuns of Schönbrunn could not presently abide him as a consulting physician in their institution.[28] Thus being reassured, the BÄK informed the AMA board that "Professor Sewering decided not to withdraw and that the German Medical Association supports his decision." This immediately caused Dr. Scalettar and Dr. James S. Todd, the AMA's senior representative in the WMA, to reconfirm their original decision to have Sewering impeached in the world council.[29]

Three days later Sewering concluded that under the circumstances his best defense would be an offense. On January 15 he granted an interview to the *New York Times* Bonn correspondent Craig R. Whitney, chiefly

24 Unedited texts for news releases, including list of distributors, enclosed with letter Kochen to author, Göttingen, Jan. 11, 1993, author's PA.
25 Seidelman to Landry, Hamilton, Ontario, Jan. 11, 1993, PA Seidelman.
26 Hanauske-Abel to Fox, New York, N.Y., Jan. 15, 1993, private archive of Hartmut Hanauske-Abel, New York, N.Y. (hereafter cited PA Hanauske-Abel).
27 Stover to Wynen, Boston, Mass., Jan. 19, 1993 (quotation); press release by Physicians for Human Rights, Boston, Jan. 19, 1993, both author's PA.
28 Steinbacher to Fuchs, Schönbrunn, Jan. 11, 1993, PA Franzblau
29 Scalettar and Todd to Wynen, Chicago, Jan. 15, 1993 (the BÄK quotation is from this letter), author's PA.

designed to counter the allegations made public by Kochen's press release. He conceded that he had been in the SS, but claimed that after his service in the army he merely belonged to a genteel cavalry SS unit, "the only part of the organization not accused of war crimes." He reiterated the falsehood he had told the Dachau denazification court in 1946, that he had been forced to join the SS when only seventeen years old. Then he said that the sisters of Schönbrunn had rejected any allegations that he had sent a patient to be euthanized. Moreover, he emphasized that the West German government had "cleared" him of all charges by awarding him three of its highest civilian honors. Finally, Sewering maintained once more that all Nazi euthanasia activities had been stopped in 1941 and, again, that the Catholic order would not have kept him on as a consultant until now had he done anything wrong. In all of this, BÄK president Vilmar said that he stood squarely behind his colleague.[30] Sewering's remarks were immediately circulated internationally.[31]

As the New York psychiatrist and medical historian Robert Jay Lifton and I made clear in a joint statement for the *New York Times* on January 18,[32] Sewering had purposely obfuscated the truth by twisting the facts in four major respects. First, he had of course never been forced to join the SS but, as was the custom then, had joined voluntarily. Second, records showed that he joined as a member of the regular (*Allgemeine*) SS and that there was no evidence he ever made contact with an SS cavalry unit, then or later. (On this, one can add today that although Sewering was technically correct in categorizing the cavalry SS before 1939 as a noncriminal organization by Nuremberg Trial criteria,[33] the Nuremberg judges had partially based their verdict on ignorance, because first of all, the Reiter-SS was predicated on the same anti-Semitic precepts as the Allgemeine SS, of which it was an institutional part, and second, cavalry divisions of the Waffen-SS, which could have drawn on the Allgemeine SS cavalry for recruitment after 1939, were implicated in crimes, such as summarily executing "bandits," that is, partisans.[34]) Third, it was clear that Sewering lied about his knowledge regarding the fate of patients transferred from Schönbrunn to Eglfing-Haar; and fourth, he tried to block out the historic facts regarding wild euthanasia after 1941.

30 *New York Times*, Jan. 16, 1993.
31 For Canada, see *Toronto Star*, Jan. 17, 1993; *Hamilton Spectator*, Jan. 18, 1993.
32 Robert Jay Lifton and Michael H. Kater, "Statement for the New York Times," Jan. 18, 1993, author's PA. Subsequent events obviated publication of the statement.
33 *Der Prozess gegen die Hauptkriegsverbrecher vor dem Internationalen Militärgerichtshof: Nürnberg, 14. November 1945–1. Oktober 1946* (1947; reprinted: Munich, 1984), 1:307, 21:473.
34 Raimund Schnabel, ed., *Macht ohne Moral: Eine Dokumentation über die SS* (Frankfurt/Main, 1957), 43; Bernd Wegner, *The Waffen-SS: Organization, Ideology, and Function* (Oxford, 1990), 11–57; Kurt Georg Klietmann, ed., *Die Waffen-SS: Eine Dokumentation* (Osnabrück, 1965), 157–64.

Sewering's chosen line of argumentation, backed by BÄK president Vilmar,[35] startled open-minded doctors everywhere. As a Canadian practitioner from Goderich in rural Ontario expressed it:"I am deeply concerned and surprised that the above physician is the president-elect of the world organization which represents my profession."[36] Göttingen Professor Kochen insisted that Sewering must have known that, through his signature on the Schönbrunn document, he was consigning Babette Fröwis to her death.[37] The entire Social Democratic-oriented Berlin section of the Federal Chamber of Physicians under the leadership of Dr. Ellis Huber protested to the Egyptian president of the WMA, Dr. Ibrahim Badran, reminding him that Sewering lacked the ability to mourn – using Alexander Mitscherlich's trenchant phrase – and that on this account alone he should resign.[38]

That Sewering finally did so on Saturday, January 23, 1993, was owing to the fact that, in quick succession, events were entrapping him. First, on Thursday, Reuter's news service reported that the World Jewish Congress (WJC), based in New York, "was considering calling on national medical groups to withdraw from the World Medical Association if it confirmed a former Nazi as its president." Reportedly, the WJC had already instructed its members in seventy-two countries to ask their medical associations to remove their support from Sewering.[39] Also on Thursday the U.S. Justice Department declared its intention of placing Sewering on their "Watch List," analogously to Austrian president Kurt Waldheim earlier, which would have meant barring Sewering from entering the United States.[40] On Friday *Die Zeit*, Germany's most respected weekly, printed New York doctor Hanauske-Abel's long protest against Sewering, repeating and documenting all the hitherto known facts, now cosigned by some hundred German doctors and sponsored by the German branch of International Physicians for the Prevention of Nuclear War (IPPNW).[41] But what must have been decisive for Sewering was that a day later, on Saturday, January 23, the Catholic order responsible for the Schönbrunn sanatorium was encouraged by Cardinal Karl Ratzinger of the Munich diocese to issue a news release, denying the doctor's

35 See Julia Albrecht, "Von der Reiter-SS zum Weltärztechef," *taz*, Jan. 20, 1993.
36 Jim Hollingworth, M.D., to author, Goderich, Jan. 21, 1993, author's PA.
37 Michael M. Kochen, "Ehemaliger SS-Mann künftiger Präsident des Weltärztebundes?" *Zeitschrift für Allgemeine Medizin* (Jan. 31, 1993): 8; see also *Süddeutsche Zeitung*, (Jan. 20, 1993); *Der Spiegel*, Jan. 25, 1993, 196.
38 Huber to Badran, Berlin, Jan. 20, 1993, author's PA.
39 Reuter's press release, "Jewish Group Says It [Is] Considering Boycott of World Medical [Assocation]," New York, Jan. 21, 1993, PA Franzblau. The veracity of this text was later confirmed by the WJC. See Steinberg to Kloiber, New York, Oct. 14, 1993, PA Franzblau.
40 *Süddeutsche Zeitung*, Jan. 22, 1993.
41 "Deutsche Ärzte protestieren," *Die Zeit*, Jan. 22, 1993.

long-standing claim that in 1943 the nuns (and, by implication, he himself) had not known what was going on with their hapless patients. Four of the sisters, still alive, testified that "it was crystal-clear that the transport occurred in the course of so-called euthanasia."[42]

At this point, had the Dachau physician admitted his involvement in euthanasia and declared that he deplored it as well as his entire Nazi past, it could have meant the end of the Sewering affair. But instead of being publicly repentant, the doctor turned the matter into a scandal by claiming that it now was his duty to divert harm from the World Medical Association, harm "which could be generated by the threat of the World Jewish Congress alone."[43] This was not a neutral phrase, for it could be interpreted as conjuring up the specter of an international Jewish conspiracy, a favorite charge of German anti-Semites in the past.[44] Nevertheless, for the time being, the leaderhip of the AMA showed itself pleased, obviously relieved that it did not have to instigate further action within the WMA.[45]

II

Observers of these events now began to shift their attention from Sewering's initial role in the scandal to two other, related questions. One was the tenacity with which BÄK president Karsten Vilmar had been supporting Sewering all along, and the other was the attitude of the American delegates to the WMA. As for Vilmar, he was immediately attacked, especially by younger German colleagues, when it became clear that he shared Sewering's suspicions toward the World Jewish Congress and maintained that Sewering had been calumniated.[46] On the very weekend of Sewering's withdrawal, the progressive *Ärzte Zeitung* stated that Vilmar had placed himself "into the public firing line," and the German branch of IPPNW told Vilmar that he no longer had the confidence of its members, because he and his BÄK had

---

42   "Die Pressestelle des Ordinariates München meldet," Jan. 22, 1993, author's PA; see also *Süddeutsche Zeitung*, Jan. 23–4, 1993.

43   BÄK press release, "Die Bundesärztekammer informiert," Cologne, Jan. 23, 1993, author's PA; see also *Süddeutsche Zeitung*, Jan. 23, 1993.

44   This is what I argued in a statement to the WMA et al., Toronto, Jan. 25, 1993, author's PA; also note Seidelman's rejection of what he perceived as a conspiracy charge in his letter to editor of the Toronto *Globe and Mail*, Hamilton, Ontario, Feb. 4, 1993, PA Seidelman. Further see Weingarten's letter to the author, Tel Hashomer, Feb. 3, 1993, author's PA; and Kochen's article, "Ehemaliger SS-Mann künftiger Präsident des Weltärztebundes?" 8; Kochen's letter-to-the-editor, March 1993, *Deutsches Ärzteblatt* 90 (1993): A-762. Kochen was justly incensed, for Sewering had polemicized against him, as a Jew, ad hominem. See Sewering's interview in *Süddeutsche Zeitung*, Jan. 21, 1993.

45   Raymond Scalettar, "AMA Applauds Withdrawal of German Official from World Medical Association," Jan. 23, 1993, author's PA.

46   See Vilmar's endorsement in BÄK press release, "Die Bundesärztekammer informiert," Cologne, Jan. 23, 1993, author's PA; see also *Ärzte Zeitung*, Jan. 25, 1993.

"severely damaged the national and international reputation of the Federal Republic's medical community."[47] On Monday, January 25, after Vilmar had once more insisted that Sewering ought to be treated as innocent until found guilty in a recognized court of law, *Ärzte Zeitung* was calling for the surgeon's resignation as chief of the *Bundesärztekammer*.[48] But Vilmar entrenched himself by arguing that the Catholic hierarchy in Munich had exculpated Sewering as early as 1978, thereby charging the sisters of Schönbrunn with duplicity. He also rejected the recent announcements by the AMA, maintaining that all the delegates at the Marbella WMA meeting in the autumn of 1992 had known about Sewering's past. Hence he saw no reason whatsoever to step down from his Cologne post.[49]

Vilmar's insinuation that the Americans in Marbella had acquiesced in Sewering's past record cast a shadow over the integrity of the AMA, and it was seized upon by the venerable *Boston Globe* on February 1, when it contended that, "as the most powerful member of the World Medical Association, the AMA must investigate why it was blind to charges against Sewering that were published in 1978. Must the old-boy network include old Nazis?"[50] Dr. Joseph T. Painter, president-elect of the AMA, immediately repudiated the suggestion that the AMA had been "at fault." Claiming that, in 1978, the year of that alleged publication, the AMA was not even a member of the WMA, he returned all the blame to the Germans, who, after all, had endorsed Sewering for his candidacy as WMA treasurer as early as 1971. The AMA had received "factually based" reports on Sewering only early in January 1993 and had acted immediately thereafter. "For the *Globe* to insinuate that the AMA would knowingly tolerate such an appointment is uninforming and insulting."[51] When *Deutsches Ärzteblatt*, the BÄK's official publication, repeated the *Globe*'s accusations, Raymond Scalettar of the AMA protested with equal vigor.[52]

47 *Ärzte Zeitung*, Jan. 22-3, 1993; Rolf Bader, executive director of IPPNW Germany Central, to Vilmar, Berlin, Jan. 24, 1993, author's PA.
48 *Ärzte Zeitung*, Jan. 25, 1993; see also *Frankfurter Rundschau*, Jan. 25, 1993.
49 Vilmar as reported in Liste Gesundheit, "Presseerklärung vom 26.01.93," Bremen, Jan. 26, 1993, author's PA; *Ärzte Zeitung*, Jan. 26, 1993. On Vilmar's attempt to discredit the Catholic order, see also Vilmar to Sirl, Cologne, Jan. 27, 1993; and Sirl to Vilmar, Schönbrunn, Feb. 2, 1993, both PA Franzblau.
50 *Boston Globe*, Feb. 1, 1993; see also note 5 to this chapter.
51 Painter to *Boston Globe*, Feb. 5, 1993, author's PA.
52 Norbert Jachertz, "Sewering–Ende einer Karriere," *Deutsches Ärzteblatt* 90 (Feb. 1993): A-239; Scalettar to Editor [Jachertz], Chicago, (Feb. 26, 1993), author's PA. This letter was printed, in the English original, in *Deutsches Ärzteblatt* 90 (March 1993): A-760. On March 23, 1993, in another letter to Jachertz, James S. Todd repeated on behalf of the AMA leadership "that no member of the American Medical Association (AMA) leadership, or of the AMA delegation to the World Medical Association meeting in Spain," knew about Sewering's case before Jan. 5, 1993 (author's PA).

Nevertheless, Norbert Jachertz, the *Ärzteblatt*'s editor in chief, remained adamant, insisting that at least some of the AMA delegates in Marbella had known about Sewering.[53] He might have had a case. For later in 1993, a solid body of evidence emerged, strongly suggesting that, in order not to know about Sewering before November 1992, the American delegates would have had to try very hard. Fact is that several former AMA officers had admitted to such damaging knowledge long before the Marbella meeting. Dr. William Rial, AMA president in 1982–83, was aware of rumors, and Dr. Lowell Steen, past AMA board chairman, had received hints of Sewering's Nazi ties. His successor, Dr. Frank Jirka, said that, when Sewering was confronted with these charges years ago, he "swore up and down he'd been wrongly accused."[54]

Even discounting the 1978 article about Sewering that, as a credible piece of investigative journalism, had appeared in German in the news magazine *Der Spiegel*,[55] there were three other English-language sources that might have been able to inform the AMA delegates: my own article "The Burden of the Past," published in 1987 in the United States; my monograph, *Doctors Under Hitler*, published with the University of North Carolina Press two years later; and, also printed in 1989, a brief article by the German physician Winfried Beck in *The Lancet*, the leading British medical journal.[56] What makes matters more serious, however, is evidence that, at the fall 1992 meeting in Marbella, Dutch and Scandinavian WMA deputies went around informing their colleagues of Sewering's Nazi record and urging them not to vote for him. Two who listened were the Australian delegates, Professor Bill Coote and Professor Priscilla Kincaid-Smith (the WMA's president-elect in early 1994).[57] In contrast, the American delegation, consisting of four AMA executives, received a superficial briefing about certain old stories haunting Sewering from a permanent AMA staff member, but this was not regarded by them as sufficiently reliable grounds for action.[58] One reason why the Americans, particularly Dr. Todd, allowed themselves to be compromised could have been the AMA's collusion with the Germans back in 1981, when South Africa had been readmitted to the WMA.[59]

53 Jachertz to Scalettar, Cologne, March 5, 1993, PA Franzblau.
54 See Howard Wolinsky, "WMA's Ex-President-Elect," *Physician's Weekly* (June 14, 1993).
55 See note 5 to this chapter.
56 See note 21 to this chapter and Winfried Beck, "The World Medical Association and South Africa," *The Lancet* (June 24, 1989): 1441–2.
57 A particularly active lobbyist was Dr. Ole Asbjorn Jensen of Denmark. See Howard Wolinsky, "WMA's Ex-President-Elect"; Wolinsky, "Ex-Nazi's World Role an Issue for AMA"; Norman Aisbett, "The SS Factor," *The West Australian*, Nov. 20, 1993.
58 Author's telephone conversation with Dr. Scalettar of the AMA and WMA.
59 Under the AMA's headship of Dr. James Sammons. See Howard Wolinsky, "The South African Connection," *Physician's Weekly* (June 28, 1993).

Such American involvement in ethically questionable WMA dealings may also have been the reason for the German delegation's self-assurance at the next large meeting of the world association in Istanbul during early April 1993. At first the German WMA accountant Adolf Hällmayr, a long-standing friend of Treasurer Sewering, uttered favorable judgments about the pulmonologist in a closed council session, along the lines that "the enormous reputation of Professor Sewering was not negotiable" and that "engagement in the SS for medical students was compulsory."[60] Vilmar himself then repeated the old canards that Sewering had been exonerated by a U.S. court in 1946 and that the German government's high rewards were enough as proof of sterling character. And with good reason and therefore not without cynicism, Vilmar reminded his listeners that, before his election to the world post, Sewering's past had been "critically discussed by various delegations" and that thereupon the doctor "was elected by a large majority." Referring to the concerns of the World Jewish Congress, Vilmar reiterated the need, on the part of the BÄK, to protect "the World Medical Association from harm."[61] And whereas Vilmar's delegation again insisted that the facts about Sewering had been "in the public domain" and that before the Marbella meeting "special notices to WMA members were not necessary," the AMA deputies still complained that before October 1992 such information should have been tabled by the Germans in a formal manner. There should have been "full disclosure at the time of nomination." By way of ultimately blaming the Germans and in order to save face amid their own bunglings, the AMA delegates, for their part, now demonstratively balloted against the proposed candidacy of Karsten Vilmar as the new treasurer of the WMA. This, however, did not prevent the Bremen surgeon from handily being voted into that position.[62]

Vilmar was now more securely anchored in the WMA than ever before and, in the mold of his predecessor in the BÄK, could with good reason look forward to becoming its president. Nonetheless, having outmaneuvred the troublesome Americans, it remained for him to shore up his position at home. This he did successfully during the ninety-sixth annual German physicians' meeting (*Deutscher Ärztetag*) in Dresden in early May. Defending his recent action before the WMA, he proceeded to lay blame on the Catholic

---

60 *World Medical Journal* 39 (March/April 1993): 23.
61 Ibid., 22–3; summary minutes, WMA 135th Council session, Istanbul, Turkey, April 1–4, 1993, author's PA. Vilmar's address was circulated at the time of the meeting in the form of an official BÄK statement, dated March 29, 1993 (PA Wolinsky).
62 Raymond Scalettar, Report of the Board of Trustees [of AMA], [early April 1993], author's PA. Scalettar himself was not present at the Istanbul meeting. The vote was a council vote, with seven in favor of Vilmar, four opposed, and one abstention.

hierarchy for misleading Sewering and the BÄK. Insisting that he was open to a critical treatment of Germany's Nazi past, he also maintained that this past had to be balanced against the more recent Communist experience in the former German Democratic Republic, whose legacy the West Germans had just acquired. On all counts, Vilmar was heavily applauded.[63]

But internationally, the indignation over Vilmar's behavior in the Sewering affair, which had long since become Vilmar's own, was still smoldering. Non-German physicians were particularly annoyed at his election to the weighty position of WMA treasurer, because they saw this as a vindication of the BÄK's past international policy. Thus William Seidelman, as member in good standing of the Canadian Medical Association, communicated to the Israel Medical Association that Vilmar's past and current defense of Sewering "disqualified" him from his new WMA posting.[64] Even less forgiving was Dr. Michael J. Franzblau, a San Francisco dermatologist and, as representative of the American Society for Dermatologic Surgery, an associate member of both the AMA and the WMA, who had become involved in the exchange of information concerning Sewering early in January 1993.[65] Referring to a proposal at the Istanbul meeting in early April that all officers of the WMA "should be of impeccable character," he postulated to the AMA that Dr. Vilmar did not meet that standard. The AMA should withdraw from the WMA for the period that Vilmar held his office.[66] But this resolution of June 1993 died on the order papers, and so, in time for the next general meeting of the WMA in Budapest early in October, Franzblau tried again. He sought a formal motion protesting Vilmar's treasury investiture, as well as an investigation into the Sewering appointment.[67] But, as Franzblau tells it, his resolution "was greeted with a firestorm of protest from the secretary-general of the WMA, the representative of the *Bundesärztekammer*, and the Belgian Medical Association. I had no support, so I withdrew the resolution before a vote, so that I can bring it back next year in Stockholm, September 1–4,

---

63 Minutes of plenary meeting, 96. Deutscher Ärztetag Dresden, Pressestelle der deutschen Ärzteschaft, Cologne, May 7, 1993, PA Seidelman.

64 Seidelman to Dr. Miriam Zangen (president of Israel Medical Association), Hamilton, Ontario, June 1, 1993, PA Seidelman.

65 Author's telephone conversation with Dr. Franzblau, San Francisco, Jan. 30, 1994.

66 Franzblau to members of AMA Reference Committee F, San Francisco, June 12, 1993, PA Franzblau. Earlier, Franzblau had asked to investigate the background of Sewering's WMA nomination. Not surprisingly, Dr. Joseph Painter, who earlier in 1993 had won the AMA presidential race against the more sceptical Dr. Scalettar and was a member of the AMA old-boy network, refused on the basis that "all the facts are out" (AMA Resolution A-93 [early June 1993], PA Franzblau; *Chicago Sun-Times*, June 15, 1993 [quotation]). See also *AM News* (July 3, 1993); *Skin & Allergy News* (Aug. 1993).

67 Text of Franzblau's resolution introduced to the Budapest WMA general meeting, Oct. 2, 1993, author's PA; see also *Der Spiegel* (Sept. 27, 1993): 284.

1994."[68] For the time being, Karsten Vilmar was firmly in control, because Michael Franzblau's motion had not even received a second.[69]

III

In order to place those developments into historical perspective, one must understand that Vilmar and Sewering are only a symptom of the German medical establishment's uniquely tarnished past and the chronic inability of its higher echelons to come to terms with it. As I have proved as early as 1987, not only were the German doctors the most heavily nazified profession in the Third Reich (with every second male doctor a Party member between 1933 and 1945),[70] but most physicians after 1945 have consistently refused to ac- knowledge this, have suppressed any attempts at enlightenment within their ranks, and have unflaggingly appointed as their leaders either former National Socialists or, in the case of Vilmar, younger colleagues obviously sympathetic to one-time members of Nazi formations. Indeed, Sewering, as president of the *Bundesärztekammer*, was the third consecutive postwar veteran of the SA or the SS, after the office of Carl Haedenkamp, who had helped the Nazi regime clear the profession of Jews, and Ernst Fromm, who had been an SS man.[71] Although on the occasion of Fromm's election as president of the WMA in October 1973 in Munich, he and Treasurer Sewering chose to speak of a hundred years of "democratic tradition" of German organized physicians,[72] the facts were contrary. Over the years it has been exhaustively documented that German doctors as a closed profession tended to be anti- democratic, antifeminist, and anti-Semitic. Very able at their jobs and capable of important contributions to the advancement of medical science, they also got caught up in an ongoing process of professionalization that led them to neocorporatism – a state where unbounded collective egotism often encour- aged practitioners to disregard their clients' concerns, while their relationship to potentially regulatory national governments remained ambivalent.[73] This

---

68 Franzblau to author, San Francisco, Oct. 14, 1993, author's PA. Franzblau further writes elsewhere: "Representatives of the German Medical Association [BÄK] met with me personally during the meet- ing and made every effort to discourage me from my attempt to get Dr. Vilmar to resign" (Michael Franzblau, "Investigate Nazi Ties of German Doctors," *San Francisco Chronicle*, Dec. 29, 1993).

69 *Deutsches Ärzteblatt* 90 (Oct. 29, 1993): C-1904.

70 Kater, "The Burden of the Past," 40; Kater, "Medizin und Mediziner im Dritten Reich: Eine Bestandsaufnahme," *Historische Zeitschrift* 244 (1987): 311.

71 *World Medical Journal* 20 (May-June 1973): 41; *World Medical Journal* 21 (Jan.-Feb. 1974): 4; Kater, "The Burden of the Past," 31-56; Kater, *Doctors Under Hitler*, passim.

72 *World Medical Journal* 20 (May-June 1973): 42.

73 For the background to neocorporatism as a phenomenon applying not only to physicians, but also other academic professions, see Konrad H. Jarausch, *The Unfree Professions: German Lawyers, Teachers, and Engineers, 1900-1950* (New York, 1990), 22-4, 220-4.

is one of the keys to understanding most doctors' rejection of the Weimar Republic, on the one hand, which tended to cast them into socialist fetters, and their bond with National Socialism and the Third Reich on the other, because the Nazis seemed in a position to meet their, at the time pressing, corporate needs, such as a unifying professional code granted to them in 1935. Hence they allied themselves with Hitler's movement even before January 1933 and thereafter remained among his staunchest supporters. As a long-term result, they acquired great wealth, and their overall prestige placed them at the top of the social pyramid for decades after World War II.[74]

After the Nazi era, the German physicians were urged by the newly founded WMA at its first meeting in 1948, supported by that confederation's membership of thirty-nine national medical associations, to render a formal statement acknowledging that during the 1930s and 1940s German physicians had violated medical ethics, had stained the professional medical honor, and had prostituted medical science by placing it at the beck and call of war and political fanaticism.[75] "Astonishment was expressed in the General Assembly of the World Medical Association that no sign whatever had come from Germany that the doctors were ashamed of their share in the crimes, or even that they fully realized the enormity of their conduct."[76] But only an incomplete declaration was issued by the German doctors.[77] In keeping with this recalcitrance, after the foundation of the Federal Physicians' Chamber and backed by the majority of German doctors who, after all, did vote them into office, Fromm, Sewering, and Vilmar as BÄK presidents have pursued what to most foreign observers has appeared as a self-serving policy for their professional peers alone, disregarding the needs of the larger commonweal.[78] Although such policies are not untypical of doctors in other present-day states, in Germany their contours appear sharper against the backdrop of quite recent history.

74 Michael H. Kater, "Ärzte und Politik in Deutschland, 1848–1945," *Jahrbuch des Instituts für Geschichte der Medizin der Robert Bosch Stiftung* 5 (1987): 34–48; Michael H. Kater, "Professionalization and Socialization of Physicians in Wilhelmine and Weimar Germany," *Journal of Contemporary History* 20 (1985): 677–701; Michael H. Kater, "Hitler's Early Doctors: Nazi Physicians in Predepression Germany," *Journal of Modern History* 59 (1987): 25–52; Michael H. Kater, "Physicians in Crisis at the End of the Weimar Republic," in Peter D. Stachura, ed., *Unemployment and the Great Depression in Weimar Germany* (Basingstoke, 1986), 49–77; Michael H. Kater, "The Nazi Physicians' League of 1929: Causes and Consequences," in Thomas Childers, ed., *The Formation of the Nazi Constituency, 1918-1933* (London, 1986), 147–81; Michael H. Kater, "Unresolved Questions of German Medicine and Medical History in the Past and Present," *Central European History* 25 (1992): 407–23; Kater, *Doctors Under Hitler*, passim.

75 Geiger and Stover to Wynen, Boston, Jan. 19, 1993, author's PA; also Jennifer Leaning, "German Doctors and Their Secrets," *New York Times*, Feb. 6, 1993.

76 "The Dedication of the Physician," *World Medical Association Bulletin* 1 (April 1949): 7.

77 Ibid., 8–10.

78 See letters to the editor by older German physicians in *Deutsches Ärzteblatt* 90 (1993): A-834, A-836; and "Im Sturzflug Abwärts," *Der Spiegel* (Oct. 25, 1993): 150–6.

Hence Vilmar's words ring somewhat hollow when he speaks of his concern about the Nazi past and writes of the "terrible events during the National Socialist dictatorship."[79] His real belief is that Nazi medical crimes were an aberration, committed only by a few deviates, and not a consequence of partially irregular developments in German mainstream scientific thought for decades.[80]

This "rotten apples" theory was rejected by the same World Medical Association of which Vilmar today is treasurer as early as September 1948, when it stated: "Since the end of the Second World War evidence has been published in several countries of the widespread criminal conduct of the German medical profession since 1933."[81] Nor has it ever been subscribed to thereafter by international medical historians.[82] Yet it formed the wellspring for two questionable actions on the part of BÄK president Vilmar during the late 1980s. In the first instance in 1987, he publicly castigated Dr. Hartmut Hanauske-Abel, a young, some-time emergency physician from Rhenish Hesse who had just assumed a prestigious research fellowship at Harvard Children's Hospital, after having published in *The Lancet* a critical article about the German physicians' role in the Third Reich.[83] At great financial cost to himself, Hanauske-Abel took Vilmar to court on several judiciary levels for many months, only to lose his case in the end.[84] Working as an assistant professor of pediatrics at Cornell Medical College in New York in 1993, the year of the Sewering scandal, and becoming actively involved in American and

79 Minutes of plenary meeting, 96. Deutscher Ärztetag, Dresden, Pressestelle der deutschen Ärzteschaft, Cologne, May 7, 1993, PA Seidelman; Vilmar to Wellhöner, Bremen, July 31, 1987, PA Hanauske-Abel (quotation).
80 See article on Vilmar's speech to the 90th Deutsche Ärztetag, Karlsruhe, 1987, "Dr. Vilmar zur Rolle der Ärzteschaft im Nationalsozialismus," *Arzt und Presse*, no. 3 (June 5, 1987), PA Hanauske-Abel; Kater, *Doctors Under Hitler*, 223.
81 "The Dedication of the Physician," *World Medical Association Bulletin* 1 (April 1949): 4.
82 See Fridolf Kudlien et al., *Ärzte im Nationalsozialismus* (Cologne, 1985); Christian Pross and Götz Aly, eds., *Der Wert des Menschen: Medizin in Deutschland, 1918–1945* (Berlin, 1989); Alfons Labisch, *Homo Hygienicus: Gesundheit und Medizin in der Neuzeit* (Frankfurt/Main, 1992), 188–246; Daniel Wikler and Jeremiah Barondess, "Bioethics and Anti-Bioethics in Light of Nazi Medicine: What Must We Remember?" *Kennedy Institute of Ethics Journal* 3, no. 1 (1993): 42–3; Götz Aly, Peter Chroust, and Christian Pross, *Cleansing the Fatherland: Nazi Medicine and Racial Hygiene* (Baltimore, Md., 1994).
83 Hartmut M. Hanauske-Abel, "From Nazi Holocaust to Nuclear Holocaust: A Lesson to Learn?" *The Lancet* (Aug. 2, 1987): 271–3. Vilmar's attack on Hanauske-Abel is in *Deutsches Ärzteblatt* 84 (1987): B 847–59; see Ulrich Stock's massive criticism of Vilmar's behavior in "Deutsche Ärzte und die Vergangenheit," *Die Zeit*, June 12, 1987, 56. An initial, critical American comment on the affair is Thomas W. Maretzki, "The Documentation of Nazi Medicine by German Medical Sociologists: A Review Article," *Social Science and Medicine* 29 (1989): 1320–21.
84 Bellinghausen to Becker, Cologne, Feb. 5, 1988; Becker to Krumsiek, Marburg, Feb. 23, 1988; "Klage des Arztes Dr. Hartmut Hanauske-Abel ... gegen ... Dr. med. Karsten Vilmar," Cologne, March 2, 1989, all PA Hanauske-Abel; Hanauske-Abel to author, Nov. 25, 1993, author's PA.

German protests against that doctor's WMA appointment, Hanauske-Abel was easily identified by Vilmar as the chief villain of an alleged anti-Sewering cabal in North America.[85]

Because he does not seem to know what drives the young, curious generation of German physicians like Hanauske-Abel, Vilmar has, in the second instance, obstructed, rather than encouraged, education about medicine under Hitler among West German physicians and students of medicine in the years after the Hanauske-Abel incident. For example, at the end of the 1980s he chastised a woman medical student who wished to know why former Nazi doctors were being allowed to sustain lucrative West German medical practices. In the pages of the BÄK's official *Ärzteblatt*, Vilmar lectured her that "your letter and the questions and conclusions contained therein give rise to the suspicion that the history and knowledge of the chief principles of our democracy have escaped you ... since you, too, are calling for the persecution of those doctors without due recourse to the law."[86] Contemporaneously, in the spring of 1989, he withheld institutional support for an exhibition, "The Value of the Human Being," intended to instruct its visitors about Nazi medical abuses. The exhibition, assembled by Drs. Götz Aly and Christian Pross of Berlin, had been adopted by the left-leaning Berlin regional section of the Federal Physicians' Chamber, under the headship of the aforementioned Dr. Huber. Because Huber's section was also the host of the annual BÄK meeting, *Deutscher Ärztetag*, the Cologne headquarters of the overarching national Chamber under Vilmar, nominally acted as cosponsor. However, events of the conference were not made to revolve around that exposition, despite a perfunctory address on Nazi medicine by a German medical historian, and Vilmar later refused to support the exhibition on a national tour of Germany, to say nothing of support for an international excursion to the United States and Canada.[87]

The example of Hanauske-Abel proves that young, progressive physicians do exist in Germany, but they belong to the minority. Michael Kochen of Göttingen University has affirmed that this minority is the driving force behind the German thrust against the BÄK, and resolutions passed against Sewering and Vilmar by left-of-center physicians' groups from Berlin and

---

85 See notes 26 and 41 to this chapter; Kloiber to Franzblau, Cologne, Oct. 18, 1993, PA Franzblau; see also *Deutsches Ärzteblatt* 90 (1993): C-1904.

86 Quoted in Kater, "Unresolved Questions," 416.

87 With the help of international universities and the Goethe Institute network, the exhibition later traveled to Boston, Toronto, and other venues. See program, "The Value of the Human Being: Medicine in Germany, 1918-1945. Exhibition: September 30-October 14, 1992, University of Toronto, Canada" (author's PA); Michael H. Kater, "Die unbewältigte Medizingeschichte: Beiträge zur NS-Zeit aus Marburg, Tübingen, und Göttingen," *Historische Zeitschrift* 257 (1993): 415n. 50; Kater, "Foreword," in Aly et al., *Cleansing the Fatherland*, vii-ix.

Bremen bear this out.[88] Dr. Pross, after publishing several enlightening studies on the dismal record of German doctors in the recent past and shepherding his educational conference to international success, is now directing a Berlin clinic for international victims of rape and torture. According to the clinic's annual report for 1992, this commendable project "was born out of the history of Nazi medicine and the subsequent refusal of a large part of German doctors after 1945 to allow a confrontation with the Holocaust survivors and to support them in their quest for recognition, rehabilitation and reparation." The report states that the treatment center is primarily funded by the German Federal Ministry for Family Affairs and Senior Citizens, as well as the secretariat-general of the German Red Cross. In the credits, the *Bundesärztekammer* is not mentioned.[89]

It appears that, whatever those younger German doctors today are doing to the credit of present-day medicine, they have not been motivated by proper instruction in medical ethics at Germany's universities, which subject, after 1945, should have been closely linked to a history of Nazi medical abuse. It can be assumed that if such teaching in German medical schools after the war had existed, Fromm, Sewering, and Vilmar would never have been elected to national office. Yet despite representations to the contrary by the German establishment, medical ethics, as it should be taught, is currently not a matter of concern for the country's medical curriculum planners, nor has it ever been.[90]

Nor, for that matter, does the subject of medical history – taught unevenly in German medical faculties[91] – include systematic instruction about Third

88 Kochen's observation in Howard Wolinsky, "A Question of Guilt," *Physician's Weekly* (Aug. 9, 1993). Further, see Huber to Badran, Berlin, Jan. 20, 1993; Liste Gesundheit, "Presseerklärung vom 26.01.93," Bremen, Jan. 26, 1993, both author's PA. See also letters to the editor by the following concerned physicians: Kappauf (Nuremberg), Sticherling (Grevenbroich), Dessauer (Hamburg), Pilz (Karlsruhe), all in *Deutsches Ärzteblatt* 90 (1993): A-758–59, A-834.

89 Behandlungszentrum für Folteropfer, Berlin, *Annual Report 1992* [Berlin, 1993], 2 (quotation), 25. Christian Pross has had a long-standing concern for the victims of human rights violations. See Christian Pross and Rolf Winau, eds., *Nicht misshandeln: Das Krankenhaus Moabit* (Berlin, 1984); Christian Pross, *Wiedergutmachung: Der Kleinkrieg gegen die Opfer* (Frankfurt/Main, 1988); Pross and Götz Aly, eds., *Der Wert des Menschen*; Pross, "Nazi Doctors, German Medicine, and Historical Truth," in Annas and Grodin, eds., *The Nazi Doctors*, 32–52; Pross's introductory chapter in Aly et al., *Cleansing the Fatherland*, 1–21.

90 This has been the recent observation of a medical critic writing in *Der Spiegel* (Oct. 25, 1993): 151. Professor William Seidelman, himself an internationally recognized authority in the field of medical education, after an official visit to German universities in 1991, noted "the absence of a formal curriculum on medical ethics in German medical schools," with the federal government blaming the universities and vice versa. The German Foreign Ministry ultimately informed him that "[t]here is no immediate need to change successful and established practice" (William Seidelman, "Current Problems of Medical Ethics and Practice," critical comment delivered at the conference, "Medicine in 19th- and 20th-Century Germany: Ethics, Politics, and Law," German Historical Institute and Goethe Institut, Washington, D.C., Dec. 1–4, 1993 [MS in author's PA]).

91 Ulrich Tröhler, "Graduate Education in the History of Medicine: Federal Republic of Germany," *Bulletin of the History of Medicine* 63 (1989): 435–43.

Reich medical crimes, and, related, on what counts German doctors, as a profession, went astray. Because currently few regular historians of medicine teach the history of medicine in Germany from 1933 to 1945 with any degree of consistency,[92] specialists in other disciplines sometimes jump into the breach to make amends. Although they mean well, they generally meet with the resistance of their colleagues and often botch their attempts for lack of proper historiographical training. When in 1988 a Marburg anatomist, together with a colleague, tried to organize a lecture series in remembrance of persecuted German Jews, he approached his medical faculty dean, referring to "the brown spots on our white physicians' smocks." The dean was visibly annoyed. Today this anatomist complains about the magnitude of the "resistance against a public discourse regarding the Nazi theme among professors of medicine, now as in the past."[93] A few years ago this scholar had been involved in a new and extended series of lectures about Nazi medicine at Marburg, organized not by the faculty, but by student representatives. Similar series were started at the universities of Tübingen and Göttingen.[94] Yet overall the contributions were so badly researched and the scope was so ill defined that subsequent publications of these lectures stood to do more harm than good. As these and other volumes made clear, those German medical historians – the properly schooled ones not excluded – shared many weaknesses: their chronic unfamiliarity with foreign-language critical literature, their awkwardly insular perspective, obsession with local detail and, resulting from all of this, as well as their ultimate inability to produce a comprehensive and fully documented history of medicine in the Third Reich in their native tongue.[95]

It must be attributed to a general lack of information about, and ongoing interest in, the ramifications of medical practice and scholarship during the Third Reich if, only a few years ago, a number of German universities were found to be using pathoanatomical specimens possibly deriving from Jewish victims of the Nazi era. To this day, although the University of Munich has

---

92 The most dedicated institutions in that regard in the past have been the universities at Kiel (Prof. Fridolf Kudlien), Mainz (Prof. Gunter Mann), and Berlin (Prof. Rolf Winau), and, very recently, Düsseldorf (Prof. Alfons Labisch). Because of recent retirements and deaths, there has, on the whole, been an attenuation of those efforts.

93 Prof. Gerhard Aumüller to author, Marburg, Jan. 19, 1994, author's PA.

94 *"Bis endlich der langersehnte Umschwung kam … ": Von der Verantwortung der Medizin unter dem Nationalsozialismus* (Marburg, 1991); Jürgen Peiffer, ed., *Menschenverachtung und Opportunismus: Zur Medizin im Dritten Reich* (Tübingen, 1992); Hannes Friedrich and Wolfgang Matzow, eds., *Dienstbare Medizin: Ärzte betrachten ihr Fach im Nationalsozialismus* (Göttingen, 1992).

95 See my critique of the above-mentioned titles in: "Die unbewältigte Medizingeschichte," 401–16. Equally flawed anthologies are: Johanna Bleker and Norbert Jachertz, eds., *Medizin im "Dritten Reich"*, 2d ed. (Cologne, 1993); and Günter Grau and Peter Schneck, eds., *Akademische Karrieren im "Dritten Reich": Beiträge zur Personal- und Berufungspolitik an Medizinischen Fakultäten* (Berlin, 1993).

not been able to dispel suspicion that some of its specimens originated from the Holocaust, the University of Heidelberg's assurances that this was not the case, although plausible, are based merely on an internal, not an external commission's report.[96]

This chronicle of the Sewering and Vilmar affairs would not be complete without an attempt to situate what I have identified as a problematical medical culture within the larger context of Germany's political climate. Against the canvas of politics and society from 1945 to the present, the course of the medical establishment, with its teaching institutions, professional subgroups, and forms of sociopolitical organization such as economic lobbies has on the whole been negative. Since the end of the Third Reich, sociopolitical reaction has often characterized the medical establishment. In the decade from 1945 to 1960, when denazification and democratic reintegration of many professional groupings were haphazard and extreme-right-wing parties could still flourish, the corps of physicians, many veterans from the fronts as well as Nazi Party members or worse, was not effectively cleansed through denazification proceedings (as Sewering's own case exemplifies), because it was desperately needed in the public health-care system.[97] In a second phase, from the middle of the 1960s to the middle of the 1980s, when democracy in Germany made impressive headway, many physicians, rather than participating in these processes, stood apart in corporatist egotism, focusing instead on their very own microempires, some of them multimillion-dollar businesses. But although their collective self-centeredness became proverbial, their earnings grew and, perversely, so did their social prestige. All of this meant a tremendous concentration of power in their hands.[98] Politically, a plurality of physicians tended to favor the conservative CDU or CSU or, from an enterpreneurial perspective, the right flank of the Free Democratic Party (FDP), Vilmar's own. Since the late 1980s, with the increase of right-radical extremism having affected representative sectors of society, this dichotomy of the second phase of the republic, between those conservative doctors and society in general has been somewhat neutralized – to the extent that more citizens have drifted to the right, in the direction of these physicians, whose position has not changed.

96   Kater, "Unresolved Questions," 421–3.
97   See Kurt P. Tauber, *Beyond Eagle and Swastika: German Nationalism Since 1945*, 2 vols. (Middletown, Conn., 1967); Hans-Ulrich Sons, "'Bis in die psychologischen Wurzeln': Die Entnazifizierung der Ärzte in Nordrhein-Westfalen (britisches Besatzungsgebiet)," *Deutsches Ärzteblatt* 79 (1982): C-60-2; Michael H. Kater, "Problems of Political Reeducation in West Germany, 1945–1960," *Simon Wiesenthal Center Annual* 4 (1987): 99–123; Kater, "The Burden of the Past," 41.
98   See Ralf Dahrendorf, *Gesellschaft und Demokratie in Deutschland* (Munich, 1967), 97–8, 382–3, 387–8; see also the global criticism in Julius Hackethal, *Nachoperation: Noteingriff zur Korrektur eines patientenfeindlichen Gesundheitssystems* (Vienna, 1977); Kater, *Doctors Under Hitler*, 224; *Der Spiegel* (June 6, 1994): 88–97.

It is in the current sociopolitical milieu, which appears to have encouraged new outbursts of xenophobia,[99] that Sewering's and Vilmar's behavior strikes foreign and national critics as simply devastating. In point of fact, the connection, however tenuous, between the rise of neo-Nazism on the one hand and the possible enthronement of a former SS man as German head of an international curative institution on the other has not been lost on keen observers. Thus the American cardiologist Professor Bernard Lown judged that, "at a time when ever more doubts are arising worldwide, whether the Germans might possibly have forgotten their 'dirty past,' the cover provided by the Federal Chamber of Physicians for Sewering confirms the necessity of serious contemplation of Germany's future development."[100] In Berlin, Dr. Winfried Beck, president of the Union of Democratic Physicians, voiced the, perhaps alarmist, opinion that at a time when in Germany human beings were once again persecuted and murdered just because they were foreigners, the candidacy of a former SS and Nazi Party member might revive National Socialist ideas.[101] Karsten Vilmar was told by IPPNW of Germany that he had displayed "a grotesque lack of judgment and sensitivity. These virtues, however, are crucial for any president of the *Bundesärztekammer*. This is particularly true today, as our country suffers from a severe resurgence of nationalistic and antisemitic activities."[102]

This chapter began with Kochen's personal involvement in the Sewering–Vilmar affair, and appropriately it shall end with it. In November 1992 Kochen had been touched not just by the bizarre modalities of the case at hand, which he then decided to become involved in personally. Insofar as Germany was concerned, he perceived a greater danger when he wrote to his Israeli colleague Michael Weingarten: "I don't want to finish this letter without telling you my increasing concern about the political development in Germany. Almost every day there are attacks against foreigners, asylants and Jewish monuments (and it is also starting against people!). I think we should tell the colleagues in all the world that the situation is much more dangerous than you can read in international newspapers."[103] Ironically, it was a German newspaper, the very "left-liberal" Munich daily that had had a hand in bringing Sewering to his knees,[104] that in early 1994 compromised Kochen. In November 1993 the *Süddeutsche Zeitung* had organized a health forum in Nuremberg to discuss disease prevention and had invited, among others, Dr.

---

99   *Der Spiegel* (April 11, 1994): 18–22.
100 Paraphrased in *Ärzte Zeitung* (Jan. 25, 1993).
101 Beck as quoted in ibid.
102 Bader to Vilmar, Berlin, Jan. 24, 1993, author's PA.
103 Kochen to Weingarten, Göttingen, Nov. 23, 1992, PA Seidelman.
104 E.g., see notes 4 and 44 to this chapter.

Sewering in his capacity as honorary chairman of the Bavarian panel practitioners' union. Reportedly, Sewering's presence, who by this time had relinquished almost all of his other manifold offices,[105] angered at least three of the forum participants. When Kochen inquired about the incident, expressing his incredulity that as disqualified a person as Sewering had been solicited by the very agency that helped cause his downfall, the paper's lawyer, one of the two forum hosts, repeated the very tired arguments Sewering had used in his attempts to exonerate himself. To add insult to injury, attorney Klaus Wagner informed Kochen that "at a meeting of the membership at large of the health forum Professor Dr. Sewering was able to clear himself of most of the accusations you had mentioned."[106] Kochen, quite convinced by now that "nothing had changed" from a year ago,[107] accused the paper of actively contributing to Sewering's rehabilitation, and he wryly added that without the pressure applied by the foreign media in the past twelve months nothing at all would have happened inside Germany.[108] The Munich daily retorted that perhaps the time had come to forgive and forget. Kochen's last contribution to the debate has been the salient point, which fittingly serves as the conclusion to this essay. He said there were certain preconditions for forgiveness, one being that the culprit express regret for past mistakes. Sewering, on the other hand, suggested the existence of an international Jewish conspiracy.[109]

That such a liberal and internationally respected daily newspaper as Munich's *Süddeutsche Zeitung* could be drawn to the side of a man with a past like Sewering's presently is deeply disturbing and augurs badly for the future. Indeed, the Sewering affair might technically be over and the Vilmar scandal may run its course, albeit without much improvement in the country's medical culture. But the conception of democracy and universal humanity on the part of initially well-intentioned Germans may be at risk, if they allow themselves to fall prey to corporate lobbyists who, in the interest of their profession, elect to forego important lessons from the not so distant past.

---

105 *Der Spiegel* (Dec. 6, 1993): 260.
106 Kochen to Schröder (editor in chief of *Süddeutsche Zeitung*), Göttingen, Dec. 9, 1993; Wagner to Kochen, Munich, Dec. 22, 1993, both in private archive of Michael M. Kochen (hereafter cited as PA Kochen).
107 Kochen to author, Jan. 4, 1994, author's PA.
108 Kochen to Schröder, Göttingen, Jan. 10, 1994, PA Kochen.
109 Wagner to Kochen, Munich, Jan. 17, 1994; Kochen to Wagner, Göttingen, Jan. 19, 1994, both PA Kochen.
*   I am grateful to Hellmuth Auerbach, Brewster Chamberlin, Michael J. Franzblau, Hans Halter, Hartmut Hanauske-Abel, Michael M. Kochen, Raymond Scalettar, Howard Wolinsky, and, especially, William E. Seidelman, for their abiding assistance during the course of my research. The Social Sciences and Humanities Research Council of Canada is, yet again, sincerely thanked for unwavering financial support during my work for this chapter.

Index

235